T0187446

Medical Therapeutic Yoga

Biopsychosocial Rehabilitation and Wellness Care

Medical Therapeutic Yoga

Biopsychosocial Rehabilitation and Wellness Care

Ginger Garner PT, DPT, ATC/LAT, PYT

Foreword by Shirley Telles PhD

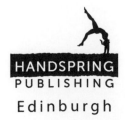

HANDSPRING
PUBLISHING
Edinburgh

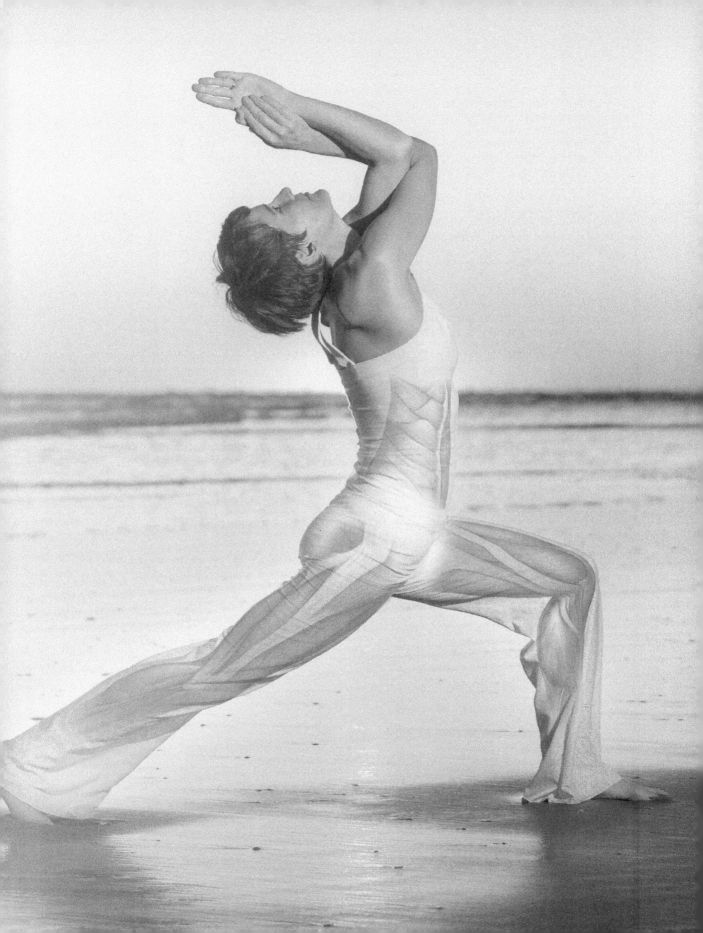

HANDSPRING PUBLISHING LIMITED
The Old Manse, Fountainhall,
Pencaitland, East Lothian
EH34 5EY, United Kingdom
Tel: +44 1875 341 859
Website: www.handspringpublishing.com

First published 2016 in the United Kingdom by Handspring Publishing Limited
Reprinted 2018

Copyright ©Handspring Publishing Limited 2016

Photographs and drawings copyright ©Handspring Publishing Limited 2016

All rights reserved. No parts of this publication may be reproduced or transmitted in any form or by any
means, electronic or mechanical, including photocopying, recording, or any information storage and retrieval
system, without either the prior written permission of the authors and publisher or a license permitting
restricted copying in the United Kingdom issued by the Copyright Licensing Agency Ltd, Saffron House, 6-10
Kirby Street, London EC1N 8TS.

The right of Ginger Garner to be identified as the Author of this text has been asserted in accordance with the
Copyright, Designs and Patents Acts 1988.

ISBN 978-1-909141-13-1

British Library Cataloguing in Publication Data
A catalogue record for this book is available from the British Library

Library of Congress Cataloguing in Publication Data
A catalog record for this book is available from the Library of Congress

Notice
Neither the Publisher nor the Author assumes any responsibility for any loss or injury and/or damage to persons or property arising out of or relating to any use of the material contained in this book. It is the responsibility of the treating practitioner, relying on independent expertise and knowledge of the patient, to determine
the best treatment and method of application for the patient.

All reasonable efforts have been made to obtain copyright clearance for illustrations in the book for which
the authors or publishers do not own the rights. If you believe that one of your illustrations has been used
without such clearance please contact the publishers and we will ensure that appropriate credit is given in
the next reprint.

Commissioning Editor Sarena Wolfaard
Project Manager Stephanie Pickering
Cover and Design Direction by Bruce Hogarth, Kinesis Creative
Illustrations by Bruce Hogarth
Photography by Brad Styron (cover), Jeff Jablonski, Naomi Byerley (content)
Index by Dr Laurence Errington
Typesetter DSM Soft, India
Printer CPI Group (UK) Ltd, Croydon, CR0 4YY

The
Publisher's
policy is to use
paper manufactured
from sustainable forests

CONTENTS

To the greatest gurus, my children
Michael, William, James,
and to Jeff,
my intellectual soul mate

REVIEWS

Medical Therapeutic Yoga *makes a unique contribution to effective interprofessional partnerships in healthcare. Replete with exceptional expertise, understanding, and care, it provides a detailed biopsychosocial model for using yoga in both preventive and rehabilitative healthcare. I applaud and highly recommend this important book.*

Riane Eisler

President, Center for Partnership Studies, author of *The Chalice and the Blade*, co-author of *Transforming Interprofessional Partnerships.*

Ginger Garner's book fulfills the need of healthcare professionals who are interested in medical therapeutic yoga, as well as yoga teachers and therapists who are working with people with medical conditions. The book is researched like an academic book, but also contains easy to use step-by-step practical suggestions that will be of great value for a large variety of healthcare and yoga practitioners.

Staffan Elgelid PhD, PT, GCFP, C-IAYT

Associate Professor of Physical Therapy at Nazareth College; editor of *Yoga Therapy: Theory and Practice*, and co-author of *Yoga Therapy for Stress and Anxiety.*

Dr Ginger Garner has masterfully explored the bio in the biopsychosocial model of healthcare while simultaneously embracing the psychosocial contributions of yoga philosophies. By weaving the richness of the yoga tradition with the modern postural-structural-biomechanical model of medicine, she delivers a practical and relevant text exploring how we may better treat the whole person during stages of physical distress and dis-ease.

Jules Mitchell MS, CMT, ERYT500

Los Angeles. Yoga Biomechanics: Redefining Stretching.

This book is an incredible accomplishment of integrating physical therapy and yoga. Ginger not only provides complete details of the theory behind Medical Therapeutic Yoga, but also includes detailed descriptions of assessment and therapeutic interventions.

Neil Pearson PT, MSc, BA-BPHE, ERYT500, CYT

Penticton, Canada. Author of the chapter "Yoga therapy", in *Integrative Pain Management*, Handspring Publishing, 2015.

Medical Therapeutic Yoga *is a comprehensive and scholarly book that effectively bridges the gap between allied medical fields and yoga. This landmark volume documents the continuity of yoga with our contemporary understanding of neuromuscular function.* Medical Therapeutic Yoga *is a well-written, beautifully illustrated, and scientifically documented volume that provides an in-depth knowledge of the physiological, anatomical, and neurophysiological links to the evolved historical traditions of yoga.*

Stephen W. Porges PhD

Distinguished University Scientist, Indiana University, Bloomington, Indiana; author of *The Polyvagal Theory: Neurophysiological Foundations of Emotions, Attachment, Communication, and Self-regulation.*

It is no small task to be able to integrate the different approaches and language that exist between modern healthcare and yoga; yet, Dr Garner succeeds in establishing this important bridge by developing a creative paradigm for rehabilitation and wellness care. Medical Therapeutic Yoga *is a paramount contribution to our current healthcare system's acceptance and welcoming of the use of yoga as an effective, safe and much needed biopsychosocial addition to the complementary rehabilitation therapies.*

Shelly Prosko PT, PYT, CPI

Physical Therapist, Professional Yoga Therapist; www.physioyoga.ca.

Medical Therapeutic Yoga *offers health care professionals a thorough roadmap to understanding how yoga might be used in their practices – and the "how-to" as well. The dense citations create a comfortable foundation for even the most conservative provider that this work is grounded in the best evidence. Rather that patching yoga onto a healthcare practice, Garner guides the reader into how they can seamlessly weave the healing power of yoga into the very fabric of their vocation.*

Matthew J. Taylor PT, PhD

Past-president of the International Association of Yoga Therapists, author of *Fostering Creativity in Rehabilitation*, expert witness for yoga injuries, and director of www.smartsafeyoga.com.

FOREWORD

"Each soul is potentially divine. The goal is to manifest this divinity by controlling nature, external and internal."

– Swami Vivekananda (1863–1902)

Rehabilitation involves dealing with people who are either born with, or due to circumstances later in life develop, special needs. It is essential to engage with anyone with special needs with sensitivity and optimism, so that their rehabilitation program can be a realization of their full potential.

This aspect of healthcare has been covered comprehensively by Doctor of Physical Therapy Ginger Garner, in her book *Medical Therapeutic Yoga: Biopsychosocial Rehabilitation and Wellness Care*, which synthesizes information from both traditional texts and contemporary literature in a unique approach to therapeutic yoga for rehabilitation. Throughout the text, her emphasis considers all dimensions of an individual's functions, including their physical, emotional, intellectual and social wellbeing, and also their spiritual beliefs.

The reader is introduced to the approach gradually through the twelve chapters of the book. Dr Garner begins with specific principles for the integration of yoga and rehabilitation in a conventional healthcare setting, and continues with an examination of the 10 precepts that form a solid foundation for Medical Therapeutic Yoga for rehabilitation. Among these precepts are the importance of considering an individual as a "whole person" in the context of their environment and other factors, including recommendations that the individual's breathing is checked and corrected as a starting point, and creating a safe therapeutic environment. The last point is especially interesting as the author discusses both the internal environment (the body and mind) and the external environment, which includes ambient lighting and level of noise. Interestingly, these descriptions are close to those described in traditional yoga texts. When considering each individual, their physical,

intellectual, psycho-emotional-social, energetic and spiritual dimensions are considered. Before discussing practice, the author provides an evidence base for yoga in healthcare based on physical principles such as kinesthetic awareness, respiration, the biomechanics of neuromuscular changes and meditation.

The author begins describing practice with an emphasis on breathing correctly, which is something traditional yoga texts strongly emphasize. The dynamics of breathing and the importance of diaphragmatic breathing are described with clarity. There are numerous informative illustrations that make the functional anatomy very easy to follow and understand. Dr Garner also provides an interesting functional movement algorithm to ensure evidence-informed, biomechanically safe yoga practice. Detailed descriptions with illustrations and videos ensure that these principles can be grasped with ease.

In the practice chapters, Dr Garner leads the reader through different yoga practices or *asanas* in standing, sitting, supine, and prone positions and in semi-inversions. For all postures, she has covered the biomechanics, the way a posture should be synchronized with the breath, the therapeutic intention and the contraindications. Possible modifications required for therapeutic yoga in rehabilitation, using props, have been illustrated and described, as are all the postures.

The author concludes the book with two chapters which are of great importance to a healthcare provider, and indeed to anyone who receives therapeutic yoga for rehabilitation. In the first of these, Dr Garner discusses an important principle for therapeutic yoga, namely the FITT principle (Frequency, Intensity, Time and Type (Specificity)). She also describes some practices for specific conditions. The concluding chapter gives medical providers and yoga professionals all the information they require to provide a successful intervention. It also includes standard outcome measures useful for assessment of progress after therapeutic yoga as well as other information for an integrated, informed and evidence-based practice.

I believe that this book is a valuable addition to the knowledge of therapeutic yoga as it (1) combines certain principles of healing which are present in the ancient yoga texts along with knowledge from contemporary medicine, and (2) the practices covered are particularly useful for rehabilitation. The principles Dr Garner provides would apply to any application of therapeutic yoga. Readers will particularly appreciate the way she has blended and explained essential, yet often neglected concepts from traditional yoga texts (such as emphasizing correct breathing before starting *asana* practice) with concepts from biomechanics and functional anatomy in a way that is easy for anyone to comprehend. This knowledge will undoubtedly stimulate students of yoga to consider further therapeutic applications of yoga in health and rehabilitation, beyond those described in the present book. These concepts have been elucidated by Dr Garner's clear descriptions and skillful use of illustrations, photographs and case histories throughout the book. I am sure it will help a great deal in making rehabilitation through yoga more successful and acceptable.

Shirley Telles PhD

Director, Patanjali Research Foundation, Haridwar, India

August 2016

PREFACE

The very nature of science is change. And to change requires asking questions. This book does that.

Quantum physics questions the nature of the observer. Samkhya philosophy, found in Ayurveda and yoga, does the same, albeit its inquiry began some 5000 years ago.

Meanwhile, the nature of humanity is to seek comfort and make a human connection, often in the midst of self-doubt. Even the most assured introvert, is not, as John Donne wrote, an island. Martin Luther King, Jr. agreed, declaring, "Whatever affects one directly, affects all indirectly. I can never be what I ought to be until you are what you ought to be. This is the interrelated structure of reality." We must create, together. This book is an invitation to that.

Medical Therapeutic Yoga invites both the biomedical and yoga fields to question the nature of the observer through science while seeking the comfort, connection, and creativity of medicine and yoga through art. Both invite transformation and require partnership.

We are intimately connected as a civilization, in a universe surrounded by countless others, and yet we still inhabit a binary mode of thinking that posits one can only be "this" or "that," for example, Christian or Buddhist, Chinese medicine or Native American philosopher, or the obvious, medical practitioner or yoga devotee.

I felt the pain of that social conditioning for decades. I was not fully accepted in either the medical or the yoga community. I was viewed with skepticism on both sides – perceived as too scientifically rigid for yogis and too "woo- woo" for the biomedical sect, from both of which I was born. I was homeless and nameless.

And so, I wandered. On purpose. And during all of that, life went on – in all its poverty and loss, grief and trauma.

It is from within that condition of poverty and loss, grief and trauma that I came to yoga, some 25 years ago. I stayed with yoga because yoga saved my life. And it saved not just mine, but also my patients' lives.

For many, this salvation may seem like common sense. After all, everyone knows yoga is helpful. But how much and in what ways?

Common sense informs much of the mundane decision-making required for daily life. In fact, one may say that common sense is cultivated through our ability to experience "everyday life." Stephen Hawking challenges this notion in *The Grand Design* (Hawking and Mlodinow, 2010), saying that all knowledge is not gained through direct observation because it is tainted by our senses. Therefore, modern physics clashes with everyday experience – and the very notion of common sense. Here again is an invitation to question the nature of the observer. Hawking goes on to say that "model-dependent realism handles this paradox" (p. 7), which resonates strongly with one of yoga's oldest philosophies, Samkhya. Samkyha philosophy gives tangible credence to questioning the nature of the observer and exactly how we sense, perceive, and interpret information. It also gives us insight to the ultimate questions everyone asks, "What is reality?" and "Why are we here?"

For me, these questions have been answered through my active struggle to shed the binary social conditioning that would have me be either a scientist, by way of physical therapy, or an artist, by way of music and yoga.

Art and science butt heads beginning in elementary school, where oftentimes physical education and art are abandoned as unnecessary topics expendable in the face of subjects such as math and reading. However, art allows our species to learn. Art makes sense of the unspeakable, and gives us insight when there are no words.

There have been three distinct times in my life where the confluence of art and science has moved me, not just to tears and chills (or "dopamine dump"), but to an involuntary and deep simultaneous rapturous and liberating grief, sometimes silent and without movement, sometimes wracking me with heaving motion, all in public.

The first was in 2004, when I happened upon a concert with my travel companion (who I had no idea would become my future life partner) at the church of St Martin-in-the-Fields in London's Trafalgar Square. The conductor played the harpsichord while he directed, and I sat in silent awe by candlelight, motionless, while tears collected in my lap.

The second occasion was in 2010, at Lincoln Center's jazz club. I was pregnant at the time, and, alongside my husband, I listened to what I was hearing. No more than two bars into Terrell Stafford's first trumpet solo, pure scat and high energy, and tears escaped from somewhere deep inside, a place I knew I'd likely never visited, at least not lately. I was blown away by the paradox of crying hopped up on jazz instrumental improvisation. It was blindingly enlightening.

The third was at the military funeral of a dear family friend's father. I sang at the funeral, as I am often asked to do, and when Taps was played at the conclusion of the service, I had to suppress powerful, heaving sobs that came up from that same deep place, only because I did not want to interrupt the service by letting a wail escape. In those sobs I felt the grief of losing my own grandfather, a WWII veteran, and so many other loved ones who had died too soon. In all cases the emotion was surprising but welcome, and most of all, healing.

The point is, Stephen Hawking's discussion of quantum physics and Stephen Porges' polyvagal theory, part of the underlying theory which girds this text, provide an opportunity for confluence that Daniel Goleman says results in "neural harmony." And at the heart of all those seemingly separate variables: quantum mechanics, polyvagal theory, and yes, God, there is yoga.

Because of that confluence, I no longer have to fight, flee, or freeze from the social conditioning of a binary existence. I can be a physical therapist, a musician, a teacher, a scientist, a woman, a wife, a mother, and a yogi.

Yoga allows me to unify all these variables into one equation: one of creativity, gratitude, nonviolence, and welcomed introspection.

Yoga has allowed my divergent, dualistic humanity to bring the sacred biology and chemistry of movement, music, and even food together in one Divine meditation, while honoring my own (and everyone else's) spiritual foundations.

Yoga saved my life because it healed me and continues to heal me, while it does the same for each of my patients.

Even as I wrote this book, I grappled with the polytrauma not just of my past, but also of my present and future. I have never written or spoken about what I am about to say. But I share it because it is my testimony to yoga's transformational potential. I also share it because yoga has been the chief vehicle and reason for my positive outcomes in clinical care for over two decades, and nurtured the creation of this book.

Sharing my story

I wrote this manuscript in spite of, and through, great trauma. During the last three years I have crested the mountainous obstacle of overcoming chronic pain, a hip reconstruction and recovery from childbirth trauma, and most bittersweet, receiving my son's special needs diagnosis. All of this happened while I was a postpartum new mother for a third time (my third son), maintaining my day job of teaching, blogging, advocacy work, traveling to give lectures, seeing patients, and being a CEO, and last but not least, working on my doctorate and writing this book. Being able to accomplish all of that is my present day testimony to my victory, via yoga, over trials, trauma, and the demands of everyday life.

My past life includes, in hindsight, what was likely PTSD, coupled with HPA axis dysregulation and a cocktail of its systemic comorbidities, such as infertility, polycystic ovarian syndrome, adrenal burnout, and weight management issues, just for starters. The implosion of my life, at one point, put me on a track as an abused wife, both sexually and emotionally. But the saddest part was that it only mirrored my previous history as a witness and victim of sexual abuse, suffered alongside a deep-seeded sense of low self-worth and confidence that subjected me to men who thought violence against women was okay.

My future trauma is societally induced, largely a result of cultural conditioning that would have women think all we need to do is "lean in" to receive equitable treatment as "the other half of the sky" in the workplace. While well meaning, the pressure that a mother can "do it all," particularly in the absence of social policy to support it (doing it all), exacts a devastating effect, not just on my family, but on entire generations of women and families who are forced to exist in a society that lacks an inherent partnership model and instead functions on an antiquated system which favors domination of one gender over another. This is why Riane Eisler's work in *Caring Economics* (Eisler, 2007) is a third underlying theme in this text. We cannot move forward as a civilization and culture without working in partnership.

Through all of this – from victimization to healing – yoga has carried me, empowered me, and yoked my faith and beliefs through the actions and practice that has ultimately allowed me to birth this book. I am sure that what I suffer has never been in vain, but through it I have found the courage to use my voice to help others through similar struggles, and through their own pain experience, trauma, and triumph. Just as we all want to strive for love, joy, peace, patience, kindness, goodness, faithfulness, gentleness, and self-control, the Fruits of the Spirit I learned as a child, so yoga allows us to resurrect the creativity in our soul. What we do in healthcare is both an art and a science. One cannot exist without the other.

This book strives to strike unity and balance between the two, and to serve as a beacon of hope to those who have been seeking a compassionate, sustainable method and safe space to optimize patient care and self-care.

References

Eisler RT (2007), The Real Wealth of Nations: Creating a Caring Economics. Berrett-Koehler, San Francisco, CA.

Hawking S, Mlodinow L (2010), The Grand Design. Bantam Books, New York.

Ginger Garner
Emerald Isle, North Carolina
June 2016

ACKNOWLEDGEMENTS

A major impetus for this book is to show medical professionals of any background, but especially in therapy fields, just how important yoga is to resurrecting creativity in rehabilitation, compassion in medicine, empathy in patient care, and empowerment and self-care in both the person and practitioner. It also serves to create a needed dialogue between yoga teachers, yoga therapists, and healthcare professionals who use yoga in clinical and wellness care.

Conquest, insight, self-searching, honesty, and spiritual devotion have allowed me to ask questions that led to the birth of this book, which started more than 15 years ago. I want to thank all of those who have helped me ask and answer those questions. It truly does take a village.

That village includes giving thanks first to my husband, Jeff, whose undying support, belief in equitable partnership, and shared intellectual curiosity forms the cornerstone of my inspiration and strength; to Naomi Satterfield Byerley, without whose willingness to master any task I could throw at her during book editing and post-production I could not have completed this book. To Matthew Taylor, PT, PhD, who always brought me back to task on simplicity and clarity and who was always there to cheer me on, even as he edited alongside me from thousands of miles away; to Stephen Porges, PhD, and his elegant polyvagal theory (PVT); his PVT bridges the elusive gap between human connection and neurophysiology, and his personal inputs to this text are invaluable.

Enormous gratitude goes to a long list of colleagues who peer edited and skewered each chapter with love: the PT team, Julie Spencer, cross referencing extraordinaire, and also Stefanie Foster, Liz Duncanson, Meagen Satinsky, Sharon Anoff, Paige Raffo, Libby Trausch, Barbara Rabin, Shari Ser, Kathy McKinney, Patricia Oyarce, Neil Pearson, Kristina Dorkoski, Lonnie Poland, and Matt Erb; the OT team, Kristin Biggins, Annie Dundas, Leigh Crowder-Bierman, LJ Taylor, and Natalie Bishop. To my cross-cultural sounding boards, Sensei Joyce Trafton, EdD, and Sanskrit guru, Nauka Joshi. To colleagues in instructional design for our conversations on optimizing learning experiences and to interdisciplinary editors, Teddie Potter, RN, PhD, and Stephen Porges, PhD, who reviewed specific sections based on their expertise in cultural transformation and PVT, respectively. And, to the hardworking creative team at Handspring Publishing, Ltd., without whose vision and dedication this book would have not be possible.

Finally, to the Professional Yoga Therapy Institute family and its network of healthcare professionals who now stretch across the globe, your belief and support of me and this methodology is invaluable. To this global village, I offer you all my deepest gratitude and eternal thanks.

Ginger Garner
Emerald Isle, North Carolina

INFORMATION ON INSTRUCTIONAL VIDEOS

Instructional videos

Medical Therapeutic Yoga, in addition to being a textbook, is accompanied by a companion guide of videos, accessible via QR codes, offering a multimedia platform for therapeutic yoga application in the clinic or home.

How to use the codes

QR codes that can be scanned with a smartphone can be found throughout the text. Some of these are **free codes**; these are listed below and indicated in the text by the words "free code" in parentheses after the code number. In addition, **subscription codes** are also included for your clinical reference if you want to complete your video library to include all the codes in the book. These are indicated by the words "subscription code" in parentheses after the code number. As an added **bonus**, the subscription also includes additional videos that will complement the book. The video library can be used for both patient education and personal practice. Visit www.medicaltherapeuticyoga.com to subscribe to the full library and learn more.

Free codes

There are 29 companion videos included with the purchase of this book. The codes are for the book owner's use only and not to be shared or copied. Free codes occur in Chapters 4, 5, 6, 8, 11, 12, and in the Glossary. Free codes are:

Code 4.1 Abdominodiaphragmatic breath with tri-diaphragmatic action (p. 80)

Code 4.2 Transversus abdominis-assisted thoracodiaphragmatic breath (p. 82)

Code 4.3 Three-part breath (p. 88)

Code 4.4 Four-part breath (p. 89)

Code 4.5 Sandbag breath (p. 90)

Code 4.6 Victorious/overcoming breath (p. 90)

Code 4.7 Alternate nostril breath (p. 92)

Code 4.8 Bee breath (p. 93)

Code 4.9 Femoral version screen/Craig test (p. 103)

Code 5.1 Three tier approach – "yoga couch" (p. 112)

Code 5.2 Capsule test (p. 113)

Code 5.3 Windshield wipers (p. 117)

Code 5.4 Arm spiral (p. 121)

Code 5.5 Scapular repositioning test (p. 122)

Code 5.6 Scapular assistance test (p. 122)

Code 5.7 Hook lying knee lifts (p. 126)

Code 5.8 Anterior/posterior non-articulation and segmental spinal articulation (p. 127)

Code 5.9 Lateral segmental spinal articulation (p. 129)

Code 5.10 Moon salute composition (p. 136)

Code 6.4 Modified Gillet test in tree pose (p. 171)

Code 8.1 Yoga couch (p. 223)

Code 11.1 More resources on back pain management (p. 296)

Code 11.2 Lateral knee drops (p. 300)

Code 12.1 Resources on meditation practice (p. 316)

Code 12.2 Resources on vocal training (p. 328)

Code G.1 Two-tier approach to yoga couch (p. 334)

Code G.2 Three-tier approach to yoga couch (p. 334)

Code G.3 Ganesha fold (p. 334)

Code G.4 Accordion fold (p. 334)

Visit www.medicaltherapeuticyoga.com to subscribe to the full library and learn more about Medical Therapeutic Yoga.

Yoga is a practical perspective on, and low-cost solution for, improving healthcare, especially given the planetary pandemic of chronic disease. Yoga is also far more effective when combined with familiar medical practices. Medical Therapeutic Yoga (MTY) is such a method of yoga prescription: it takes existing evidence-based practice and streamlines clinical assessment and management to improve patient satisfaction and outcomes. Practicing MTY can also lower overhead costs while reducing or preventing practitioner burnout as a more holistic, person-centered model for care. Because physical yoga practice represents the majority of transnational yoga practice, and physical transformation is often the first entry point for feeling better, this text will focus on the physical breath and postures as a means for using yoga medically.

The difference between delivery of therapy in the medical model and delivery of therapy using yoga is found in the term "biopsychosocial model." The biomedical model is identified as allopathic, conventional, traditional, mainstream, or Western medicine. The biopsychosocial (BPS) model that yoga embodies can describe integrated, integrative, complementary, alternative, functional, or Eastern medicine. Use of the BPS model in medicine is supported and encouraged by the World Health Organization and the Institute of Medicine, as well as numerous studies and professional organizations. Yoga, delivered through the BPS model, elicits a neurochemical response mediated by the neurophysiological mechanisms of yoga. In this text, this mechanism is introduced through explanation for application of the breath and posture.

The use of yoga in healthcare offers providers and patients "another way of being in the world" (Anderzen-Carlsson et al., 2014), a phenomenological perspective. Phenomenology captures how we view things based on our experience, and is described as the study of the structure of consciousness experienced through a first-person point of view (Smith, 2013). The central themes of this text are based on shifting our thinking toward a new model of practice in rehabilitation using proposed common psychotherapeutic and physiological factors that affect rehabilitation outcomes. This new model for practice, detailed via MTY, is guided by the BPS model and undergirded by the "10 precepts" (see later in this chapter). The result for clinicians is familiarity with how yoga physical practices can be safer and more efficacious through application of the evidence base, as well as blend with current procedural guidelines and scopes of practice in healthcare.

Overview of this book

- Chapter 1 introduces the background for yoga in healthcare and lays the groundwork for the 10 practice precepts

- Chapter 2 introduces the biopsychosocial model of practice and the historical evidence base that supports MTY as a method for using yoga in rehabilitation

- Chapter 3 builds an evidence base to inform the practice of yoga in healthcare based on seven physiological principles

- Chapter 4 provides instruction in respiration as the primary prerequisite to posture prescription and safety, as detailed in Chapter 5, as well as the inclusion of assessment tools for the orofacial, respiratory, and yogic locks system, in addition to an overview of orthopaedic screening tools and instructions for femoral version testing

- Chapter 5 explains the use of the functional movement assessment (FMA) algorithm in adult and geriatric forms to streamline clinical decision-making in rehabilitation

- Chapters 6–10 present options for biomechanical alignment and orthopaedic considerations for yoga postures:

  - Chapter 6 — Standing postures

  - Chapter 7 — Seated postures

Chapter 1

Outline of Chapter 1

- Leadership in medicine
- Leadership in yoga
- Nomenclature and legal status
- Medical Therapeutic Yoga
- Yoga in healthcare
- Yoga's perennial philosophy
- Ten precepts
- Review

Leadership in medicine

The ancient wisdom of yoga has offered generations a compassionate method for conscious living and psychophysiological transformation. The medical model we use today perhaps evolved from a similar intention, one of helping others live a safer, healthier, and more fulfilled life.

Hippocrates, credited as the "father of modern medicine," set forth a gentle, natural, non-diagnosis-driven intervention model that sought to determine the source of a problem, rather than focus on the end diagnosis of a condition. Hippocratic proverbs such as "let food be your medicine and medicine be your food" remain with us today. In today's diagnosis-seeking, pharmaceutical- and procedural-heavy biomedical model, opinions such as this underscore the need for further evolution toward medicine's original philosophy.

Today's biomedical model is still incredibly beneficial and absolutely necessary for acute care. Excellence in handling acute care and crisis-based disease management is a strong point of today's allopathic medicine. Its weaker record with chronic disease prevention and management, though, is well established (Elliott et al., 2002; Pomeroy, 2012; Van Hecke et al., 2013).

The collective inability to proactively prevent or address chronic disease has led millions of sufferers to seek more integrative methods of healthcare. Yoga's inclusion in healthcare can improve medicine for the future.

The collective inability to proactively prevent or address chronic disease has led millions of sufferers to seek more integrative methods of healthcare. Yoga's inclusion in healthcare can improve medicine for the future. The result of this evolutionary union is described in *Medical Therapeutic Yoga*.

Leadership in yoga

Historical perspective

To move forward with positive change, it is helpful to understand what came before. An understanding of the history of yoga can be beneficial to honor its origins, but to also make way for an integrated future.

The word yoga, translated from its Sanskrit origins, can be broken down into its root "*yuj*," which means to join, to yoke, to bind, to attach, to direct and concentrate one's attention on, and to use and apply (Iyengar, 1976). Yoga is one of six systems of Indian philosophy systematized by Patanjali in the *Yoga Sutras* (Iyengar, 1976). The *sutras* comprise between 185 and 196 (texts differ on the exact number) aphorisms for daily living and are said to have been written down by Patanjali between 195 and 200 BC, after having been passed down verbally for generations (Iyengar, 1976, 1993; Satchidananda and Patanjali, 1990; Mohan and Mohan, 2010). The *sutras* are based on the *Ashtanga* path of yoga, or eight-limbed yoga practice, and *Samkhya* philosophy (Iyengar, 1993).

Patanjali claimed only to be the compiler of the *Yoga Sutras*, not the author. Universally recognized as the father of *Raja yoga*, or "royal yoga," which encompasses the eight-limbed yoga practice, Patanjali stated the "aim of yoga was to calm the chaos of conflicting impulses and thoughts" (Satchidananda and Patanjali, 1990). A path to self-realization, yoga is said to bring the mind and its actions under conscious control. Each chapter of the *sutras* deals with the difficulties and joys of daily living, corresponding to the eight-limbed path and teaching aspirants how to master overcoming obstructions (*kleshas*) to practice and aspire to well-being.

Yoga is an ancient art but perhaps an even more powerful subtle science. Even so, identifying it as an "art and science" is a modern descriptor (De Michelis, 2005), less related to its ancient roots where there was less distinction between postural yoga and meditation. Yoga has an expanded role identified as "yoga therapy" defined by the International Association of Yoga Therapists as "the process of empowering individuals to progress toward improved health and well-being through the application of the philosophy and practice of Yoga" (Taylor, 2007).

> Yoga is more than a form of physical movement.

Yoga is more than a form of physical movement. The physical nature of today's familiar practice does not suggest that physical and spiritual growth are mutually exclusive (Singleton, 2010). Yoga is also an accessible method for living well.

Historically, the practice of yoga has been associated, in the modern era (19th and 20th centuries), with "stretch and relax" principles (Singleton, 2005), although there was considerable overlap and influence from British colonialism, English bodybuilding, and even association with "freedom-fighting" martial practices disguised as "yoga" (Singleton, 2010). This makes the modern practice of yoga, termed "modern postural yoga" by De Michelis (2005), perhaps discontinuous from, but not independent of, the Vedic practice of yoga occurring prior to British colonial occupation of India.

A final important note is offered via the early 20th-century era of modern yoga, identifying the phrase "yogic therapy." The term was already being utilized by yoga teacher K. V. Iyer in 1927 (Singleton, 2010), chiefly to describe male pursuit of "yogic physical culture," closely resembling bodybuilding of the day. Krishnamacharya likewise recognized three parallel therapeutic purposes of yoga: (1) yoga for people who are healthy (*siksha*), (2) yoga as therapy (*cikitsa*), and (3) yoga for personal transformation (*upasana*), or spiritual practice, maintaining that yoga should be individualized and teachers should "teach what is appropriate for the individual" (Mohan and Mohan, 2010).

Yoga's historical therapeutic roots are well established (Mohan and Mohan, 2010), making yoga applicable in healthcare through utilization of the evidence base while recognizing that new postures and movements or breath within postures will be "invented" on an ongoing basis. This marked evolution is evidence of yoga's "living" science and underscores its accessibility and adaptability for all populations. The need for "brands" of yoga, then, may be rendered unnecessary when yoga is available to everyone and can be medically adapted for use by anyone. This is not to minimize the importance of the forerunners of yoga, as mentioned earlier, such as Swami Vivekananda and Krishnamacharya and his students B. K. S. Iyengar, Indra Devi, A. G. Mohan, and Pattabhis Jois. They are, in large part, collectively responsible for the gift of transnational yoga we have today.

Despite Indra's presence, yoga, like allopathic medicine, has followed a distinctive patriarchal lineage. But in the 21st century, patriarchal domination has begun to give way to a more egalitarian practice of yoga. A survey conducted by Harris Interactive Bureau in 2012 for the *Yoga Journal*, the largest circulated yoga magazine worldwide, reported that in the United States alone, of the 20 million people practicing yoga, 82.2% are women. What is more, yoga teachers in the 21st century are mostly women. Yoga will continue to evolve and become more accessible to all populations, and this is a process to which this text hopes to contribute in a spirit of partnership and egalitarian pursuit.

However, from the late 20th century forward, what have existed as brands or lineages of yoga should be reconsidered. Yoga as a whole is more important than one type of yoga, since a single prescription cannot be used as a "recipe" or defined as a singular methodology or path for pursuit of yoga. In the 21st century the irrelevance of dogmatic lineages is poignant when we are faced with the epidemic proportions of chronic pain and disease internationally (WHO, 2005) which provide the impetus for using an accessible, holistic or BPS approach for pain management (Pergolizzi et al., 2013). The BPS approach, discussed in Chapter 2, offers a template for yoga prescription in healthcare.

Nomenclature and legal status in complementary and integrative medicine

Practices that do not quite fit under the realm of allopathic medicine were historically organized and categorized under the term "complementary and alternative medicine" (CAM). CAM is a group of therapies that covers an "array of healthcare approaches with a history of use or origins outside of mainstream medicine" (NCCAM, 2013), and is also known as complementary and integrative medicine (CIM). There are two major groups of CAM defined by the National Center for Complementary and Alternative Medicine (now known as the National Center for Complementary and Integrative Medicine; NCCIM, 2015). Those categories include "natural products" and "mind/body practices." A third category, which does not fit precisely into one of those groups exclusively, is recognized as "other complementary health approaches" (NCCAM, 2013). The Indian system of philosophy and medicine, which includes the practice of yoga and Ayurvedic medicine, falls under the categories of "mind/body practices" and "other complementary health approaches," respectively (NCCAM, 2013). Medical Therapeutic Yoga is designated as a "complementary" therapy according to NCCIM's definition (2015) of the word because yoga, as a non-mainstream practice, is combined with (rather than replaces) a conventional medical practice, in this case, rehabilitation. CAM is widely practiced and accepted throughout the world by governments, healthcare systems, and individuals. There is a range of regulations and systems in place for recognizing the practice of CAM. What follows is a brief overview of European, Australian, and North American legal practices on the use of CAM and the chief factors involving leadership and evolution of yoga in the biomedical model today.

Europe

Approximately 65% of people in Europe report that they have used some form of CAM (CAMDOC Alliance, 2010): "Post-graduate training courses in specific CAM therapies are provided to doctors at several universities in the majority of EU Member States, and in other countries at private teaching centers only" (p. 3). Both obligatory and elective preparatory or introductory courses in CAM are provided in the medical undergraduate curriculum in many countries. In most countries in Europe, CAM legislation has a consistent presence dictating specific therapies that can be performed by medical doctors or other regulated practitioners. CAM legislation is government-administered in Belgium (1999), Bulgaria (2005), Denmark (2004), Germany (1939 and 1998), Hungary (1997), Iceland (2005), Norway (2004), Portugal (2003), Romania (1981), and Slovenia (2007) (CAMDOC Alliance, 2010). Countries with CAM legislation in preparation include Ireland, Luxembourg, Poland, and Sweden. Partial CAM legislation exists in Cyprus, Finland, Italy, Lithuania, Latvia, Liechtenstein, Malta, Romania, and the United Kingdom. No CAM legislation exists in Austria, Estonia, France, Greece, the Netherlands, Spain, and Slovakia; while CAM legislation is present in Switzerland's national constitution (CAMDOC Alliance, 2010).

United Kingdom

The United Kingdom has long-established public sector hospitals for CAM. The British Research Council on Complementary Medicines was established in 1982, more than 10 years before those in America; it is also recognized that complementary and alternative medicine reduces the costs of the healthcare system (Maddalena, 1999). The British Medical Association supports the incorporation of CAM into undergraduate medical school curricula and the creation of accredited postgraduate training programs. A reported 2.5 million people practiced yoga in Britain in 2004 (Singleton and Byrne, 2008). The majority of the yoga population in Britain is officially represented by the organization British Wheel of Yoga.

Australia

Because of its strong Chinese heritage, dating from the 19th century forward, Australia has long recognized the importance of CAM. In 1974 the Australian Parliament established the Committee of Inquiry into Chiropractic, Osteopathy, Homeopathy, and Naturopathy (Parliamentary Paper, no. 102/1977). A reported 1 billion Australian dollars is spent on CAM annually (World Health Organization, 2001). The majority of yoga practitioners (85%) are women (Penman et al., 2012). Most yoga practitioners report using yoga for a specific health or medical reason, and reported yoga to be successful in management of the problem (Penman et al., 2012).

North America

United States

In 1991 the US Congress began the work of encouraging research in the field of integrative medicine by establishing the Office of Alternative Medicine (OAM) within the National Institutes of Health. In 1993 the National Institutes of Health Revitalization Act of 1993, Public Law 103-43 (NIH, 1993) increased the size of the OAM office in order to accommodate the growing demand for research and practice (WHO, 2001).

The number of Americans practicing yoga jumped by 87% to an estimated 16.5 million from 2004 to 2008, putting it in the top 10 CAM modalities used according to a National Health Interview Survey conducted in 2009. The NCCAM reports that Americans spent $34 billion on CAM therapies and just under $6 billion on yoga and yoga-related products alone (Nahin et al., 2009). Currently there is no legal regulation or third-party accreditation of yoga or yoga therapy in the United States. There is a voluntary registry known as the Yoga Alliance and an organization that is adopting preliminary self-regulation for lay trained yoga therapists, the International Association of Yoga Therapists (IAYT). Both organizations are based in the United States. The American Occupational Therapy Organization does acknowledge that yoga, as CAM, can be used as a "preparatory method or purposeful activity to facilitate the ability of clients to engage in their daily life occupations"

(AOTA, 2011, p. S27) as a therapeutic modality which addresses biomechanical and rehabilitative frames and the motor control and motor learning frames.

Canada

Canada has multiple CAM training programs and professional organizations related to CAM. Among the earliest legislation was the Quebec Medical Act of 1973, which required the annual registration of allopathic physicians practicing acupuncture, in addition to establishment of rules for training and practice by physicians and non-physicians (International Digest of Health Legislation, 1993). In 1996, the Canadian Complementary Medical Association was formed by those physicians interested in traditional and CAM therapy (Gray, 1997).

Medical Therapeutic Yoga: mindfulness and partnership in medicine

Early biopsychosocial model pioneer Engel (1977) described effective pain management as an interactive psychophysiological and behavioral phenomenon that requires the clinician to address psychological and social factors during treatment. In contrast, biomedical medicine often views the patient as someone who receives care, rather than as a decision-maker and stakeholder in his/her healthcare. This level of involvement by patients is called "self-management," a term first coined by Thomas Creer (Creer et al., 1976; Novak et al., 2013).

Under the current system, patient satisfaction, patient outcomes, patient–provider relationship, chronic disease and injury prevention, and public health education suffer. Occupational hazards are also high for healthcare providers, including therapist disability, compassion fatigue, and high rates of suicide (Wallace et al., 2009; Devi, 2011; Fiabane et al., 2012; Iliceto et al., 2013).

In their article "Interdisciplinary education and teamwork: a long and winding road," authors Hall and Weaver (2001) state that interprofessionality needs more attention in healthcare, while a multidisciplinary approach is essential in decreasing patient catastrophizing, self-reported patient disability, aiding pain relief, and improving physical functioning, emotional stress, depression, and quality of life (Pergolizzi et al., 2013).

The reasons for biomedical myopia are multifaceted; yet, they are faulted by a common denominator, which is the lack of interprofessional partnership. The MTY program began in 2001 (Garner, 2001) as a continuing education certification, working to address difficulties healthcare providers struggle with to deliver quality BPS care; it was from this program that this text was evolved. Interdisciplinary partnership was a central mission for MTY, with a vision to decrease barriers to yoga receipt and use in healthcare and to facilitate healthy dialogue between healthcare fields and the yoga community at large. The vision is in alignment with the Institute of Medicine, which states that interprofessional partnership is vital for improving patient adherence and patient outcomes (IOM, 2013).

Healthcare systems in the United States can thrive and be more innovative if a paradigm shift toward partnership is considered (Garner, 2014). Partnership values historically marginalized qualities attributed as stereotypically feminine, including compassion, softness, nurturing, empathetic listening, and non-violent collaboration. These qualities have largely been treated as inferior to perceived "masculine qualities" such as dominance, toughness, conquest, power, authority, force, and strength of will (Eisler, 2007). In medicine, these qualities are often personified in the "power of the white coat."

Adopting a partnership model for collaborative practice in healthcare may improve access to and coordination of healthcare services, promote appropriate use of specialist clinical resources, improve chronic disease outcomes, increase patient safety, reduce length of hospital stays, patient complications, the number of hospital readmissions, clinical error rates, and mortality rates. Additionally, partnership-based healthcare may increase patient satisfaction, improve career satisfaction for healthcare professionals, reduce care costs, the rate of suicides, the number of outpatient visits, and improve access to mental healthcare (WHO, 2010; Eisler and Potter, 2014).

Medical Therapeutic Yoga (MTY) works to contribute to partnership in healthcare and yoga through:

- Fostering safety and clinical efficacy in rehabilitation and injury prevention
- Offering the potential for cultivation of mindfulness in medical practice and daily living
- Encouraging active patient participation and encouraging "person–provider" relationship over "patient–provider" relationship
- Embodying slow medicine
- Fostering interprofessional collaboration
- Adopting the biopsychosocial (BPS) model of assessment (introduced in Chapter 2)
- Teaching continuing education and graduate level medical education via an interdisciplinary model.

MTY works to contribute to research and scholarship of yoga in healthcare through:

- Provision of inter-rater and intra-rater reliability via biomechanical analysis of yoga postures and breath
- Provision of evidence-based therapeutic rationale for biomechanical alignment and execution of postures and breath techniques
- Addressing a gender context for teaching in a time when research in women's healthcare is still largely neglected. A gender gap in healthcare expenditures still remains, while women continue to suffer from more chronic diseases and a woman in the United States is more likely to die in childbirth than a woman in any other industrialized nation in the world (US DHHS, 2007; Hellwig, 2013; Save the Children, 2013). Connective tissue properties and neuroendocrine function undergo a vast range of fluctuation and resilience in the female during different seasons of her life, including being at higher risk for connective tissue injuries (Kjaer and Hansen, 2008; Fitzgerald

and Mallinson, 2012) or changes in pain and impairment that are cycle-dependent. Therefore, yoga when used as medicine, should be adapted to women's needs

- Provision of interdisciplinary educational competencies for graduate and postgraduate level curriculum (IOM, 2013; Pergolizzi et al., 2013) that honor yoga's origins and complexity

- Facilitating interdisciplinary relationship and subsequent creativity in rehabilitation through a BPS five-faceted model using a partnership model (Garner, 2014)

- Broadening yoga's reach in medicine for physiological stability in the individual rather than limiting yoga to only flexibility, mobility, mindfulness, or relaxation training

- Facilitating adoption of traditionally feminine characteristics known to improve patient outcome and satisfaction

- Increasing awareness of a partnership system in healthcare and of egalitarian principles in the care of patients and practitioners alike.

Yoga in healthcare

Yoga is an experiential, not just an academic practice. Yoga philosophy is the interaction between an individual and his or her own biology as a personal biofeedback system. This means the *sadhaka*, the practitioner of *sadhana* (a means to accomplish something), should have a regular yoga practice. The clinician who practices yoga pursues direct experience over exclusive intellectual experience, somewhat akin to medical doctors' or therapists' completion of residencies and clinical internships before being allowed to sit for their board exam and receive a license to practice.

Yoga provides the healthcare provider a container to experience and apply the BPS model, allowing yoga to be used in healthcare in a clinically meaningful way. Yoga recognizes that pain arises from a lack of unity. If a person has physical pain, the yogic model acknowledges the pain is present because one part of the system (in the BPS model) is not communicating

well with other parts of the system. Therefore, yoga is also a systems-based approach to assessment in healthcare.

For example, in order to treat back pain, a clinician must look at every system in the person, which in medicine is recognized as systems review. A clinician must make sure that the low back pain his or her patient is experiencing is not actually a functional gastrointestinal disorder or tumor. But yogic evaluation takes the medical practice of systems review to a new level. The cause of the low back pain is considered to be five-faceted (physical, psychoemotional, intellectual, energetic, and spiritual) and cumulative, rather than arising from a single accident, incident, system failure, mechanical failure, or inherent weakness or atrophy.

Yoga also cares for the practitioner by preventing or managing burnout or caregiver fatigue. A heavy toll is exacted on caregivers due to heavy caseloads, limited control over the work environment, long hours, as well as organizational structures and systems in transition. These variables are directly linked to increased stress and symptoms of burnout, and in turn, have adverse consequences for clinicians and the quality of care that is provided to patients. Irving et al. (2009) cite that the overwhelming presence of stress in healthcare providers provides clear justification for the "development of curriculum aimed at fostering wellness and the necessary self-care skills for clinicians" (p. 61). Yoga techniques such as meditation are cited in the study to "enhance well-being and coping with stress in this population" (p. 61). Guidelines to the practice of yoga in healthcare are found in Chapter 12.

Yoga's perennial philosophy

There is a fair amount of discussion as to whether or not yoga is a religion. This discussion is germane to utilizing MTY as it is apt to come up in practice. Here is how MTY responds.

Yoga indirectly addresses religion without being a religion. Swami Bharati, alongside other yoga leaders such as Georg Feuerstein and T. K. V. Desikachar, demystify yoga by dispelling the notion that yoga could be considered a religion. Yoga is contained within religions but religion is not contained within yoga (Bharati, 2013). Seven qualifying statements support yoga as separate from religion (Bharati, 2013). Yoga has:

1. No deity to worship

2. No worship services to attend

3. No rituals to perform

4. No formal statement of religious belief

5. No requirements for confession of faith

6. No clergy, nor is there an institutional structure of overseers or leaders

7. No system of temples or churches.

Yoga is defined by several popular figures and fore-runners in yoga culture today:

- *Light on Yoga*: "Yoga is not for him who gorges too much, nor for him who starves himself. It is neither for him who sleeps too much, nor for him who stays awake. Yoga is … moderation" (Iyengar, 1976).

- *Yoga for Body, Breath, and Mind: A Guide to Personal Reintegration*: "Yoga removes obstacles to clear perception, therefore achieving personal reintegration. Reintegration is the process of changing a wandering mind into a centered one, a wanting mind into a contented one, a self-indulging mind into a self-fulfilling one. It is yoga" (Mohan and Miller, 2002).

- *Yoga, The Poetry of the Body*: "Yoga is a way to be with whatever is, it isn't always about getting better or changing things from what they are" (Yee and Zolotow, 2002).

- *Fire of Love: Teaching the Essence of Yoga*: "Yoga doesn't care about the shape of your body, but the shape of your life" (Palkhivala, 2006).

Patanjali provided a beautiful analogy for yoga in the Yoga Sutras: "yoga is like a forest filled with variety and color. Every tree in a forest has the same goal, to reach toward the light. When practiced with awareness, the tree grows. Practice is the only method of feeding it."

Ten precepts

The yoga in this text follows 10 precepts grounded in the current evidence base and follows recommendations from the World Health Organization and Institute of Medicine on the use of the BPS model for effective person-centered care and pain management (WHO, 2002; IOM, 2011; Pergolizzi et al., 2013).

The 10 precepts operate from the primary neurobiological mechanisms exercised and subsequently achieved via meditation through postures and the breath. As a result, the neurochemical response or consequence of stress, as explained below in the concept of allostatic load, can be mediated via these mechanisms. MTY is a neural exercise of physiological structures often involved in breathing and posture that have a neural, endocrine, and immune consequence. Guidelines for achieving these responses are outlined below.

Medical Therapeutic Yoga:

1. *Views the person and their potential for injury or disease through a BPS model of assessment (WHO, 2002; IOM, 2011) in order to affect all-health outcomes through reducing allostatic load.* The phenomenon of allostatic load and its impact on health directly affects pain (Goldberg and McGee, 2011), stress, sleep, and fatigue (Rohleder et al., 2012), age-related disease (Taylor et al., 2011; Danese and McEwen, 2012), and epigenetic impact, including longevity (McEwen et al., 2012). First mentioned in the *Archives of Internal Medicine* by McEwen and Stellar (1993), allostatic load is defined as "the cost of chronic exposure to fluctuating or heightened neural or neuroendocrine response resulting from repeated or chronic environmental challenge that an individual reacts to as being particularly stressful" (p. 2093). McEwen (1998) and McEwen and Seeman (1999) simplified the term by defining it as wear and tear on the body systems due to physiological adaptations to repeated stressors.

These early descriptions of allostatic load represented a new shift in the medical model – one of refocusing attention on internal responses to a perceived hazard (McVicar et al., 2014). Logan and Barksdale (2008) describe allostatic load as the failure that occurs due to unsuccessful adaptation (allostasis), which ultimately results in pathophysiology and chronic disease. McEwen and others' early research on intracellular homeostasis and its critical influence on cognitive and biological response underscores the concept of stress as a "genuinely psycho-biological phenomenon" (Beckie, 2012; McVicar et al., 2014).

Goldberg and McGee (2011) propose that persistent exposure to deleterious social and economic conditions perpetuates the fight-or-flight response. The chronic accumulation of stress hormones, such as cortisol, is strongly correlated with many diseases and negative health outcomes (Goldberg and McGee, 2011). This phenomenon, primarily attributed to the HPA (hypothalamic–pituitary–adrenal) axis and its relationship with cortisol dysregulation, is well documented (Logan and Barksdale, 2008; Ross and Thomas, 2010; Beckie, 2012; Friedman et al., 2012; Streeter et al., 2012; McVicar et al., 2014).

Allostatic load is determined, in the heuristic model, as a result of genetic, environmental, biographical, psychosocial, behavioral (lifestyle choices such as diet, activity, and sleep), and clinical variables in the individual (Beckie, 2012). The multivariable nature of the allostatic load further underscores the need for a multifaceted BPS approach, or one that "bridges the fields of biomedical and psychosocial stress" (WHO, 2002; Beckie, 2012; Pergolizzi et al., 2013).

Paine et al. (2012) corroborate evidence that supports the powerful influence of chronic mental stress to trigger myocardial infarction. Other physiological biomarkers of psychosocial stress include the well-documented phenomenon of pro-inflammatory markers in the bloodstream, including cytokines and tumor necrosis factor (IL-1β, TNF-α, and IL-6), and the failure of glucocortiocoid receptors, leading to conditions such as endothelial dysfunction (Paine et al., 2012), depression, diabetes, autoimmune diseases, upper respiratory infections, and impaired wound healing (Cohen et al., 2012). A meta-analysis cited yoga's positive effect on reducing biomarkers of inflammation to improve immune function (Morgan et al., 2014). Therefore, the use of a yogic BPS model to reduce allostatic load through patient-centered care is the first and most important precept in MTY practice.

2. *Exists to establish interdisciplinary integrative yoga education in healthcare in order to protect the consumer of yoga* (IOM, 2000; Pergolizzi et al., 2013).

3. *Recommends the breath be attended to prior to teaching postures or movement.* Neuroendocrine regulation and effect of cortisol regulation, psychoemotional epigenetics, and GABA (gamma-aminobutyric acid) system and HPA axis regulation are directly affected by diaphragmatic breath (Brown and Gerberg, 2009; Streeter et al., 2010, 2012). The diaphragm is implicated in trunk stabilization, pelvic floor health, and postural control (Kolar et al., 2010, 2012; Bordoni and Zanier, 2013), with greater fatigability found in individuals with recurrent low back pain (Janssens et al., 2013). For this reason, the transversus abdominis (TA)-assisted thoracodiaphragmatic (TATD) breath is recommended for use during dynamic yoga posture performance. The TA has historically been identified as having an important function in provision of regional stability for the trunk (Hodges et al., 1996; Hodges and Richardson, 1997; Jull and Richardson, 2000). Contemporary support for TATD breath, which addresses both neurophysiological and psychobiological mechanisms, will be presented in Chapter 4. From a strictly mechanistic perspective, TATD breath provides lumbopelvic and concomitant synergistic regional stability through sufficient timing and control of the TA, increased intra-abdominal pressure for increased trunk stiffness, and neurophysiological training, which allows the TA to function independent of, and prior to, limb movement. Its synergistic role with efficient use of the respiratory diaphragm and its contribution to postural control, pelvic floor muscles, and multifidus, not forgetting the addition of other hip synergists, allows the TATD breath to create a more

stable yoga pose and ultimately, a safer and more clinically effective yoga prescription.

4. *Advocates for biopsychosocial stability as a primary focus with mobility as a secondary focus.* Structural alignment of postures is guided by six physiological principles and four principles of biomechanics, discussed in Chapter 3. Application of the current evidence base of neuromechanics and common motor synergies that determine mapping of motor intention and, ultimately, action is required to establish the safety of the individual (Torres-Oviedo and Ting, 2010; Ting et al., 2012), and for the creation and prescription of safe yoga programs for wellness and/or rehabilitation. This stability focus also includes creating a safety net for movement and social engagement which can affect autonomic and psychobiological functioning and tissue response via polyvagal theory, which will be discussed in Chapter 3.

- *Stabilization as a primary focus.* The primary physical focus of posture practice should be creation of a safe movement therapy environment through protection of proximal anatomical structures, chiefly the nervous system and spinal column/cord, via stabilization. Protection of the mind–body complex should target neuromechanical and synergistic function in balance control (Ting et al., 2012; Chvatal and Ting, 2013) and neuroendocrine regulation via allostasis (McEwen et al., 2012) to promote safe movement and outcomes in yoga. Lumbopelvic stabilization through the canister or cylinder model and multiplanar functional mobility with provision of spinal unloading via intra-abdominal pressure changes offered by abdominal wall function (Stokes, 2010; Lee, 2011) is a focus, along with prioritization of stabilization in a proximal to distal fashion. As a result, secondary and tertiary foci include upper quarter (shoulder complex) and lower quarter stabilization via functional postural training, respectively. Exceptions to this precept are discussed in Chapter 5.

- *Mobilization as a secondary focus.* The secondary physical focus of posture practice should be mobility, with flexibility following as a distant third focus. The only exception to this precept would include addressing fascial restriction that may inhibit muscular contraction and thus preclude neurophysiological stability. Fascial mobilization can improve regulation of state allostasis in those individuals where there is a clear absence of weakness or faulty neuromotor patterning in a muscle unit or complex. In these cases, prescription of restorative postures and exclusive use of (1) breathwork and/or (2) manual therapies (within the rehabilitation professional's scope of practice) could facilitate gentle myofascial release that would support the return to stability.

5. *Informs dynamic execution of breath and postures via instructing: (1) internally supported postures (asana) or (2) passive rehabilitation methods via externally supported postures (asana)* based on functional carryover to ADL (activities of daily living) such as walking, for example. Common muscle synergies for walking and balance require muscle synergy analysis, which assists in discerning motor deficits of spatial or temporal muscle activity quality (Chvatal and Ting, 2013). Muscle synergy analysis (in this case, yoga postures) may also provide more generalizable assessment of motor function because it (muscle synergy analysis) can identify impairment across multiple motor task performances (Chvatal and Ting, 2013).

6. *Combines Ayurvedic (sister science or medical side of yoga) clinical evaluation methods for analysis in yoga prescription.* Although this assessment is beyond the scope of this text, early evidence does support the epigenetic effects of yoga, which creates a relationship between genomic mapping and the Ayurvedic doshas (Bhushan et al., 2005; Hankey, 2005; Sharma et al., 2007; Prasher et al., 2008; Rastogi, 2010; Ghodke et al., 2011; Morandi et al., 2011).

7. *Includes evidence-based sound, music, and voice analysis as therapy for anti-inflammatory*

properties and ventral or myelinated vagus nerve stimulation (Porges, 2011) via the auricular nerve branch (Bernard, 2004; Levitan, 2007; Brandes et al., 2008, 2009; Nilsson, 2008; Bella et al., 2009; Bengtsson et al., 2009; Conway et al., 2009; Murrock and Higgins, 2009; Thaut et al., 2009; Thaut and McIntosh, 2010), trigeminal, and/or phrenic nerve connections.

8. *Teaches non-weight-bearing headstands (sirsasana) and non-cervical-weight-bearing shoulderstands (salamba sarvangasana), emphasizing protection of vulnerable joints that include the small joints of the hands, feet, and the spine and pelvis.*

9. *Is non-dogmatic and welcoming to all disciplines of yoga and respects all spiritual belief systems.*

10. *Teaches the student to seek the self pursuant to one's duty/mission (dharma).*

Table 1.1 summarizes the 10 precepts of Medical Therapeutic Yoga.

Review

Chronic disease is an epidemic problem internationally (WHO, 2005). The health benefits yoga can confer to both patient and practitioner are encased in a compassionate, holistic, and person-centered BPS model and have significant implications for improving health and healthcare. Using scientifically tested methods of rehabilitation to deliver yoga is a natural segue to transforming clinical practice and personal health.

Table 1.1
Ten precepts of Medical Therapeutic Yoga

Medical therapeutic yoga:
1. **Views** the whole person through a yogic biopsychosocial (BPS) model
2. **Establishes** interdisciplinary integrative yoga education in healthcare
3. **Recommends** attention to breath prior to teaching postures or movement
4. **Advocates** for BPS stability as a primary focus with mobility as a secondary focus, guided by principles of neurophysiology and biomechanics
5. **Informs** dynamic execution of breath and postures via instruction of internal or external support
6. **Combines** Ayurvedic clinical evaluation methods for analysis in yoga
7. **Includes** sound, music, and voice analysis as therapy
8. **Teaches** non-weight-bearing headstands and non-cervical-weight-bearing shoulderstands and emphasizes protection of vulnerable joints
9. **Welcomes** all disciplines of yoga and spiritual belief systems
10. **Guides** the student to seek the self pursuant to one's duty/mission

The biopsychosocial model for yoga in healthcare

This chapter provides the basis for culturally sensitive partnership of the yogic (*panca maya*) biopsychosocial model (BPS) with the World Health Organization's (WHO) International Classification of Functioning, Disability and Health (ICF) (WHO, 2001). Maximizing their interrelationship can help manage obstructions to health, wellness, and precursors of "dis-ease," which will be discussed in a case study format for practical application. Evidence for blending rehabilitation and yoga continues in this chapter, and methods for operationalizing a yogic BPS model are also reviewed.

Outline

- Challenges facing 21st-century healthcare
- The biopsychosocial model
- Using the yogic biopsychosocial model
- Biopsychosocial assessment
- Influencing change behavior
- Crossing the threshold into effective chronic disease management and health promotion: what medicine needs to thrive
- Defining disability and health functioning models
- Determining competence and considering sensory integration
- Case study: ICF and obstructions model synergy
- Conditional observations for overcoming obstructions
- Review: cultural competence

Challenges facing 21st-century healthcare

In 1948 the World Health Organization confirmed its definition of health as being "a state of complete physical, mental, and social well-being and not merely an absence of disease" (WHO, 1948). Yet healthcare systems in many countries still struggle to embrace its full meaning amidst rising healthcare costs that are inversely proportional to health outcomes. The 20th century required a shift in medicine, away from acute disease toward chronic and lifestyle disease management (Wahdan, 1996; Dean et al., 2011), underscoring a real need for a shift in thinking in healthcare (Elliott et al., 2002; Pomeroy, 2012; Van Hecke et al., 2013). The WHO estimates that out of 58 million deaths in 2005, 35 million could be directly attributed to chronic disease (WHO, 2005).

Chronic pain is also on the rise. The International Association for the Study of Pain (IASP) and the European Federation of IASP Chapters estimate 20% of the world population suffer from pain, while 1 in 10 adults are newly diagnosed with chronic pain each year (Goldberg and McGee, 2011; IASP, 2012). A reported one in three adults has trouble living independently due to chronic pain (IASP, 2012). The IASP reports the major categories of chronic pain are cancer, osteoarthritis and rheumatoid arthritis, surgeries and injuries, and spinal problems. The diversity of causes and their comorbidities make pain management a multifaceted and interdisciplinary task (Goldberg and McGee, 2011; Pergolizzi et al., 2013). Some of the comorbidities correlated with chronic pain include diabetes, arthritis, depression, irritable bowel syndrome (Bonaz and Bernstein, 2013), and asthma (Bair et al., 2003; Krein et al., 2005; Arnow et al., 2006; Hestbaek et al., 2006; Kato et al., 2006; Piette and Kerr, 2006; Goldberg and McGee, 2011).

Patient satisfaction is also affected, with the Institute of Medicine (IOM) endorsing the BPS approach in their 2011 report *Relieving Pain in America: A Blueprint for Transforming Prevention, Care, Education, and Research*, suggesting that the patient-centered BPS model of care has been shown to be the most effective and cost-effective way to address pain. IOM committee member Myra Christopher states:

"Effective pain management is a moral imperative, a professional responsibility, and the duty of people in the healing professions" (Tawoda, 2012).

With the chronic disease rate projected to increase another 17% over the next 10 years (WHO, 2005), yoga is a viable low cost option for intervention. A 60-year meta-analysis supports yoga as a possibly superior intervention to conventional standard physical activity in the geriatric population (Patel et al., 2012), while a 2010 literature review (Ross and Thomas, 2010) supports yoga as being as effective as or superior to exercise for both healthy and diseased populations. Yoga is also effective for a range of chronic disease processes and addiction issues through affecting biomarkers for inflammation such as C-reactive protein (CRP) and cytokines, cardiovascular, psychoemotional and physiological health, and immune function (Bijlani et al., 2005; Kochupillai et al., 2005; Pullen et al., 2008; Kuntsevic et al., 2010; Ross and Thomas, 2010; Streeter et al., 2012; Tekur et al., 2012).

Yoga's multifaceted methodology, including breathwork, meditation, movement, and lifestyle counseling, can affect what the WHO (2005) identifies as the largest risk factors for premature aging and mortality, which include the following:

- Unhealthy diet
- Physical inactivity
- Poor lifestyle
- Choices that lead to obesity
- Cardiovascular disease
- Diabetes
- Several types of cancer.

Personal responsibility also affects health outcomes, even more so than medical intervention (Kaufman, 2012; Pomeroy, 2012). Therefore the positive influence of yoga philosophy to affect variables that improve patient adherence and outcomes, including self-management and increasing health locus of control, confidence, and self-efficacy (Cramer et al., 2013), could serve two chief purposes in chronic disease prevention and management.

The biopsychosocial model

The BPS conceptual model (Fig. 2.1) proposed in this text is based on recommendations from the Institute of Medicine, the WHO's ICF model, and an evolution of the five-limbed yogic BPS (*panca*

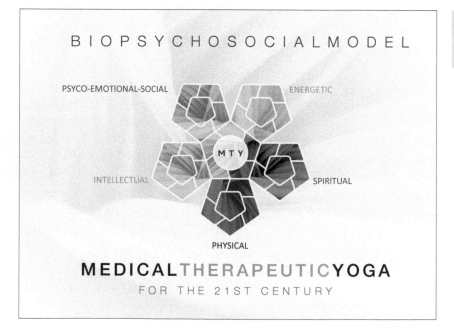

Figure 2.1

The yogic biopsychosocial model

(five) *maya* (pervading)) model (WHO ICF, 2002; Easwaren, 2007; IOM, 2011). The BPS model has been validated with a multitude of populations, including:

- Cerebral palsy (Rosenbaum and Stewart, 2004; Jonsson et al., 2008; Andrade et al., 2012)

- Diabetes (Awad and Alghadir, 2013)

- Bipolar disorder (Ayuso-Mateos et al., 2013)

- Multiple sclerosis (Conrad et al., 2012)

- Stroke (Glassel et al., 2014)

- Low back pain (Glocker et al., 2013)

- Distal radius fracture (Harris et al., 2005)

- In general physical therapy and rehabilitation (Bartlett and Lucy, 2004; Jette, 2006)

- Breast cancer (Khan et al., 2012)

- Morbid obesity (Lin et al., 2014)

- Osteoarthritis (Oberhauser et al., 2013)

- Hand conditions (Rudolf et al., 2012; Scorza et al., 2013).

The WHO ICF model (Fig. 2.2), a BPS template for delivery of healthcare, recognizes that the metric of the human condition, including personal and environmental factors, does play a role in determining a person's level of disease or functioning, and, therefore, must be considered in patient care. The BPS model offers (Bartlett and Lucy, 2004; Rosenbaum and Stewart, 2004):

- A range of entry points for intervention in medicine

- Inclusion of social support and community resource health promotion

- A more holistic, patient-centered template for clinical decision-making

- The opportunity for more effective communication between patient and practitioner

- Improved patient satisfaction and patient outcomes through addressing the whole person, instead of just a diagnosis

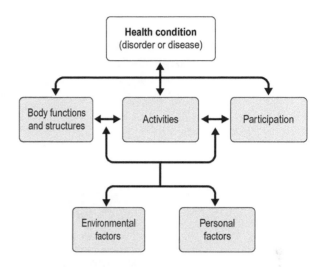

Figure 2.2
World Health Organization's International Classification of Functioning, Disability and Health (ICF) model (reproduced with permission from the World Health Organization)

- Evidence-based medicine and research in a compassionate and individualized way

- A "universally accepted conceptual framework to define and classify disability" (Scorza et al., 2013, p. 1).

Using the yogic biopsychosocial model

When the BPS model (Fig. 2.3) is used in the yogic system, the clinician should recognize that personal and environmental factors intimately affect psychobiological health and well-being, as outlined in the WHO's ICF model, as well as the following:

- It addresses all five dimensions, recognizing that each one is valuable and critically interrelated in a circuitous relationship rather than a hierarchical one.

- It acknowledges that change is an inherent part of developing awareness. The yogic model fosters questioning one's frame of reference and habits of thought in order to come to or appreciate a new understanding (Mezirow, 2003). In other words, freedom requires transformation or the willingness to change. Mezirow's transformational learning

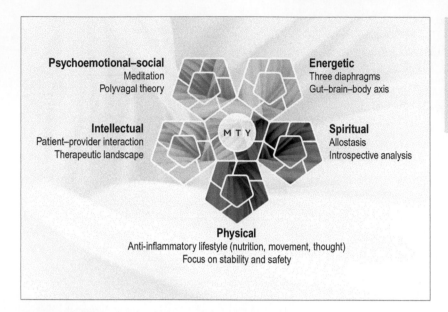

Psychoemotional–social
Meditation
Polyvagal theory

Energetic
Three diaphragms
Gut–brain–body axis

Intellectual
Patient–provider interaction
Therapeutic landscape

Spiritual
Allostasis
Introspective analysis

Physical
Anti-inflammatory lifestyle (nutrition, movement, thought)
Focus on stability and safety

Figure 2.3
Biopsychosocial model overview. Empowering patients to take responsibility for their health depends on focused, biopsychosocial assessment

theory (TLT) allows for questioning the way social roles are inhabited, how clinical findings are interpreted based on those past experiences and concepts of personal authorship, and in what context patients are viewed (hopefully as a whole rather than a diagnosis, which is only part of a whole).

The five dimensions of the yogic model, as described in the *Taittiriya Upanishad*, known as "Ascent to Joy" or degrees of happiness, are as follows (Easwaren, 2007):

1. Material body, physical and nutritional sheath (*annamaya [ahn-nuh mah-yuh]*)

2. Vital sheath, energetic body, life force, breath (*pranamaya [prah-nuh mah-yuh]*)

3. Mind, emotional, social body, discrimination (*manomaya [mahn-noh mah-yuh]*)

4. Intellectual body, wisdom/discrimination (*vijnanamaya [vignyah-nuh mah-yuh]*)

5. Bliss body, spiritual, individual connected with the divine/soul (*anandamaya ([ahn-nahn-duh mah-yuh]*).

Biopsychosocial assessment

Because each of the five dimensions is interrelated, assessment takes place on a continuum rather than in a vacuum. Psychobiological stress and allostatic load can be directly influenced by yoga (Bijlani et al., 2005; Yang, 2007; Kuntsevich et al., 2010; Streeter et al., 2010; Anderson and Taylor, 2011; Tekur et al., 2012) through multimodal yoga prescription, but not least, via influencing vagal nerve activity and parasympathetic nervous system interaction with the hypothalamic–pituitary–adrenal (HPA) axis (Ross and Thomas, 2010; De Couck et al., 2012; Noggle et al., 2012). These discoveries make yoga a powerful, if not necessary, modality for use in medicine, especially for the plethora of diseases influenced by stress.

Subjective intake

Assessment begins with subjective intake. This typically occurs via patient interview, observation, and a thorough review of intake forms to screen for systemic red flags. Factors to review and discuss include:

• Previous medical history (PMH) – review of general systemic health

• History of present illness (HPI) including current medications, diagnoses, and treatments

• Pain (pain analog scale, or PAS) patterns

• Patient's personal goals for therapy.

Subjective intake should also consider the patient's report, including their daily routine, that includes:

- Activity (previous, current, and preferred level, type)

- Nutritional habits – a 3-day food diary is recommended

- Social support system

- Psychoemotional health, including inter- and intrapersonal relationships

- Environmental surroundings and effects on health at work and home, including climate and ergonomic factors.

Objective intake

The objective intake includes five facets:

1. and 2. *Physical and energetic assessment* through the functional movement algorithm (FMA) — The FMA offers a method for global BPS assessment based on individual interaction with, and stress response to, yoga postures and breath. It is driven by four major objective domains concerned with regulation of allostatic load, discussed in Chapter 5, that also consider the non-tangible and more esoteric philosophy of energy anatomy and life-force, or "*prana*."

3. *Psychoemotional or stress response observation* — The psycho-emotional-social limb or pentagon corresponds with mindful practice of not only postures and breathing, but interaction with the self and others. Yoga, through breathing, meditation, or posture practice, can affect all-health outcomes through modifying our perception of stress and stress response. Ability to change the stress response, through a meditative state, can be responsible for neural plasticity and cerebral cortex thickening, which can "improve memory, attention, thought, and language" (Khalsa, 2013).

4. *Intellectual observation* — The intellectual pentagon of the model, the gateway for transformation, is aptly translated as the "transformational body" in yoga (Easwaren, 2007). Our duty as healthcare providers is to discern the individual's

needs and help them change behavior through genuine, motivational interaction and communication with them (Lundahl et al., 2013; Benarous et al., 2014). The intellectual limb or pentagon ultimately determines the health of the person since it determines willingness, motivation, and readiness for change behavior. The majority of health problems in the 21st century are preventable or remediable by health behavior change (Rollnick et al., 2008; Dean et al., 2011), which means the future of healthcare will focus on behavior change and is largely concerned with patient adherence and motivation in order to affect chronic lifestyle-related conditions (Dean, 2009).

5. *Spiritual inquiry* — Impacting spiritual readiness includes fostering directed action for mind/body connection and introspective awareness that is commensurate with the individual's personal belief system. Easily the most avoided aspect in healthcare, the spiritual facet of health can be correlated with religious belief, non-theistic groundings, and/or the ability of a person to connect meaningfully with the world around them.

Other assessment that can occur separate from, but in concert with, administration of the FMA includes:

- Systemic differential diagnosis

- Lifestyle assessment via constitutional testing (Ayurvedic analysis, nutrition and epigenetics of nutrition, and a systems approach to gut microbiota management)

- Environmental analysis (consideration of therapeutic landscape, including ergonomics or home safety) — An important variable influencing treatment outcomes is the therapeutic landscape and actual physical intervention. The conceptual framework provided by Miciak et al. (2012) addresses the idea, and importance, of providing a safe, therapeutic landscape and setting where healing can take place, something that is of great importance in using yoga as medicine. The physical qualities of the therapeutic environment and the intervention logically represent the physical pentagon of the BPS model and occur through consideration of green space on health, well-being, and social safety (Groenewegen et al., 2006). Further, the consideration of therapeutic landscape in yoga is of particular interest in the medical or clinical setting, where access to natural, serene, or calm environments can be scarce (Hoyez, 2007). An ideal landscape can be achieved in many settings, despite the globalization of yoga, through making simple changes such as eliminating overhead fluorescent lighting, changing wall or flooring colors or coverings, and generally considering green space in clinical settings

- Blood chemical analysis including CRP (C-reactive protein) level, vitamin D, and diurnal cortisol level, for example — Vitamin D deficiency has been connected to sleep apnea, metabolic syndrome, obesity, diabetes, osteoporosis, pre-eclampsia, and cardiovascular disease (Kienreich et al., 2013; Ryan et al., 2013; Scholl et al., 2013; Erden et al., 2014), while skewed cortisol and CRP levels have been well established, earlier in this text, as increasing chronic disease and mortality risk

- Use of standardized outcome psychometric measures with a BPS context (Chapter 12), such as the Short Form (SF)-36 — The SF-36 measures functional health and well-being from the individual adult's point of view (Quality Metric, 2013) and is a likely candidate for use because of its BPS framework (versus biomedical) and support from the WHO (2001), and its ability to measure self-efficacy, readiness for change, and health beliefs. The SF-36 does not screen for sleep and nutrition, so they must be assessed separately since lack of sleep and poor nutrition (Morris et al., 2009) are well established to influence health. Lack of sleep is associated with altered cortical synaptic function, GABA levels, and hippocampus function (Cirelli, 2013) while inadequate sleep in adolescents is associated with a decline in neurocognitive function and in emotional regulation and attention, specifically problem-solving, verbal memory, auditory attention, visual sustained attention, psychomotor speed, and computational accuracy (Fallone, 2002; Shochat et al., 2014).

Influencing change behavior

The intellectual pentagon could emerge as the most critical dimension to address in the BPS model because it identifies barriers to learning and change, critical for achieving whole health. The process of affecting intellectual health should be, in every sense of the word, an emancipatory process (Kitchenham, 2008).

Patient education and counseling are hallmarks of effective intervention in medicine. Patient adherence (DiMatteo et al., 2007), satisfaction, and outcomes are determined by an individual's health beliefs and literacy, ultimately dictating their willingness and ability to change, especially in vulnerable populations (Green et al., 2014). Low health literacy is a recognized public health problem (Kutner et al., 2006; US Department of Health and Human Services 2010), correlated with:

- Increased hospitalizations (Baker et al., 2007, 2008)

- Decreased preventive care (Scott et al., 2002; White et al., 2008)

- Poorer overall health (Bennett et al., 2009)

- Racial disparities in healthcare (Saha, 2006)

- Higher mortality rates (Sudore et al., 2006; Baker et al., 2007, 2008; Peterson et al., 2011).

The difficulty in promoting behavior is multifaceted and can include:

- Neurocognitive status of the patient and somatosensory status (Dunn, 2009)

- Readiness to change, self-efficacy, social support status, perceived threat of disease or severity of illness (DiMatteo et al., 2007)

- Perceived locus of control (Turiano et al., 2014).

Motivational interviewing (Abramowitz et al., 2010) techniques such as authentic and compassionate communication skills via non-violent communication (Rosenberg, 2003; Nosek, 2012) can make communication more productive by addressing individual variations which affect communication, such as age, cognition, motivation, or psychoemotional status, for example. Creation of mindfulness and awareness in both the provider and patient is perhaps best addressed through the lens of transformational learning theory, which allows the patient, as an adult learner, to question his or her own beliefs and frame of reference, as opposed to just accepting or learning new information without reflective discourse (Mezirow, 2003; Kitchenham, 2008). Transformational learning theory provides a container for that liberation through allowing "transformation of problematic frames of reference – fixed assumptions or expectations – to make them more inclusive, discriminating, open, reflective, and emotionally open to change" (Mezirow, 2003, p. 58).

One entry point for fostering health behavior change is through improving provider–patient communication. Improving provider–patient communication (Green et al., 2014) through a partnership relationship (Eisler, 2007; Garner, 2014) in both general and psychotherapy medical settings has been correlated with improved pain, decreased disability, and patient satisfaction (Hall et al., 2010).

Strategies for influencing changes in health behavior are summarized in Table 2.1. Strategies include the following:

- Rollnick et al.'s (2008) motivational interviewing technique suggests following the "RULE" principle: R – *resist* the urge to correct, noted as "resisting the righting reflex," U – *understand* your patient's motivations, L – *listen*, and finally, E – *empower* with gentle, permission-based questioning, that is, posing questions in a way that asks permission of the patient and conveys respect through partnership, rather than through an authoritarian or "provider as expert" relationship.

- Informing the patient about evidence-based care. In a trial of patients with low back pain, patient adherence, physical functioning, and outcomes improved when this facet was included (Rutten et al., 2014). Providers should be able to explain, in general terms, the scientific rationale and support for a recommended treatment, or in this case, yoga intervention.

- Increasing perceived locus of control (Turiano et al., 2014) by validating patient experience and not dismissing it as subjective or mood-oriented (Doyle et al., 2013).

Table 2.1
Strategies for influencing health behavior

Strategies for influencing health behavior include:
1. Establishing a partnership relationship
2. Informing the patient about evidence-based care
3. Validating patient experience
4. Identifying somatosensory threshold

- Identifying somatosensory threshold (Dunn, 2009), which is described in the literature as the amount of sensory input needed for an individual to learn and function psychoemotionally–socially (Dunn, 2009). Sensory integration and processing is a concept traditionally grounded in occupational therapy; however, the interdisciplinary nature of applying the BPS model for optimal outcomes requires sensitivity to all aspects of the individual's constitution and in this case, includes sensory processing (Garner, 2001; WHO, 2002; Dunn, 2009; IOM, 2011; *The Patient Patient*, 2013). For example, if a patient is a low threshold passive sensor, then he or she would respond to the smallest introduction of information in the therapeutic setting. This would require a more sensitive and subtle approach than the high threshold active seeker, who naturally needs more sensory input for learning (Dunn, 2009). Occupational therapist Winnie Dunn offers a model for somatosensory classification that would place the patient in one or more of the following categories (Dunn, 2009):

- High threshold active – seeker (energetic) – needs more input for learning

- High threshold passive – bystander (quiet) – waits for others to present sensory information for learning

- Low threshold active – avoider (fussy) – avoids sensory input and requires limited sensory information for best concentration

- Low threshold passive – sensor (distractable) – most sensitive and a small amount of information overwhelms the individual and makes concentration difficult.

These suggestions, of course, represent the ideal; however, our current healthcare system has crumbled under the high pressures of expediency and profit. Although patient education and counseling are perhaps the most important aspects of patient-centered intervention (Miciak et al., 2012), they are services that have low or no reimbursement rate in insurance-based healthcare models, especially in the United States. Hence, lack of reimbursement creates significant barriers to adequate receipt of patient education.

Quite often in medicine, healthcare is driven through creating fear and issuing ultimatums in the name of "efficiency," expedited patient management, or to avoid legal action or threats of negligence. This is described as a dominator model relationship that is driven by pitting one profession or gender over another (Eisler, 2007). Drug companies also shoulder responsibility for improving healthcare. Pharmaceutical marketing tactics through television and print advertising can cause individuals to request, and even demand, drugs and diagnostic tests from their physicians. As a result, physicians may feel they are obligated to respond to patient demands, for fear of litigious action on the part of their patient populations.

> If the transformative process does not lead to an outcome, modern "progress" is stunted and negative social and economic repercussions will be felt.

For patients to thrive, the BPS ideal must be continuously kept in our collective vision. It is through facilitating growth in the transformative sheath or intellectual pentagon that this model can help improve education in patients and foster a higher locus of control, both of which are undeniably linked to decreased mortality risk and improved longevity for patients (Turiano et al., 2014). After all, if the process does not lead to an outcome, modern "progress"

is stunted and negative social and economic repercussions will be felt. Therefore, acknowledging the artistic side of medical practice has implications for quality of healthcare delivery (Lane, 2010).

The yogic BPS model provides a template for empowerment of patients through active participation, self-reflection, and critical analysis of assumptions (Kitchenham, 2008), which is a unique quality not present in other types of CAM and certainly not readily accessible in the biomedical model. Healthcare must recognize that conservative care provides a sustainable method of seeking health instead of continuing to subscribe to invasive biomedical care that is far more costly and, in the case of low back pain, yields poorer short- and long-term outcomes (Mafi et al., 2013; Saltychev et al., 2014). Healthcare providers must persist in pursuit of what is best for the patient and individual, because ultimately the financial prosperity and security of a nation is determined by the health of its citizens.

> Healthcare providers must persist in pursuit of what is best for the patient and individual, because ultimately the financial prosperity and security of a nation is determined by the health of its citizens.

Crossing the threshold into effective chronic disease management and health promotion: what medicine needs to thrive

There are two areas of disease prevention that are, by far, the most important modifiable lifestyle variables. Those areas are diet and lifestyle. Yoga addresses them both in the BPS model via the principle of non-violence (*ahimsa*).

Yoga is an ancient lifestyle practice, not just one that provides physical exercise and meditation. The yogic BPS inherently embraces, due to the individual code of ethics assigned in the eight-limbed (*Ashtanga*) yoga practice, a non-violent lifestyle toward the self and all things (Easwaren, 1985), which also includes consideration of non-violence in nutrition for all-health outcomes (Fig. 2.4). Exercise will be addressed in Chapters 4–10, but one factor less often considered in yoga is nutrition.

This attention to non-violence is where the historic vegetarian lifestyle of yoga arises from; however, not all yoga practitioners need to be, or should be, vegetarian. The traditional diet of a yogi or yogini (one who practices yoga) historically was, and still is today, vegetarian. This diet was adopted as a result of yoga's philosophy that kindness and non-violence (*ahimsa*) toward all living creatures is requisite as part of recognition of the best and healthiest self.

However, there are conditions where being a vegetarian may not always be possible or ideal. For this reason, yoga does not require vegetarianism but instead determines a person's nutritional needs based on their individual characteristics, called a constitution. In other words, nutrition in Indian medicine, similar to the philosophy of other cultural systems of medicine such as traditional Chinese medicine or Native American medicine, is not addressed through a single one-size-fits-all approach, as in Western medicine.

Regardless, vegetarianism and its health benefits are widely embraced throughout Western medicine and culture, and science has provided us with overwhelming evidence of its health benefits. Adopting a plant-based diet can be optimal for health, but it is only part of making healthy lifestyle choices. Nutritional habits are an important and integral part of the yoga lifestyle, and can directly contribute to systemic health and outcomes. Digestion plays a critical role in the natural healing process. As far back as the ancient Greeks, the philosopher Epicurus declared that sound digestion was "the basis of all human goodness" and poor digestion was so morally destructive that "everything possible should be done to avoid it."

Beyond nutrition, the other important facet of non-violence toward the self is physical activity and weight management. The three most important risk factors cited in developing persistent grades of low-level inflammation in the body include poor nutritional choices, physical inactivity, and obesity (Nathan, 2008; Dean, 2009). The inflammatory processes caused by this trio contribute to chronic diseases and pathophysiologies such as cardiovascular disease, breast cancer, colorectal cancer, dementia, chronic lung diseases, osteoarthritis, and diabetes (Watzl, 2008; Jin, 2010; Serafini et al., 2010).

Proactive behavior which prevents and reverses states of inflammation in the body depends on lifestyle choices,

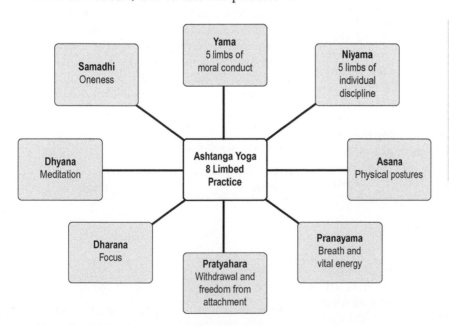

Figure 2.4

Ashtanga yoga: eight-limbed practice. Pranayama and asana are, in Medical Therapeutic Yoga methodology, reversed in order. Breath is recommended to be addressed before movement, according to the precepts

chiefly diet and exercise. A diet high in flavonoids can diminish the presence of pro-inflammatory gene expression (ICAM1, ILR1, TNF-α, and NF-κB1) and significantly lower circulating white blood cells (Elenkov et al., 2005; García-Lafuente et al., 2009; Hermsdorff et al., 2010). Physical activity provides a strong protective anti-inflammatory effect in the body through lowering resting levels of inflammation in the body that contributes to chronic inflammatory disorders, obesity, and other chronic non-communicable diseases (Pedersen, 2006, 2011; Petersen and Pedersen 2006; Wilund, 2007; Mathur and Pederson, 2009; Brandt and Pedersen, 2010). In essence, skeletal muscle acts as an endocrine organ, possessing immunologic function that contributes directly to our health.

Although a full discussion of nutrition is outside the scope of discussion in this book, the lack of modeling of good health habits by healthcare professionals has a detrimental impact on influencing patients. An unhealthy healthcare provider decreases the chance that he or she will promote healthy lifestyle behaviors to patients (Dean, 2009).

Therefore, the importance of a healthcare professional having a personal yoga practice cannot be overemphasized. *Living Your Yoga*, as Judith Hanson Lasater discusses in her book of the same name (2000), can directly impact our influence as healthcare providers. Healthcare providers can improve their clinical efficacy by adopting a regular yoga practice. A cumulative effect of 10 minutes of practice, three times per day, can be beneficial to exact positive systemic effects, as recommended by the WHO (2010). Focusing on non-violence and nurturing the self and the planet is a first step toward completing the paradigm shift in healthcare from biomedical to biopsychosocial. Experientially embracing yoga makes for better teachers and healers through improving chronic pain management and health promotion.

Defining disability and health functioning models

To make the yogic BPS model relevant, a synthesis of health functioning models via the WHO's ICF model is needed. In 2001 the WHO established what has become an internationally accepted model that guides the healthcare professional's determination of, and definition for, health due to recognition that "the scope of health extends beyond the realm of disease to the wider domain of overall human functioning" (Scorza et al., 2013).

The ICF framework provides a container for interpretation of health, illness, function, and healthcare professional roles (WHO, 2001). The ICF model has been validated by numerous studies to be effective with a wide range of patient populations including orthopaedic, neuromuscular, and psychoemotional/ mental health ranging from pediatric to geriatric (Harris et al., 2005; Conrad et al., 2012; Rudolf et al., 2012; Ayuso-Mateos et al., 2013; Glocker et al., 2013; Oberhauser et al., 2013; Scorza et al., 2013).

Ancient yogis also realized the importance of "wholistic" or person first care. The model of the obstructions (*kleshas*) could exemplify the yogic model for recognition of impairment and factors responsible for impeding or preventing health and well-being (Table 2.2). The five obstructions (*kleshas*) recognize that an individual's life experiences can ultimately shape their health outcomes.

There are five obstructions: ignorance (*avidya*), the first obstruction, is said to give rise to the remaining four obstructions, egoism (*asmita*), attachment (*raga*), hatred or aversion (*dvesha*), and clinging to life (*abhinivesha*) (Iyengar, 1976). The interrelationship of the obstructions with the WHO's ICF model can provide a cross-culturally sensitive and holistic method for addressing individuals' needs. The

Table 2.2
Obstructions to practice

Kleshas	Obstructions
Avidya	Ignorance
Asmita	Egoism
Raga	Attachment
Dvesha	Hatred/aversion
Abhinivesha	Clinging to the body

WHO also identifies the ICF as a BPS model because it considers environmental and personal factors as part of the "disablement" process and health functioning. As a result, the obstructions together with the five pentagons of the yogic BPS model, are both intimately related to, and congruent with, the ICF model.

There are multiple positive variables to consider in the convergence of yoga philosophy with today's medical model. Some of those considerations include a practitioner's ability to function in a "dynamic systems" model, one where there are multiple points of entry for intervention in medicine (rather than just the physical), seeing the patient as an active (rather than passive) participant in his/her health and healthcare, and finally, the utilization of neutral (rather than disabling) language to describe a person's health and well-being.

Overcoming obstructions to health is not the goal in yoga. Rather, being aware of, and attending to, the obstructions (ignorance, egoism, attachment, hatred or aversion, and clinging to life) and their many forms is given higher priority. B. K. S. Iyengar, in the quintessential text of early Western yoga instruction, *Light on Yoga*, states that the obstructions can be active, latent, or hidden; they are never absent (Iyengar, 1976). This statement supports the ICF model for provision of a deeper understanding of a disease process (or how to prevent disease and disability). The inherent wisdom of recognizing obstacles to wellness acknowledges that if we can understand a person's likes, dislikes, fears, and loves, then we can plan more effective medical intervention.

Using yoga to facilitate health and wellness depends on more than just conceptualization of an academic model. Yoga's efficacy in medicine depends on the practitioner's ability to experience yoga, rather than just pursue scholarly study and theoretical analysis. A regular yoga practice will largely determine the effectiveness of the medical professional's clinical efficacy in patient practice. The five obstructions to practice and integration of both BPS models presented in this text (ICF and the *panca maya/koshic* model), provides an integrative template for achieving better patient outcomes, increasing patient satisfaction, and improving intervention in preventive care, health promotion, and disease management.

Determining competence and considering sensory integration

Still, there is more to the BPS model and the five obstructions than simply adopting a consistent yoga practice. How is competency determined within application of the models? Physical competency of the yoga postures and breathing techniques have been widely debated, as evidenced by the number of yoga anatomy texts currently in publication; however, physical mastery of postures will be discussed in later chapters. Primarily, what should be considered before discussing posture mastery is identification of a range of interventions based on a measure of the individual or patient's consciousness, competency, and self-efficacy. The original "conscious competence matrix" was introduced by Mitchell and Savage in 1979 and was used to describe the four stages of skill acquisition (Folkins, 1992). The four stages (Fig. 2.5) progress as follows:

1. Unconscious incompetent action (you do not know that you do not know)

2. Conscious incompetent action (you know that you do not know but can assimilate the information and understand why it is important for health)

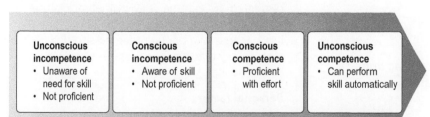

Unconscious incompetence	Conscious incompetence	Conscious competence	Unconscious competence
• Unaware of need for skill • Not proficient	• Aware of skill • Not proficient	• Proficient with effort	• Can perform skill automatically

Figure 2.5

Conscious competency matrix (based on the work of Mitchell and Savage, 1979)

3. Conscious competent action (you know that you know)

4. Unconscious competent action (it just seems easy).

Although "unconscious competency" could be misinterpreted as "thoughtless movement or action," it describes a movement, behavior, or action in which the individual achieves total absorption without distraction. This has also been referred to as "second nature" or reflective ability. The matrix can be applied to teaching yoga, which underscores the importance of having a personal yoga practice. If a teacher of yoga cannot convey, with open-ended and inspirational language, the deeper potential of a yoga posture, breath, or philosophical teaching with unconscious competence, the patient is not likely to gain unconscious competence with his/her new skillset in yoga.

This can also describe Patanjali's ultimate intention for practicing yoga, "super-consciousness" or "*samadhi.*" Both Eastern and Western psychology approaches recognize the importance of practice, whether dealing with physical and/or emotional blocks to health and happiness. Continuation of the explanation of competency determination with an illustrative case study follows, as well as inclusion of sensory threshold considerations based on the work of Winnie Dunn (2009), discussed earlier in the chapter.

Case study: ICF and obstructions model synergy

Disability is described in the ICF as "a difficulty in functioning at the body, person, or societal levels, in one or more life domains, as experienced by an individual with a health condition in interaction with contextual factors" (WHO, 2001). See Dina's story, which illustrates the synergy between the ICF and obstructions models.

Case study

Internal Classification of Functioning and obstructions models – Dina's story

This case story shows how the ICF and obstructions models overlap in order to provide vital information for helping the patient, Dina,*

toward recovery from disability and to establish competency in yoga based on her sensory perception (sensory perception is discussed further in Chapter 3).

*Please note that the patient's name has been changed to protect her privacy.

Patient's health condition

Dina K. is a pleasant 63-year-old woman of Native American descent who suffers from chronic pain related to childbirth trauma experienced 30 years ago and due to various microtraumas over the years; this limits her activities of daily living. Dina retired early, about 13 years ago, because of her pain and dysfunction. She continues to have functional limitations at present.

Body functions/structures

Dina experiences difficulty with pelvic pain that contributes to sexual dysfunction. She has pain with attempted intercourse secondary to suspected vaginismus/pelvic myalgia and inability to have gynecological exams completed secondary to suspected hypertonicity of the pelvic floor. Additionally, she has related sacroiliac joint pain and a diagnosis of fibromyalgia. All of the conditions together limit her work and life tasks.

Environmental factors

Dina is very active in her church and community, donating her time freely to various humanitarian efforts. She is the primary caregiver for her father, who has dementia and was recently placed in a skilled nursing facility. Dina, due to her low sensory threshold, is admittedly easily distracted by external environmental circumstances (such as laundry that needs completing, or caretaking or volunteer tasks to do). Her low sensory threshold also creates sensitivity to noise and light.

Personal factors

Dina readily gives of her time, often in neglect of self-care, and has a difficult time saying "no" to volunteer work. She avoids medication whenever possible, eats organic and non-GMO (genetically modified organisms) food due to her work with local healthcare providers, and regularly receives Medical Therapeutic Yoga via physical therapy and acupuncture for management. Her main obstructions to wellness are her lack of compliance with her physical therapy plan of care, in addition to lack of boundary setting and her distractibility. She feels that she is consciously competent with safely performing her prescribed yoga program; however, follow-through and consistent compliance is an issue. With a constitution that is recognized in Ayurvedic medicine as an air/ether constitution (*vata*), Dina can lose focus easily or forget to take care of herself, including forgetting to eat regular meals and complete her therapy program. However, she is tirelessly motivated to be well again, and is able to maintain, at a minimum, passive therapies such as regular massage and acupuncture.

Activities

Her therapist and family alike have regularly counseled Dina on the importance of being an active participant, rather than a passive recipient, of medical therapies. For example, active physical therapy combined with medical therapeutic is more likely to yield long-term results than reliance on pain medications or passive therapies alone.

Obstruction overview

Lack of education (avidya)

Lack of education (knowledge) about her own condition can perpetuate Dina's pain experience and disability. The yogic model would focus on patient education and empowerment with the right tools for self-management and advocacy (this would include educating her to ask relevant questions and self-advocate for appropriate services at other doctor and therapy visits). This education could also be extrapolated for her other family members

undergoing medical treatment, such as her father, in order to help her manage her overall stress, burden of care, and worry about what is best for her father's well-being and health. Additionally, she acknowledges her preoccupation and distractibility, yet they continue to be a prominent reason for noncompliance with active therapies.

Egoism (asmita)

Her decision to retire early to caretake her health is a demonstration of setting aside the ego of "career" to seek long-term well-being. However, attachment to the identity of her career could perhaps be one reason that she constantly overcommits to volunteer activities and helping others. Volunteerism is not a bad thing in itself, just as the ego is not "bad." However, when the ego identifies with things in your life that are a long-term detriment to your well-being or those you love, then boundaries must be set to avoid self-destructive patterns.

Aversion to change (raga)

Aversion to change in general and a fear of pain can sometimes drive individuals to make fear-based decisions. This means Dina may be avoiding movement therapies such as Medical Therapeutic Yoga because she is afraid of pain or afraid of other consequences, such as neglect of family or friends or community. But this fear comes at a price, since Dina has lost her own health, perhaps, due to unrealized fear.

Clinging to life (abhinivesha)

Lastly, clinging to life is perhaps the least significant issue with Dina, because she readily sacrifices her mind and body for her faith as a devout Christian lay minister and mission-oriented volunteer. However, her identity for the last decade has been associated with disability and pain, and this could make detachment from disability and a movement toward being proactive for wellness more challenging.

Chapter 2

Conditional observations for overcoming obstructions

There are a number of ways in which both clinicians and their patients can benefit from study and application of the yogic "obstructions" (*klehsas*) philosophy model. Acknowledging that growth and transformation require change, and that change requires acknowledgement is an important first step in dealing with barriers to health and wellness. Patient counseling and guidance toward making healthy lifestyle choices, which include the practices of yoga, requires compassionate interaction and self-awareness.

One method for facilitating personal growth is identification of intellectual preferences. For example, a small study group can be highly effective for many individuals; however, if that same small study group grew to a size of 30 or more individuals, its effectiveness might begin to diminish if participants were to feel uncomfortable or too vulnerable speaking in a large group setting. However, one-on-one patient education could make an individual who has difficulty with social interaction very uncomfortable and less likely to follow or listen to a provider's advice. Therefore, information sessions conducted via video, handouts, or electronic/digital handouts may be best for this patient population. The Gracious Space technique (Fig. 2.6) developed by the Center for Ethical Leadership, which creates awareness of "a spirit and setting where the stranger can learn in public," could also be considered to facilitate a successful learning environment, as found in Hughes and Nienow's text *Courageous Collaboration with Gracious Space: From Small Openings to Profound Transformation* (2011). Using the technique would consider the myriad of variables for the individual that would create a comfort zone for learning, and then try to incorporate those into the intervention or session time. Considering these practices can help further shift the paradigm of practice toward the new era of person-centered, partnership-based care.

What does not kill us makes us stronger

A second condition associated with the obstructions is the importance of recognizing that adversity, or stress, can create strength instead of illness. The

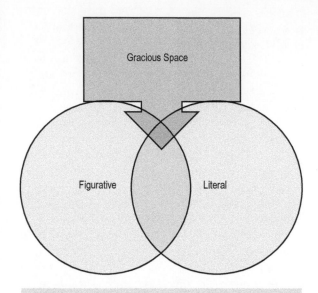

Figure 2.6

Gracious Space is found in the overlap between figurative and literal domains and is a place where a person feels comfortable learning in public

health beliefs of a person color their view of stress. An 18.5 year analysis of 7,268 men and women who reported that "stress" had "affected their health a lot or extremely" showed that they had a 2.12 times higher risk of coronary death or myocardial infarction than those who reported no effect of stress on their health (Nabi et al., 2013). A National Health Interview Study linked to National Death Index mortality data from 1998 to 2006 supports that the 33.7% of adults who perceived that stress negatively affected their health or reported higher levels of stress were more likely to have worse health and mental health outcomes (Keller et al., 2012). Further, those same people also had a 43% increased risk of premature death (Keller et al., 2012). Our attitude toward stress, then, has a direct impact on all health outcomes and risk of premature death. Additionally, adults who survive natural disasters, such as 574 adults who survived the 2004 tsunami in Southeast Asia, have less likelihood of suffering from post-traumatic stress disorder and a higher reported quality of life if "they believed that life was meaningful and that they had value as a human being" (Nygaard and Heir, 2012).

In other words, whether or not an individual suffers from mental or physical conditions depends on their attitude toward adversity.

Viewing stress and pain as a teacher or friend, instead of the enemy, can improve long-term health outcomes, health status, and quality of life (Keller et al., 2012; Nygaard and Heir, 2012; Nabi et al., 2013).

Stress reduction, then, is as much of a misnomer as trying to achieve homeostasis (instead of allostasis) in the body, since we are not trying to reduce stress or find a static homeo"stasis" in the body, rather we are trying to change how our body perceives stress and actively adapt (allostasis) to how our mind and body responds to it. In short, if "you are what you eat," then also "you are what you think."

Stress as "contagion" also carries great implications (Kaplan et al., 2013). The belief that stress is contagious begs to address the potential for individuals to engage in avoidance behavior, become complacent toward healthy lifestyle choices, or engage in outright self-destructive behavior. Shifting one's perspective toward constructive attitudes and coping mechanisms to address health beliefs and behaviors, then, can have an impact on preventing premature aging and death (Keller et al., 2012; Nygaard and Heir 2012; Kaplan et al., 2013; Nabi et al., 2013). Yoga that is designed with sensitivity to nomenclature and attitude(s) toward stress should focus on building stress resilience, rather than stress reduction.

Review: cultural competence

There are three socially sensitive components that influence application of the model to improve cultural competence in mindful healthcare delivery (Table 2.3):

1. Person first language (Folkins, 1992) — The use of "person first language" identifies the individual first, rather than allowing a disability to define or precede identification of an individual. For example, in the case of diabetes, a person is not "a diabetic" but the "person with diabetes"; or, in

Table 2.3

Culturally sensitive components of care

Culturally sensitive care component	Description
Person first language	Identify the individual first
Person-centered culture	Work together with the individual
Partnership theory	Individual is an active participant in his or her health

the case of cerebral palsy, a child with cerebral palsy has a disability, rather than being labeled a "disabled child."

2. Person-centered culture — Shift from "patient-centered" terminology to a person-centered culture. In other words, the patient–provider authoritative relationship, where "doctor knows best," evolves into a person–provider partnership where the physician or therapist works together with the individual to establish a plan of care.

3. Partnership theory — In partnership theory, a person becomes an active part of his or her healthcare instead of a passive recipient. Relationship drives partnership theory and is recognized as moving from a domination-based interaction to a partnership (Eisler and Potter, 2014). This would allow the individual to take responsibility for his or her care instead of just being a passive recipient of "doctor's orders," and would also foster creativity in rehabilitation (Garner, 2014).

Improving healthcare requires an evolution of both medicine and yoga. This text offers a contribution to the international effort to create a cross-cultural system of medicine that is sensitive to other cultures and practices. The clinical implication, then, is anyone can do yoga. But to practice yoga deserves careful attention. It is a subtle science that deserves respect as a part of healthcare and for its complexity, and as such, should require advanced study in biomedical and biopsychosocial studies.

Yoga is deserving of the constant theoretical inquiry and ongoing scientific scrutiny that all biomedical science receives. Chapters 4 and beyond establish a model for prescribing yoga therapeutically and in wellness populations, from a biomechanical and orthopaedic viewpoint.

Healthcare providers bring a unique knowledge to the yoga paradigm of practice, while yoga educators can do the same for healthcare professionals. There is room for everyone in the practice and prescription of yoga both in and as medicine, so long as there is interdisciplinary research and mutual respect to advance the study of yoga as a valid, reliable, and viable method for BPS assessment and intervention.

Neurophysiological foundations for evidence in practice: historical and contemporary support

The premise of merging yoga with rehabilitation and preventive care acknowledges that our biomedical system is moving from a mechanical model (local system and tissue intervention cause and effect) to a neurophysiological model (in this case a single yoga posture or breath affects global change in multiple body systems). For example, prescription of respiratory diaphragm work through yogic breathing can affect not only local tissues such as visceral function and fascia or transversus abdominis (TA) or pelvic floor length/tension, but also emotional well-being through biochemical influences known to exist through cortisol and hypothalamic–pituitary–adrenal (HPA) axis regulation and polyvagal response. This chapter addresses six neurophysiological foundations that inform physical yoga prescription to affect global neurophysiological change. These variables are guiding principles for fostering clinical safety and efficacy in rehabilitation and wellness populations and represent evidence-based benchmarks for evolution of yoga prescription. They, like those in the other chapters, have been compiled through a review of the literature and refined through clinical practice and didactic field testing in both graduate and continuing/postgraduate education since 1998. Vitality and health depend on the systems-based evidence that supports the role of these neurophysiological principles for yoga prescription, and the interrelationship they have with pain science. Foundations for safety, stability, motor control, respiration, and multimodal support in yoga postures are conceptualized via these neurophysiological phenomena for systems-based intervention (listed in the outline below). Finally, with respect to the myofascial effect of each pose, realize that fascial tensile force cannot be simply applied in such a linear or reductionistic fashion. All fascial meridians could be affected by a single pose, depending on the person's condition or disability, including their state of hydration, phase of healing or injury, stress response, psychoemotional or autonomic nervous system status. The guidelines provided for fascial tensile force in Chapters 6–10, in context, serve as a general guideline for attending to fascial plane(s) most likely affected in a pose, and for evolution of future theory.

Outline

- Neurophysiological foundations for evidence-based practice
- Kinesthetic awareness
  - Reflexes
  - Sensory modulation
    - Tactile
    - Balance: vestibular and visual
    - Pain and trauma
- Respiration
- Stabilization
- Support
- Mobilization
- Meditation
- Review

Neurophysiological foundations for evidence-based practice

This section establishes six neurophysiological foundations that offer healthcare providers a framework for yoga prescription, as summarized in Table 3.1.

Kinesthetic awareness

Kinesthetic principles are used in teaching consciousness and proprioceptive awareness. The neuroscience of reflexes, which includes the myotatic stretch reflex (MSR), Golgi tendon organ (GTO), and implications for stretch in yoga, are basic principles important for application of yoga as a movement therapy.

Chapter 3

Table 3.1

Six foundations of neurophysiology

Kinesthetic awareness	• Reflexes
	• Sensory modulation
	• Tactile
	• Balance: vestibular and visual
	• Pain and trauma: mapping the somatosensory, limbic, and cognitive highway
Respiration	• Diaphragmatic anatomy
	• Respiratory physiology
	• Systemic implications: neuroanatomical implications in diaphragmatic breathing
Stabilization	• General joint stabilization requisites
	• Controlled flexibility theory
	• Historical relevance of lumbopelvic research
	• Four planes of control
	• Scapulothoracic and glenohumeral
	• Femoroacetabular and tibiofemoral
Support	• Internal/intrinsic control
	• External/extrinsic control
Mobilization	• Joint positioning
	• Closed kinetic chain
	• Open kinetic chain
	• Open-packed joint
	• Close-packed joint
	• Arthrokinematics
	• Spinal kinematics
	• Fascia
	• Skin interruptions and adhesions
	• Neural mobilization
Meditation	

Reflexes

The neuroscience of cortical reflexes has continued to evolve (Kistemaker et al., 2013) since English physiologist Sir Charles Sherrington's original work on the monosynaptic reflex response in 1924 (Liddell and Sherrington, 1924; Marcus and Jacobson, 2003; Pruszynski and Scott, 2012; Yavuz et al., 2014). The current evidence base on the MSR and the GTO informs neuromuscular intervention, tendon compliance, and sensorimotor control and feedback in practical yoga posture prescription.

Myotatic stretch reflex

The monosynaptic myotatic stretch reflex (Fig. 3.1) is characterized as a deep tendon reflex dependent on afferent stretch velocity input which is directly proportional to muscle spindle activity; meaning muscle spindle activity increases with stretch velocity (Schuurmans et al., 2009). The thickly myelinated structure ensures that the muscle spindle is one of the fastest conducting fibers in the body, creating a contraction of the muscle at approximately 100 m/s via motor fibers in the muscle spindle located within the muscle unit (Mense, 2010).

In yoga, the evidence can be interpreted in two ways: in a fixed posture, requisite control of limb stiffness in static postures is required for attaining joint or multijoint stability, and can be regulated via (1) voluntary muscle activation through feedforward mechanisms related to patterns of co-contraction (Franklin, 2004) or (2) changes in reflex sensitivity (Shemmell et al., 2010). Yoga postures have potential to train the individual for heightened reflex sensitivity. If this is true, then joint stability could theoretically be achieved at a lower metabolic cost and energy expenditure, which is an absolute goal of the central nervous system (Franklin, 2004).

Gender differences in clinical application of the MSR and GTO also exist. Connective tissues of men and women differ physiologically. Women demonstrate lower collagen synthesis response in exercise than men, attributed to estradiol's weakening effect on tissue (Kjaer and Hansen, 2008; Hoge et al., 2010). MSR response likewise varies by gender, with the

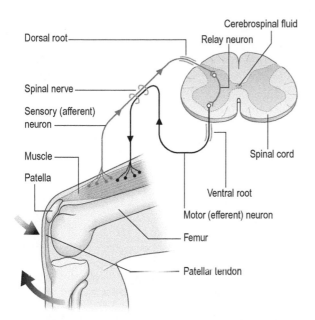

Figure 3.1
Myotatic stretch reflex

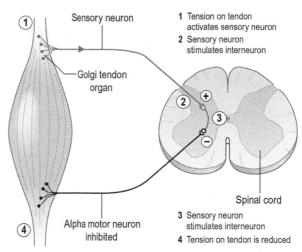

Figure 3.2
Golgi tendon organ reflex

lower MSR response for women occurring around the time of ovulation, correlated with peak levels of estrogen (Casey et al., 2014). Passive stretch changes range of motion (ROM) for women but not men after a 20-minute session (Hoge et al., 2010). Stretch does not affect musculotendinous stiffness overall, a finding confirmed by previous studies (Magnusson et al., 1996, 1998) and which underscores the findings of Weppler and Magnusson (2010), who posited that flexibility may not be an entirely mechanical phenomenon.

These results require two conclusions: (1) MSR can be voluntarily influenced to elicit higher athletic performance and potential; (2) gender differences exist which should influence yoga prescription. To further complicate the theory, the GTO has been implicated in contribution to muscle spindle response (Kistemaker et al., 2013), meaning the MSR potentially does not act alone.

Golgi tendon organ

The Golgi tendon organ (GTO) (Fig. 3.2) consists of myelinated Ib fibers with quick velocity potential

and is identified in the literature as an inverse MSR or autogenic inhibition (Mense, 2010). The GTO is a bisynaptic, slower reflex activated by contractile tension of the sensory receptor, which, overall, results in an inhibition of muscle activity (Mense, 2010). The difference between the MSR and the GTO lies in the location of the sensory axons. GTO sensory axons are located near musculotendinous junctions and end on inhibitory neurons that decrease the activity of motor neurons. Muscle spindles, by contrast, end on motor neurons that increase muscle activity (Mense, 2010; Yavuz et al., 2014).

A brief history of stretch

To synthesize the relevance of the MSR and GTO in yoga, the types of stretch that implicate these reflexes should be addressed (Table 3.2). The majority of stretch types are based on viscoelastic deformation and include two stretch types (Weppler and Magnusson, 2010): (1) static (Magnusson et al., 1995, 1996, 1998) and/or (2) repeated cyclical stretches (Taylor et al., 1990; Gaoa et al., 2011), the latter of which reportedly employs hysteresis and achieves flexibility through sustained active stretch (Magnusson et al., 1998). Three remaining stretch types are: (1) constant joint angle stretch (Taylor

Chapter 3

Table 3.2
Overview of five types of stretch

1. Static
2. Repeated cyclic – Employs hysteresis to achieve flexibility reportedly through sustained stretch
3. Constant joint angle
4. Constant load/passive stretch via creep – Creep = constant force (compressive or tensile) issued over time which causes the material to continue to deform (or lengthen) until its limit (state of equilibrium) has been reached
5. Proprioceptive neuromuscular facilitation

et al., 1990; Duong et al., 2001; McNair et al., 2001), (2) constant load or passive stretch to evaluate creep (Ryan et al., 2008), and (3) contract/relax proprioceptive neuromuscular facilitation (PNF) with or without pre-isometric contraction (Magnusson et al., 1996).

Gains in ROM plateau at about 6 weeks of stretching (Cipriani et al., 2012), with nine supporting studies found in Weppler and Magnusson (2010); however, no studies for stretch programs lasting more than 8 weeks (with a single session of stretch) have been undertaken (Ben and Harvey, 2010; Weppler and Magnusson, 2010), which necessitates further investigation into the role of sarcomere length changes in flexibility. Another gap in research that should be considered is yoga's flexibility utility in sensory modulation.

Sensory modulation: muscle length dimensions and biomechanical properties

Muscle length measure has, in the past, stood as the global indicator for flexibility. However, this represents a single dimension that considers only a muscle's ability to arrive at a predictable endpoint (Weppler and Magnusson, 2010). Muscle length measure does not differentiate between single and multidimensional concepts in flexibility, allowing for the conclusion that flexibility is not necessarily only a biomechanical phenomenon, but may include a sensory adaptation

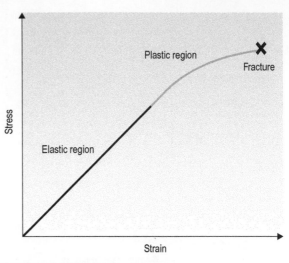

Young's modulus or modulus of elasticity
The modulus represents mechanical properties that can also exist in human building materials
The elastic region – Area of deformation of material(s) which returns to their original shape once load is removed
The plastic region – Area where materials under stress/strain conditions will no longer return to their original shape once the load is removed. This region is the end of the elastic region
Beyond plasticity – Area between the plastic region and failure point where permanent deformation occurs. The material will continue to deform until it reaches its failure/fracture point
Fracture point – Point of failure. The material can no longer tolerate the load, which could include bone, ligament, tendon, muscle, or cartilage and can also include not just fracture, tearing, or splintering, but also shearing

Figure 3.3
Young's modulus

potential (Folpp et al., 2006; Ben and Harvey, 2010; Weppler and Magnusson, 2010).

The role of elastic deformation versus plastic deformation in achieving flexibility, which influences length/tension relationship and is represented in Young's modulus (Fig. 3.3), is unclear. Ten studies cite plastic deformation as the reason for increased flexibility yet none of these used evidence supported by the classic model (Weppler and Magnusson, 2010). Instead, short-term elastic or viscous flow was supported. As a result, flexibility must consider not only the role of mechanical deformation, but also that of sensory adaptation potential. Table 3.3 gives an overview of biomechanical factors that influence tissue extensibility. Flexibility is

Table 3.3

Biomechanics and structural alignment principles that influence tissue extensibility

1. Connective tissue properties
2. Load/deformation and stress/strain
3. Length/tension relationship of muscle
4. Joint function

inherently tied to stability, and as a result, the discussion on flexibility will be completed later in this chapter (see below, Controlled flexibility theory).

Tactile sense

Tactile perception, or exteroception, is one of the five senses and involves the mechanoreceptors for vibration, light touch or distortion, pain, temperature, and pressure (Swenson, 2006; McGlone and Reilly, 2010). In contrast, interoception describes how we perceive our well-being from the inside out (Craig, 2002). Exteroception is controlled by the cerebral cortex in the dorsal column–medial lemniscus system (Puce, 2010), a tract providing a connecting point with the thalamus (Fig. 3.4) (Swenson, 2006).

Tactile sense describes the ability to perceive the sense of touch. As part of perceptive ability (*manas*) in yogic universal structure, tactile sense is part of the subtle body mastered by direct experience or, in the absence of input, by inference. Somatosensory modalities provide a sense of placement in space and a sense of the size, shape, and texture of things on the body surface, and are required in order to inform movement through space. Decision-making, control strategies for object manipulation, and haptic interface (nonverbal communication via tactile input) planning are all essential functions that involve the tactile sense and require development of consciousness as well as healthy motor control strategies. Both proprioceptive and cutaneous reception affect neural discharge, which is implicated in normal movement and also in bioengineering of devices such as limb prosthetics, where there is an absence of somatosensory information (Weber, 2011).

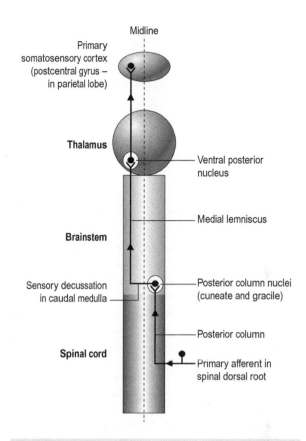

Figure 3.4

Medial lemniscus system

Immediate clinical application in yoga prescription relies on the ability to cultivate yogic language and manual therapy skills necessary to improve movement quality, tactile acuity, and pain management (Luomajoki and Moseley, 2011), by helping the individual attain proprioceptive intelligence via provision of tactile cues for location of the body in space. Mindfulness, in fact, begins with cultivation of a somatosensory skillset (Kerr et al., 2013).

Knowledge of the five types of tactile sense (Table 3.4) affords the clinician the ability to provide specific manual cuing that is evidence based. Provision of a point of contact for safe yoga posture execution is threefold with respect to tactile sense. First, the clinician must recognize that touch, specifically two-point discrimination, is less sensitive on the back and may require additional cues

Table 3.4
Five types of tactile sense

1.	Vibration
2.	Light touch or distortion
3.	Pain
4.	Temperature
5.	Pressure

beyond tactile. The placement of the hands or fingers for manual cuing and biofeedback should be at least 40 mm apart (Kitada, 2010), compared to other areas of the body, which require only 1 mm of distance for two-point discrimination (Johnson et al., 2000). Second, deep touch, or pressure, is directed by receptors in the internal organs and fascia, and requires a force of between 0.02 and 0.06 g at the fingertips, but approximately 0.2 g on the thigh (Kitada, 2010), to influence the ability to sense position and movement of the body through space (proprioception) (Swenson, 2006). Third, development of an instructional "yoga" language that addresses each of the five types of kinesthetic tactile sense maximizes biofeedback and fosters development of proprioceptive intelligence, postural control, and body consciousness or awareness.

Qualitative movement and pain management determinants: the "magic bullet" of sensory poetry

Flexibility end-limits are typically determined by the sensory system and are influenced by pain onset, maximal stretch, and maximum pain tolerated (Weppler and Magnusson, 2010). Using yoga in medicine requires a language that is both distinct from and more poetic than normal medical terminology. It involves something more than telling a patient or student to "put your arm there and move your spine like this." That type of instruction might perhaps be adequate in physical therapy or rehabilitative medicine but it is not yoga. Teaching yoga requires more than simply relaying instructions on

how to align a pose. To use yoga therapeutically to affect biopsychosocial (BPS) outcomes, an academic knowledge of kinesthetic sense must be merged with yogic tactile sense. What emerges is a new language informed by science, a kind of "sensory poetry."

The breath can be used as an example of how to inform medical language with yogic poetry. It is generally accepted that the breath can be used as the vehicle for meditation. If a person utilizes the respiratory diaphragm properly, the central nervous system should, in somatosensory theory, have to process less information about the process of breathing, referred to as unconscious competence in skill acquisition theory. If an individual is processing less sensory information, the central nervous system (CNS) sends less input and can decrease sympathetic activity. In theory, deep breathing should kickstart the process of healthy neuroendocrine regulation via influencing vagal activity, which is posited to upregulate parasympathetic activity (Jerath et al., 2006). This dichotomous theory that pits parasympathetic and sympathetic autonomic control against one another has been challenged by the notion of polyvagal theory (PVT) (Porges, 1995, 2007, 2011, 2012), which will be discussed in the vagus nerve section.

Knowing this is the biomedical means for explaining the end result of deep breathing, how would the healthcare provider convey this to the patient using yogic language? See the instructional "*sensory poetry*" narrative below, based on utilization of the neuroscience of tactile kinesthetic sense.

Sensory poetry narrative

To use yoga therapeutically to affect biopsychosocial outcomes, academic knowledge of kinesthetic sense must be merged with yogic tactile sense. What emerges is a new language informed by science, a kind of "sensory poetry." Based on utilization of the neuroscience of tactile kinesthetic sense, the following is an integrative kinesthetic script, a kind of kinesthetic transcendental meditation:

Touch

- In a comfortable resting position (supine, seated, or sidelying), feel how the breath moves your body.

- Notice how your body is affected by the breath. Notice the sensation in your arms, your trunk, your legs, your pelvis, your head, your face, your tongue – all as a result of your breath.

- Make a single, small, almost imperceptible movement that will allow your breath to more passively enter your lungs. Perhaps dropping the root of the tongue away from the roof of the mouth. Perhaps shifting your posture so that the air flows with less obstruction and your airway feels more open.

- One at a time, make other small movements, on an exhale, that will allow you to drop into your breath more deeply with the next inhale.

Pressure

- If you are resting on your back, feel how the earth rises up to meet you, to support you. If you are resting in seated, or seated against the wall, feel how the earth rises up under your sitting bones, to support you, to lift you up.

- Allow the earth to accept your breath, expanding the body, providing support.

Proprioception

- Feel the warmth of your breath at the tip of your nose.

- Feel how your breath expands your chest wall and creates openness, the potential for change, for energy increase.

- Feel the air on your skin, and how your breath interacts with the air in the room.

- Use the breath now, to explore any areas of the body or mind that feel dull or achy or painful. Use the breath like a light, sending the light of your breath to burn away the fog, dust away the cobwebs, and ready the mind and body for working together. Breathe positive energy.

Vibration

- Feel the subtle interaction of your breath with the subtle movement of the earth. Notice the breath, and perhaps the earth's vibrational quality.

- Allow the vibration of your breath to take on a deeper, slower rhythm. Exhale, and count the moments (seconds) of the breath. Inhale, and match the length to the exhale. Appreciate the musical quality of the breath. You are singing.

- Your breath is a song, moving in time to the vibrational frequency of the air in the room, the support of the earth's circadian rhythm, creating a flow that syncs you to the music of your breath.

- *"You are a song, a wished for song"* – Rumi (translated by Coleman Barks, 1995).

A final benefit of utilizing the divisions of tactile sense and employing reflexes is to induce meditation, the paramount intention of yoga. Sense of touch is a rapidly adapting modality in the body. The acute sense of touch will diminish in mere seconds when no new input to the touch receptors is received owing to the highly myelinated and rapidly adapting potential of the CNS (McGlone and Reilly, 2010; Roudaut et al., 2012).

This phenomenon is important for yoga because our ability to meditate depends on stability within a pose. If the pose is unstable, the CNS will continue to receive messages from the receptors in the skin, joints, and internal organs, making deep meditation and the journey to *samadhi* – or even inward relaxation – more difficult. In a stable pose the CNS is allowed to quieten as fewer signals are sent, making external and internal relaxation easier. In this way, the physical practice of yoga facilitates an entry point to meditation.

Balance: vestibular and visual sense

The receptors for our vestibular sense are located in the inner ear in semicircular canals and a reservoir called the utricle. These receptors allow us to maintain our equilibrium in space. They are sensitive to different stimuli and are involved in different reflexes:

- The horizontal canal houses the external semicircular canal and detects angular acceleration (spinning), cervical rotation, and flexion/extension, making it responsible for balance and hearing (Groves and Fekete, 2012).

- The superior canal houses the anterior semicircular canal and detects vertical movements, such as nodding the head.

- The posterior canal detects cervical sidebending.

- The utricles are responsible for detecting linear acceleration, changes in gravity, and coordination of whole-body postural adjustments (righting in space) (Saladin, 2012).

Patients sensitive to head motions in space could have a pre-existing condition, be recovering from an illness or injury, or not be acclimatized to stimulation of the utricles or semicircular canals. Dizziness or vertigo is not a preclusion or contraindication to posture practice. Indeed, carefully sequenced postures can help minimize or even resolve cases of motion sickness, dizziness, and vertigo.

Rehabilitation professionals will regularly encounter patients who have been debilitated secondary to vestibular disease or dysfunction caused by concussion, blast-induced mild traumatic brain injury, diaphragmatic dysfunction, or disorders of the inner ear.

A complete discussion of the anatomy of the vestibular system and rehabilitation is outside the scope of this text. However, yoga prescription in healthcare must consider neurological threshold and complicating vestibular factors for safe yoga prescription (see Case study: balance, vestibular, and visual sense).

Case study

Balance, vestibular, and visual sense

This case study details treatment activities and evidence-based therapies appropriate for a patient with post-concussive symptoms experiencing mild balance problems with vestibular complaints due to an orthopaedic injury.

Post-concussive symptoms and etiology

Post-concussive symptoms in sport include dizziness, vertigo, reported unsteadiness, and oscillopsia (McGrath et al., 2013). Individuals who report exertional post-concussive symptoms due to exercise or hyperthermia may also experience insidious neural deterioration in the "cerebellar and cerebral cortices," evidenced by "widespread microglial activation" during mild traumatic brain injury (mTBI), which carries major long-term implications for quality of life and health (Alsalaheen et al., 2010; Sakurai et al., 2012; Griesbach et al., 2013).

Overall, post-concussion vestibular issues can be exacerbated by pain, difficulty concentrating, attention issues, any pre-existing or new temporomandibular joint dysfunction, headache (tension type), and activity and mental task tolerance issues (Purcell, 2009; Riechers and Ruff, 2010). Vestibular issues which should be assessed include sensorimotor delays, abnormal eye movements (nystagmus), including visual acuity and target acquisition, gait instability, postural stability and balance, positional testing, and vestibulo-ocular reflex functioning, including horizontal and vertical gaze stabilization (McGrath et al., 2013). Additionally, the symptoms of concussion can be similar to, or include, post-traumatic stress disorder (PTSD) (Purcell, 2009).

Current recommendations for return to activity

The general recommendation is to avoid all activities, both mental and physical, until all symptoms are resolved (Sakurai et al., 2012; McGrath et al., 2013). Individuals must be symptom-free not just at rest but also with the introduction of full cognitive and physical activity (Aligene and Lin, 2013). Hyperthermia and exertion/fatigue are also implicated in negatively affecting neurocognitive outcomes and long-term neurological health (Alsalaheen et al., 2010; Badel et al., 2011; Griesbach et al., 2013). If vestibular symptoms such as dizziness, gait, or balance issues are not resolved by rest, then vestibular rehabilitation is indicated (Morinaka, 2009). Additionally, premorbid functioning is reported to affect recovery after mTBI (Morinaka, 2009).

Other causative factors

Other musculoskeletal issues that can be causative factors in treating post-concussion vestibular dysfunction include temporomandibular joint dysfunction (TMD) and neck pain, with the most common otologic symptoms of TMD including otalgia, tinnitus, and vertigo (Garner, 2012, 2013). Neck pain, tenderness in the sternocleidomastoid and along the nuchal line, and orthostatic hypotension can also be implicated in musculoskeletal differential diagnosis of vestibular dysfunction, especially in the 85% of orthopaedic injury-induced concussions that suffer vertigo and concomitantly present with musculoskeletal comorbidities (Gurley et al., 2013). Outcome measures for post-concussive vestibular management can be found in Chapter 11.

Treatment options

There are seven treatment options available for targeting vestibular issues in patients with post-concussion symptoms. They include: (1) canalith repositioning maneuver for benign paroxysmal positional vertigo (BPPV) (Dye, 2008); (2–4) vestibulo-ocular exercises which can include adaptation (to focus on affecting intact vestibular circuits through the use of retinal slip during head movement), habituation (enhance vestibular compensation via repetitive exercises), or substitution exercises (train ocular compensation in those with major vestibular impairment); (5) balance exercises (including static and dynamic positional exercise with and without introduction of neurocognitive tasks); (6) musculoskeletal assessment, differential diagnosis,

and management as needed of cervical spine integrity, myofascial restriction, headaches, or temporomandibular joint function; and finally (7) gait training (with and without inclusion of neurocognitive tasks and over both even and uneven terrain) and postural and trunk control and awareness, which also includes testing the patient under aerobic conditions to identify exertion-induced neurophysiological or cognitive impairment (Morinaka, 2009; Alsalaheen et al., 2010; Badel et al., 2011; Aligene and Lin, 2013; Gurley et al., 2013). Additionally it is important to note that failure to progress by the 6-month mark should warrant further neurological workup and consult (Aligene and Lin, 2013).

Vestibulo-ocular reflex (VOR) exercises

The following VOR exercises, prescribed in treating vestibular dysfunction with the yogic biopsychosocial model, have been successfully used in two case studies (Garner, 2001, 2012, 2013). View Fig. 3.5 to help patients develop self-management strategies and facilitate a patient's responsibility for their health and well-being. Yoga equipment (toys) included a yoga/sticky mat, two foam blocks, a chair, a wall, two Mexican-style blankets, and a nurturing therapeutic landscape. "Therapeutic landscape" describes the location and atmosphere of the treatment setting and is juxtaposed against the typical non-green space biomedical setting, which can often be associated with a "harsh therapeutic landscape" (Groenwegen et al., 2006). The clinical environment for these cases was a private, climate-controlled space with no outside noise or interuption; it had adjustable halogen or soft LED lighting (with dimmers available), pleasant paint colors and décor, and an overall non-sterile "hospital or clinic-like" standard setting.

VOR exercises were performed with two parameters: (1) performance for 1–2 minutes until subtle nausea is experienced and/or (2) use of variable speed until just before the target falls out of focus. The intention for exercises included: eye tracking for gaze stabilization in a yoga pose, easy seated pose (*sukhasana*), which resembles tailor sitting but on tiered blankets for support and comfort. Initially the patient sat in a chair secondary to concerns of excessive degrees of freedom imposed by lack of postural control and lumbopelvic awareness. See Figs 3.6 and 3.7 for an example.

Actions undertaken included: (1) movement of eyes in different directions (vertical, horizontal, diagonal, clockwise/counter-clockwise), (2) general tracking of finger tip or thumb (if no contraindications the upper extremity was used as related to cervical spine), and (3) tracking with candle for smooth pursuits. Also included were screening of plumb line alignment for postural awareness and pain-free active range of motion in the cervical spine.

The starting positions for therapy included progressing from seated in a chair to standing upright (mountain pose) to transitioning from stand to sit on the floor (easy seated pose) over a period of several sessions. Actions, in order of prescription, follow (Garner, 2013; Oyarce, 2013):

Case study

1. Perform 1–2 minutes until subtle nausea is experienced

2. Variable speed until just before target falls out of focus

3. Adaptation takes 6–8 weeks.

Oculomotor exercises

Intention: Eye tracking

Starting position: Easy seated two-tier approach for comfort/neurovascular and muscular protection/postural alignment lumbar spine

Action:

- Move eyes in different directions (vertical, horizontal, diagonal, clockwise/counter-clockwise)

- General tracking of fingertip or thumb (if no contraindications upper extremity use as related to cervical spine)

- Tracking with candle for smooth pursuits.

Action

- Practice of slippage of head on atlas (*mild jalandhara bandha* or chin lock)

- Eye movements while maintaining cervical retraction (*mild jalandhara bandha*)

- Nose circles while maintaining cervical retraction (*mild jalandhara bandha*)

- Atlas/axis rotation awareness

- Eye movements with cervical flexion, extension, side-bending and rotation as indicated/pain free

- Targets for cervical rotation eye level target (x) to right, center, left, right (3 times)

- Targets for cervical rotation eye level target (x) to left, center, right, left (3 times)

- Chase flashlight (pain free).

Finally, it is important to remember that recovery is often prolonged in children and adolescents, a fact attributed to their differences in biochemical and metabolic pathways; this means that return to play and sport will potentially be delayed and a longer recovery time than for adults should be allowed (Purcell, 2009; Alsalaheen et al., 2010; Aligene and Lin, 2013; Driscoll, 2013; Harmon et al., 2013).

Integrative MTY prescription for vestibular dysfunction

A review of integrative yoga prescription for vestibular issues includes the following:

1. Provision of a supportive clinical environment and nurturing therapeutic landscape (Groenewegen et al., 2006). Measures which could help bring about positive outcomes would include discussing time management with the patient to improve patient compliance with a prescribed home program, use of kinesthetic interventions that consider visual, auditory and tactile input, including light touch, deep pressure, proprioceptive sense, and vibration (Garner, 2001).

Another intervention with the potential to influence change is self-reflection activities, such as journaling, which are supported to facilitate cognitive processing and psycho-emotional-social health and well-being (Ullrich, 2002).

2. Manual mobilization with movement during yoga postures in which the spine receives priority over the extremities for facilitating postural control and awareness, and where the breath also receives priority for neuroendocrine and neurophysiological functioning (Kolar et al., 2010; Stokes, 2010; Streeter et al., 2012; Bordoni and Zanier, 2013).

3. Autogenic training and biofeedback to influence sensorimotor delay(s), abnormal eye movements, positional testing for BPPV, vestibulo-ocular reflex functioning through horizontal and vertical gaze stabilization via saccades, visual acuity, and target acquisition, gait instability, and postural stability and balance (Riechers and Ruff, 2009; Alsalaheen et al., 2010; Aligene and Lin, 2013; Gurley et al., 2013). Additionally, mirrors and yoga equipment such as bolsters and blocks are also used for biofeedback (Garner, 2001, 2012, 2013).

4. Inclusion of balance training in yoga postures is not yet well supported (Jeter et al., 2014), yet the extent to which voluntary control can be exerted over both short and medium latency automatic postural responses is open to interpretation and also requires more research (Jacobs and Horak, 2007). Nonetheless, balance training is an unwavering modality in the domain of rehabilitation, is scientifically well supported for efficacy, and is used in vestibular, neurological, and musculoskeletal conditions, and sports rehabilitation and conditioning.

Patients may accidentally neglect to completely fill out intake forms when seeking medical treatment, leading to an inability to identify precursors for fall risk. It is therefore important to thoroughly interview the patient for issues which may affect balance, including previous medical history. Factors which impact balance across the lifespan include sarcopenia, low vitamin D levels, poor proprioception, visual acuity, asymmetries in gait, vestibular impairment, sensory deficits or sensorimotor integration, reduced upper body stability and joint mobility, orthostatic hypotension, and pathophysiologies such as diabetic neuropathy, cognitive deficits, and/or neurological conditions such as cerebral palsy, Down syndrome, stroke, multiple sclerosis, or other neurodegenerative conditions (Iosa et al., 2014). Age-related gait changes which affect balance include wider stance, loss of reciprocal gait, smaller step length, and slower gait.

Lastly, an algorithm for vestibular intervention using a yogic model is provided in Fig. 3.8, illustrating the progression of a 6-week treatment period for a fifth-decade female who presented with vertigo with a 30-year history and per patient report unrelated to an accident or injury. She presented with self-reported intermittent bouts of "severe vertigo" that, when the vertigo was present, left her unable to perform activities of daily living (ADL) or complete her duties as a realtor. After the 6-week trial and with an 8-week follow-up, the patient had no recurrence of vertigo and was able to lie in full supine lying and complete all tasks on the algorithm and ADL without recurrence of vertigo. It was her first time lying supine and having 8 consecutive weeks free of vertigo in 30 years.

This case study provides early evidence that supports the use of yogic methodology in managing vestibular dysfunction after concussion via extrapolation and integration of the current evidence base in vestibular rehabilitation. Vestibular rehabilitation's well-documented effect on post-concussion outcome provides a platform for evolution of the biomedical model to embrace a biopsychosocial approach using yoga in vestibular rehabilitation.

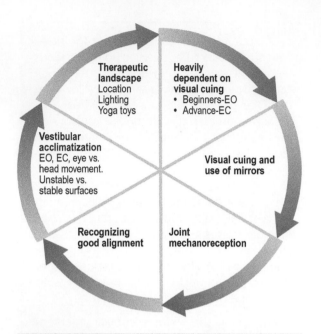

Figure 3.5

Biopsychosocial sensorimotor considerations in vestibular rehabilitation. EO, eyes open; EC, eyes closed

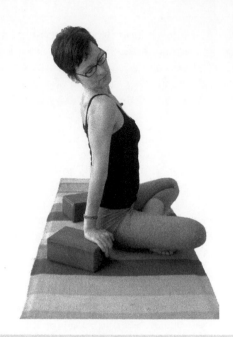

Figure 3.7

Therapist-demonstrated vestibulo-ocular reflex (VOR) exercises

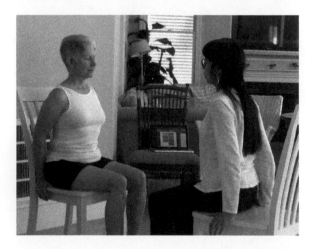

Figure 3.6

Therapist-assisted vestibulo-ocular reflex (VOR) exercises (reproduced with permission from the models pictured)

Pain and trauma management: mapping the somatosensory, limbic, and cognitive highway

Since approximately one-fifth of the population suffers from pain (Minett et al., 2014), it is important that practitioners understand how pain might affect yoga prescription. Research and scientific inquiry into pain is relatively young. Only half a century has passed since 1965, when the first theory, known as the gate control theory of pain, was proposed by Melzack and Wall (1965, 1967) (Fig. 3.9). The theory challenged the previous, simplistic notion that pain was a "reflexive response" to stimuli, with the amount of pain felt being a direct correlation to the amount of physical damage (Tan et al., 2011). The gate control theory of pain was based upon the modulation of input to the spinal dorsal horns and the dynamic role of the brain in its ability to effectively "close the gate," or block pain perception (Le Bars, 2002; Melzack and Katz, 2013), via stimulation of larger nerves whose signal is transmitted faster than unmyelinated C-fiber nerves (Tan et al., 2011). It was deduced that if synaptic transmission of pain signals could be blocked via cutaneous sensory input from the pain site's periphery, then nociceptive modulation was possible. The gate control theory has served as the chief basis for effective multimodal neural modulation via soft tissue mobilization, sensory stimulation, or therapeutic touch (Mancini

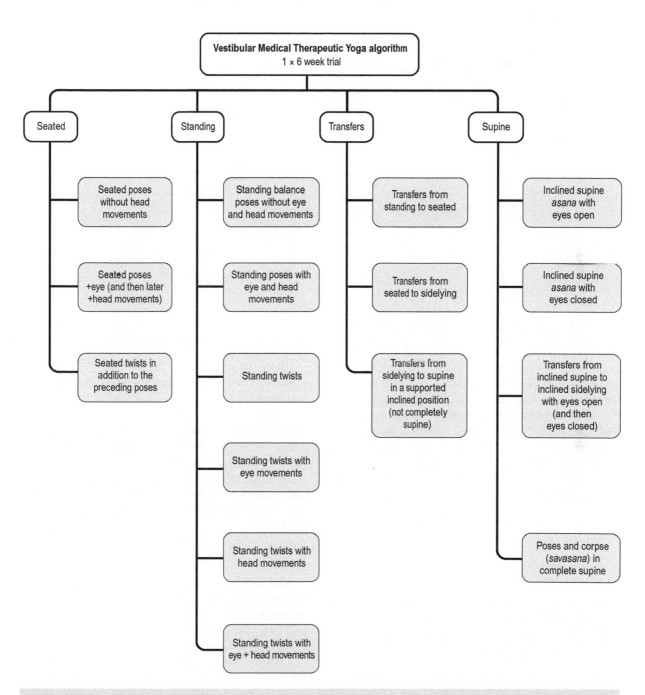

Figure 3.8
Balance: vestibular and visual sense algorithm

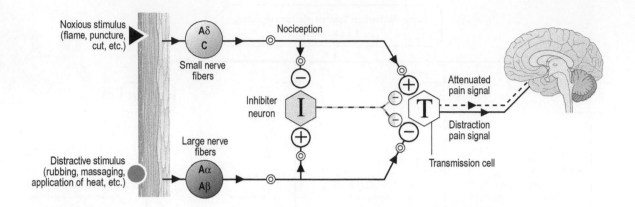

Figure 3.9
Gate theory of pain

et al., 2014), and transcutaneous electrical nerve stimulation (Kumar and Rizvi, 2014) for the last 50 years.

Biomedical medicine now recognizes the enormous influence that psychological variables, such as attention, past experience, anxiety, depression, and perspective, exert on the individual's pain experience (Melzack and Katz, 2013). Neuropathic pain is "common and complex" and is "frequently resistant to conventional medical therapies and surgical approaches" (Kumar and Rizvi, 2014, p. 5). Lewandowski and Jacobson (2013) categorize pain into three general types:

1. Nociceptive pain — Activation of primary afferent neurons via noxious stimulation

2. Neuropathic pain — Primary lesion in or damage to the peripheral or central nervous system

3. Functional — Chronic pain and discomfort referred to different regions of the body but with no agreed-upon structural, inflammatory, or biochemical abnormalities.

Historically, the evolution of the gate control theory was accelerated and evolved in large part as a result of research into phantom limb pain and the discovery that pain could be felt even without input from the spinal cord (Melzack and Loeser, 1978; Melzack, 1990). The recognition that pain theory must consider pathways above the spinal cord helped shape a new theory, looking at pain experience as a multifaceted neuromatrix (Melzack, 1990; Tan et al., 2011; Melzack and Katz, 2013).

The pain neuromatrix theory (Fig. 3.10) and its six components is also referred to as the body-self neuromatrix (Tan et al., 2011). The neuromatrix is described as a network with somatosensory, limbic, and cognitive components (Mendell, 2014), well acknowledged in the World Health Organization's (WHO) International Classification of Functioning, Disease, and Health (ICF) model that states personal and environmental factors must be assessed to address individuals' health, disability, and functioning (WHO, 2001). A myriad of factors inform the discussion and direction of future research in pain neuroscience and pain management on the frontlines of medicine.

The five-faceted BPS yogic model (see Fig. 2.1) acknowledges that pain can result from physical, emotional, intellectual, energetic, or spiritual connections, while the ICF model (see Fig. 2.2) recognizes that pain has environmental and personal substrates (WHO, 2001; Melzack and Katz, 2013). Ultimately, the experience of pain is valuable. The neuromatrix theory "guides us away from Cartesian theory that pain is a sensation produced by inflammation, injury, or other tissue pathology" and toward recognition that pain is a "dynamic process that involves ascending and descending pathways" with multiple influences (Melzack and Katz, 2013, p. 1).

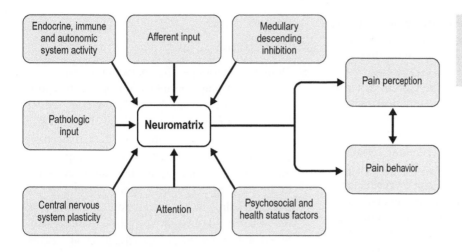

Figure 3.10

The neuromatrix theory (© R. Melzack, 1970; reprinted with permission)

Pain is _____

A simple question underscores the non-linear complexity of pain in neuroscience. Complete the following sentence: Pain is _____. Pain is experienced and felt in as many different ways as there are grains of sand on the seashore. Pain can be personal, dynamic, multidimensional, isolating, distracting, protective, informative, emotional, a teacher, a symptom, a warning sign, stigmatizing, expected as a part of life, exhausting, motivating, subjective, catastrophic, disabling, stressful, constant, infrequent, or connected to past experience. Pain is even more than these variables, which is why it is difficult to treat, or even debate, the origins and pathways of pain. Therefore, evolution in pain neuroscience is not only expected, it is absolutely necessary.

Two mechanisms thought to contribute to the overactive brain neuromatrix are "decreased GABA (gamma-aminobutyric acid) neurotransmission (Suarez-Roca et al., 2008) and long term potentiation of the anterior cingulate cortex" (Zhuo, 2007; DeCouck et al., 2014, pp. 9–10). Several considerations must be made in light of these findings:

- The first is that pain can be experienced without the presence of nociceptors (Minett et al., 2014).

- The second is that the extent that a patient can be distracted from the pain experience directly correlates with the degree that the individual's cognitive task is disturbed (Kucyi et al., 2013).

Those who can voluntarily disengage from pain have stronger anatomical links between periaqueductal gray (PAG), the opiate-rich area of the brain responsible for pain suppression, and the default mode network (Kucyi et al., 2013). Proof that the PAG could be influenced by increased GABA activity, posited to increase through yogic practices (Streeter et al., 2007, 2010, 2012), or that yoga could affect structural plasticity of the anatomical connection between the PAG and default mode network, could have serious implications for pain neuroscience and management. At present, literature favors using meditative and yogic practices to influence psychological factors that impact pain, but there is a paucity of research in this area and a great need for deeper exploration (Olivo, 2009) in order to understand the pathologic mechanisms of chronic pain.

There is also the question of vagus nerve activity in pain management. Peripheral vagal nerve stimulation of vagus afferents to relay information to the brain to treat headaches, migraines (Multon and Schoenen, 2005), epilepsy, and depression (Nemeroff et al., 2006; Daban et al., 2008) is promising.

However, could vagal nerve stimulation be delivered noninvasively through yogic meditative and deep breathing or sound practices in order to impact a wide range of patient populations? Proper employment of the respiratory diaphragm during inhalation can trigger stretch receptors in the alveoli, baroreceptors, chemoreceptors, and other sensors in the respiratory structures, and through vagal afferents, sends information to the CNS in order to "influence perception, cognition, emotion regulation, somatic expression, and behavior" (Brown and Gerbarg, 2009; Streeter et al., 2012, p. 573). Yogic breathing (particularly overcoming breath, a cyclical eccentric resistance breath that can also be performed with chanting "*om*") can increase heart rate variability (HRV, known as the beat-to-beat interval, with low HRV associated with maladaptive stress responses that adversely affect all-health outcomes), improve vagal tone, and increase parasympathetic activation (Brown and Gerbarg, 2009). HRV is, consequently, highly correlated with vagal nerve activity (Fig. 3.11) (Tan et al., 2009).

Positioned as it is midway between the brain and viscera, the effects of the primarily afferent fibers (80%) of the vagus nerve (Porges, 2011) are far-reaching and influence cardiac, musculoskeletal, periodontal, integumentary, neuromuscular, vestibular, cardiac, immune, endocrine, and visceral function (Bordoni and Zanier, 2013). In review, five mechanisms implicate the vagus nerve in pain modulation (DeCouck et al., 2014):

1. Inflammation (Tal, 1999) — Vagal nerve activity is inversely proportional to inflammation (Tateishi et al., 2007)

2. Sympathetic nervous system activity (SNSA) — SNSA can cause vasoconstriction, muscle tension, impaired microcirculation, and possible ischemia

3. Oxidative stress

4. Brain activity

5. Opioid receptors — The vagus nerve can modulate pain through influence on opioid receptors via vagal sensory nerves (DeCouck et al., 2014). Intact vagal nerve input has been identified as a requisite variable in adequate anti-nociceptive opioid analgesia, with levels of high vagal/HRV found to drop during inadequate nociception in humans undergoing surgery (Jeanne et al., 2009), leading to the deduction that low vagal nerve activity is linked to dysfunctional opioid-based anti-nociception (DeCouck et al., 2014). Opiate pharmaceuticals have remarkable side effects, including addiction and abuse, while yogic breathing via deep-paced breathing (Lehrer et al., 2003; Streeter et al., 2012; DeCouck et al., 2014) is an inexpensive, low-tech, safe modality that can influence activity in the cortex and body systems with no adverse side effects.

In the artistic vein of medicine, auricular stimulation of the vagus nerve evokes neurophysiological responses similar to those found in direct vagal nerve stimulation (Rao et al., 2013). Active listening and/or the production of vocal sounds are neural exercises of the middle ear muscles, which can influence social engagement via vagal regulation of the heart (Porges, 2015b). The vagus nerve (cranial nerve X) innervates the pharynx and larynx, in part, and its fibers travel with, and are undistinguished from, helpmeet innervation, cranial nerves IX and XI. The vibratory input around the ears and orifices of the facial anatomy results in potential stimulation of the auricular branch of the vagus nerve (Vadiraja et al., 2009). This stimulation can be accomplished through chanting/vocal toning (Rao et al., 2013). Limbic deactivation was also found in subjects who chanted "*om*" but not those who phonated the unvoiced sound "sss" (Kalyani et al., 2011). Finally, though outside the scope of this text, music, which is often used in yoga teaching, is well supported (Nilsson, 2008) to achieve pain relief and anxiety reduction and is often cited in Porges' (2007, 2011) theory for positively affecting polyvagal regulation.

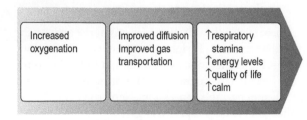

Figure 3.11
Health outcomes of yogic breathing

Often implicated in pain management is the need to address trauma and sensory processing, an area where current vagus nerve theory falls short. Polyvagal theory (PVT), however, offers strong biological plausibility that, coupled with clinical expertise, establishes new theory for evidence-based pain management and trauma therapy (Fig. 3.12). PVT accounts for an older phylogentic system, a reptilian response that we see in animals who experience fear. If an animal knows it cannot escape danger, and also knows that danger may be life-threatening, it does not fight or flee, but may start to "shut down" its responses. The animal is still, and all systems slow or even shut down, as in vasovagal syncope. This ability to detect risk or danger, including life-threatening danger, is termed "neuroception" (Porges, 2012).

Current trauma theory does not account for the "shut down" response in conditions such as PTSD (post-traumatic stress disorder) or autism spectrum disorder (ASD), for example. Additionally, there are some cases where sympathetic tone is necessary, as in the case of neonate HRV, where high variability could be an isolated unwanted vagus response. This observation led to the development of PVT, which provides an elegant theory that bridges existing scientific gaps in vagus nerve response and HRV with conditions such as ASD and cardiovagal tone through evolving "fight or flight" response to also include a "shut down" stress state.

In PVT there are two vagal systems. The first is an evolved, mammalian, myelinated, ventral vagus mediated by corticobulbar pathways linked to

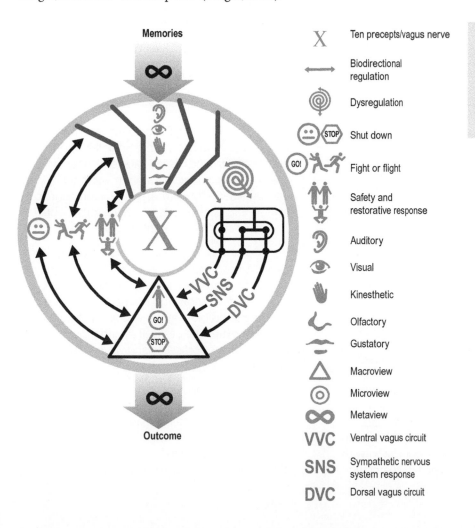

Figure 3.12

The 10th cranial nerve, the vagus, per polyvagal theory, guides the 10 precepts for the use of yoga in rehabilitation and wellness care

X	Ten precepts/vagus nerve
↔	Biodirectional regulation
	Dysregulation
	Shut down
	Fight or flight
	Safety and restorative response
	Auditory
	Visual
	Kinesthetic
	Olfactory
	Gustatory
△	Macroview
◎	Microview
∞	Metaview
VVC	Ventral vagus circuit
SNS	Sympathetic nervous system response
DVC	Dorsal vagus circuit

brainstem function that regulate supradiaphragmatic organs (lungs and heart) including the middle ear and striated muscles of the face, larynx, and pharynx. The second vagus pathway is an older, reptilian, unmyelinated, dorsal circuit that regulates the gut and subdiaphragmatic viscera.

The diaphragm is the key connecting point of the two vagal pathways, and through sound, voice, facial expression, and baroreceptor function (also a part of the myelinated vagus pathway), PVT can change the way we view and treat trauma, ASD, and conditions influenced by general allostatic load. (See the case study giving Gabriel's story for potential mechanisms of polyvagal theory in practice.)

Case study

Potential mechanisms of polyvagal theory – Gabriel's story*

Polyvagal theory (PVT) can seek to reconcile the stress response of Gabriel's autistic spectrum disorder (ASD) and his congenital heart defect.

Gabriel, at 2 years old, was diagnosed with severe developmental delays in expressive speech, as well as socio-emotional delays that were thought to result from the primary speech delay. At 26 months, the only word Gabriel could say was "gaa." The complicating factor in Gabriel's case was that he was diagnosed with a coarctation of the aorta, which had become critical and required surgery within a month of its discovery. Both diagnoses came to Gabriel's family within 24 hours of each other.

The poignant connection to PVT and the integrative approach offered in this text is that Gabriel's speech condition was considered unrelated to his heart condition by the biomedical model. However, the two were explained as being connected when a physician trained in traditional Chinese medicine (TCM) learned of Gabriel's case. The explanation posited by the physician was that depressed heart chi is associated with speech delays, and that, after his coarctation

repair, he would begin to speak. His family did follow the TCM physician's nutritional recommendations to help bolster his system and ready it for surgery. However, as for the rest, they had to wait until after the surgery to see if the physician's prediction would come true.

Gabriel went on to have cardiothoracic surgery within the month, and on the day of surgery, as Gabriel was being transferred to the pediatric intensive care unit (standard procedure for this type of surgery), the nurse came out to update Gabriel's parents. She said that although Gabriel was just fine, there was a delay in visiting him because Gabriel had awoken early, become agitated, and pulled out his intubation tube. The nurse went on to explain that they had resedated him and were making him comfortable, after which, he could have visitors.

The nurse added, *"I had to come out and tell you, because when he did wake up and pulled out his tube, the first word he said was "mama."*

Gabriel's mother was floored. She said it felt as though the wind had been completely knocked out of her. Her mind flashed back to all those times she had sung to him, taught him sign language, and provided him with a safe environment to explore and learn. But, despite her efforts, Gabriel had never said "mama" – until today.

And so the TCM physician was right. As soon as Gabriel's heart condition was fixed, which slowly began to repair his broken cardiovagal tone which had unknowingly caused high blood pressure to his brain and low blood pressure to his lower extremities, as well as putting extreme pressure on the aortic arch and valve, Gabriel did begin to speak.

Fast forward 6 years, and Gabriel was finally diagnosed with high-functioning ASD. He does present with typical social engagement traits such as flat facial affect and lack of vocal intonation, as well as the tendency to be overwhelmed in situations with too much sensory input, like sound and light. His mother also notes he was very sensitive in utero, easily startling with both sound and light input.

As a vocalist, yogi, and therapist, Gabriel's mother invests much time in the therapeutic value of sound and breath, and is learning about the triggers that may make Gabriel perceive a threat or feel unsafe. For Gabriel, this may be something as simple as going to the bathroom on his own at a restaurant, being asked to answer a question in front of other people, or attend a function that is crowded and noisy.

Porges' theory may offer insight into Gabriel's case by reconciling the stress response of Gabriel's speech delays and ASD with his heart defect and subsequent repair, given that the subdiaphragmatic or phylogenetically older vagal circuit may have been perpetuated in Gabriel owing to his congenital cardiac condition that interfered with normal baroreceptor and respiratory function controlled by the ventral vagus circuit. Porges (2015b) confirms that this theory, in Gabriel's specific case, may have neurobiological plausibility in that the "atypical neural feedback may have maintained this physiological state."

Though there is no "hard science" to support this reconciliation of cardiac impairment and socio-emotional and speech delays, PVT certainly offers a neurophysiological example of why Gabriel would "freeze" when told to go by himself to the water fountain at school or when asked to speak to a stranger. PVT maintains that the "fight or flight" response, on its own, does not entirely describe Gabriel's, or any child with ASD's, range of reactions to perceived threat. Nor does fight or flight and its associated binary ANS descriptor describe, for example, what a rape victim must feel like when she (or he) knows she cannot escape from her attacker.

The dissociation that occurs when someone has experienced too much trauma or pain for too long is beautifully reconciled with PVT. It describes the bidirectional interactions that

Porges calls, a "face–heart" connection. We must understand that in order for an individual to have healthy social-emotional engagement and allostasis, that person must feel safe.

Please note that the patient's name has been changed to protect his privacy.

The identification of two vagal motor circuits, dorsal and ventral, provides an expanded understanding of stress response modulation, which is to properly regulate the "fight, flight, or (newly defined) shut down" response through creating a safe environment for interaction. Chiefly, if the CNS processes less motor input because the breath is at ease and not labored, then a yogic breath practice should improve stress response. PVT theory, then, provides the neurophysiological explanation for why music, sound, and yogic breathing (*pranayama*) are critical in regulating physiological state and facilitating allostasis.

Ultimately, when someone is comfortable the vagal brake is functioning. The brake acts as a protector and calming agent that mediates sympathetic and dorsal vagal surge response (Porges, 2015b), of which the "gut" clenching visceral response is an example. By contrast, release of the vagal brake increases heart rate and cardiac output in response to environmental input without involving the sympathetic nervous system (Porges, 2011). In order to curb metabolic and neuroendocrine cost of "fight or flight," vagal brake regulation is a critical concept that clarifies the relationship between dynamically changing cardiac vagal tone and behavioral reactivity (Porges et al., 1996).

The bodywork of physical yoga practice alone, then, may not always be capable of achieving positive physiological states that the myelinated vagus circuit can provide. Those state traits include social engagement behaviors, positive affective experiences, relationship building, spiritual readiness, and safety (Porges, 2015a). However, through trigeminal nerve input and respiration (*pranayama*) delivered through focusing on breathwork first, which can also include sound and music, the myelinated vagus nerve circuit could be accessed. Likewise, as a therapist, your presence, breath patterns, and vocal intonation have an effect on the patient's stress response and feeling of safety, which underscores the importance of experiential learning and postgraduate education in yoga prescription as a healthcare provider.

Respiration

The beneficial role of yogic respiration in neuroendocrine regulation, mental health, cognition and attention, cardiopulmonary function, cardiovascular autonomic function (Jyotsna et al., 2013), pain management (Zautra et al., 2010), and hemodynamic function (Parshad et al., 2011) is well established (Jerath et al., 2006; Brown and Gerbarg, 2009; Kuntsevich et al., 2010; Mason et al., 2013). Yogic breathing also affects the milieu of both patients with asthma (Singh et al., 2012) and healthy patients (Tharion et al., 2012) at bronchial and avleolar levels to improve diffusion and gas transport via increased oxygenation by improving quality of life (QOL) measures, respiratory stamina, energy levels, and calm (Singh et al., 2012).

Diaphragmatic assessment and intervention through a yogic BPS lens could help manage esophageal reflux, scalene hypertonicity, subclavius dysfunction, polyvagal dysregulation, thoracic outlet syndrome, pelvic floor dysfunction, cervical/neck symptoms, dental pain, pain perception, and

cardiopulmonary health. Respiration is one of the most readily adaptable voluntary mechanisms by which to affect autonomic change, especially yogic respiration (Joseph et al., 2005; Jerath et al., 2006; Pinheiro et al., 2007; Turankar et al., 2013).

Diaphragm anatomy

The diaphragm is the main muscle of respiration (Fig. 3.13). A domed sheet mere millimeters in thickness (Bordoni and Zanier, 2013; Goligher et al., 2015), the diaphragm spans the entire torso, separates the chest cavity from the abdominal cavity, and intersects with fascia, muscle, tendon, bone, internal organs, and nerves. Small in thickness but vast in multisystem effects, the diaphragm's proper employment dictates the long-term health and well-being of the individual.

The diaphragm's three anatomical attachments comprise (1) costal, (2) sternal, and (3) lumbar portions, making it a functional part of every body system, including cardiopulmonary, neuroendocrine, periodontal, reproductive, fascial, musculoskeletal, integumentary, neurovascular, and psychoemotional. The costal portion of the diaphragm originates from the last six ribs and intersects via "digitations" with the TA muscle (Anraku and Shargall, 2009; Downey, 2011). The sternal portion of the diaphragm connects

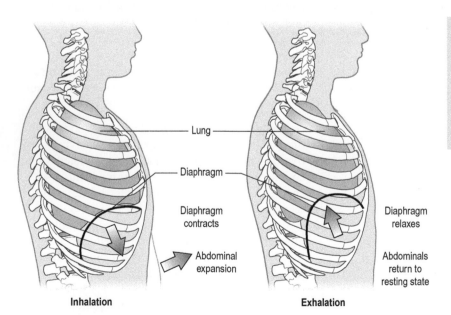

Lung

Diaphragm

Diaphragm contracts

Abdominal expansion

Diaphragm relaxes

Abdominals return to resting state

Inhalation **Exhalation**

Figure 3.13

The diaphragm spans the entire torso and separates the chest cavity from the abdominal cavity, intersecting with fascia, muscle, tendon, bone, internal organs and nerves

the preperitoneal and pericardial connective tissue (Dakwar et al., 2012). The lumbar portion has visceral fat connections that are correlated with proprioceptive function of the diaphragm (Bordoni and Zanier, 2013).

The three diaphragmatic attachments also implicate two other diaphragms, the thoracic and the pelvic. Through fascial connections, the hyoid area houses the vocal folds and the glottis (the thoracic diaphragm), and connects the respiratory and pelvic (pelvic floor) diaphragms. Pressure above and below the corresponding thoracic and pelvic diaphragms must maintain a certain length/tension balance, depicted by Young's modulus, to achieve allostasis health in polyvagal, HPA axis, visceral, and orthopaedic mechanisms.

Respiratory physiology

A respiratory rate above 20 breaths/minute is abnormal and categorized as hyperventilation, while a rate of 24 breaths/minute and over indicates likely critical illness (Cretikos et al., 2008). Hypoventilation is defined as inadequate alveolar ventilation, which is excessive CO_2 and O_2 deficit in alveoli, arterial blood, venous blood, and body tissues. Hyperventilation is not an issue of excessive O_2 levels but unbalanced levels of CO_2. Unbalanced levels cause arterioles to decrease in size until the blood supply to the tissues is so restricted that the amount of O_2 consumed becomes irrelevant. This phenomenon provides the rationale for "paper bag breathing," theorized to increase CO_2 levels. Patients with symptomatic paroxysmal atrial fibrillation, for example, improve arrhythmia burden, heart rate, blood pressure, anxiety and depression scores, and quality of life domains, through yogic intervention (Lakkireddy et al., 2013).

Systemic implications

Neuroanatomical implications in diaphragmatic breathing

Systemic dysfunction screening should be included to recognize clinical red flags for visceral involvement (Fig. 3.14).

Periodontal, cervical, and upper thoracic

Use of secondary muscles of respiration, such as the scalenes or subclavius, function in improper

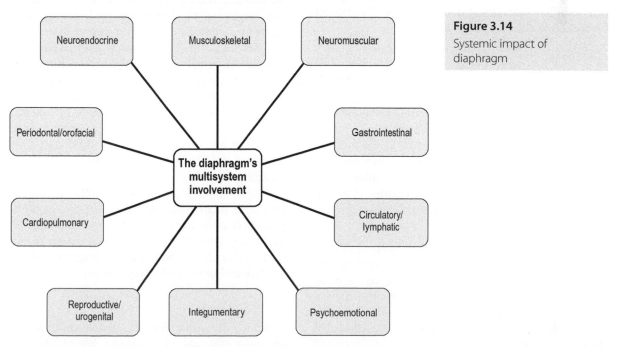

Figure 3.14

Systemic impact of diaphragm

respiratory diaphragm strategy via chest breathing, which carries implications for the periodontal, cervical, and upper thoracic regions. Elevation of the first rib via the subclavius secondary to clavicular/chest breathing or phrenic nerve disorder is also an etiology of thoracic outlet syndrome (Zhang and Dellon, 2008; Laulan et al., 2011). Non-typical postural habits, such as a forward head posture, sloping shoulders, and excessive thoracic kyphosis, also work in a cause–effect relationship with the suboccipital region. Diaphragmatic dysfunction can affect proprioceptive sensitivity in the greater occipital nerve (C2) at its cranial entry point via the vagus or hypoglossal nerve (Kemp et al., 2012), which has implications for headache management. The rectus capitis posterior minor blends with the deep cervical spine fascia and connects to the dura and reciprocal tension membranes (Kahkeshani and Ward, 2012), as well as the nuchal ligament and its direct dural connection and innervation by C2, and further connects the diaphragm with bidirectional kinetic chain impairment at terminal ends. Finally, diaphragmatic dysfunction, through the trigeminal ganglia via its connecting point with the phrenic nerve and termination at the periodontal ligaments, can be an etiology of dental pain, temporomandibular joint (TMJ) dysfunction, and vestibular dysfunction (Bordoni and Zanier, 2013).

Cardiac

Respiration is the neglected vital sign (Cretikos et al., 2008; Gandevia and McKenzie, 2008). Respiratory rate is a significant predictor of serious events such as cardiac arrest and admission to intensive care (ICU) (Hodgetts et al., 2002; Goldhill et al., 2005). It is also a constant, powerful modulator of cardiovascular control (Porges, 2011; Bordoni and Zanier, 2013) with vagus nerve regulation in part achieved via the sinoatrial node, which is accessed chiefly through respiratory habits (Porges, 2011).

Specifically, the myelinated vagus is effective during exhalation in that the myelinated vagal efferent pathways slow the heart and downregulate sympathetic influences and the HPA axis (Porges, 2015b). Abdominal breathing stimulates the vagal afferents in the diaphragm that enhance vagal efferent influences (Porges, 2015b).

Additionally the trigeminal nerve, through its direct connection to the diaphragm via the phrenic nerve, could contribute to cardiac arrhythmia, arterial pressure decrease, and bradycardia (Meng et al., 2008; Adeeb et al., 2012; Kemp et al., 2012). Venous stasis necessitates diaphragmatic evaluation by a physical therapist to aid in peripheral blood flow (Chiappa et al., 2008), based on the finding that lymphatic absorption depends on rhythmic diaphragmatic stretching and the influence of intraperitoneal pressure and postural awareness (Moriondo et al., 2008). Proper diaphragmatic breathing then, is critical for improved baroreflex sensitivity, reduced systolic, diastolic, and mean blood pressures, and improved HRV in patients with hypertension (Pinheiro et al., 2007). In short, cardiac autonomic function can be attenuated by yogic breathing (Turankar et al., 2013) through PVT (Porges, 2015a).

Gastrointestinal

The diaphragm receives efferent (motor) input from the vagus nerve (Chapleau and Sabharwal, 2011). Because the phrenic nerve anastomoses with the vagus nerve (Drake et al., 2009; Messlinger et al., 2011; Bordoni and Zanier, 2015) and its efferent esophageal connection, diaphragmatic dysfunction could feasibly contribute to swallowing or reflex problems (Eherer et al., 2012; Da Silva et al., 2013). Gastrointestinal physiologists recognize that the diaphragm acts essentially as two muscles, crural and costal, thereby functioning to prevent gastric reflux (Eherer et al., 2012) as well as in provision of mechanical respiration (Pickering and Jones, 2002). The lower esophageal sphincter and diaphragm are also synergistic, "collaborating as a functional unit" (p. 150), which explains why breath retraining improves gastroesophageal reflux disease (GERD) symptoms, quality of life, and pH-metry in those with GERD (Eherer, 2014). The phrenicocolic ligament also connects the diaphragm to the descending colon (Netter, 2014) as an extension of the peritoneum and could implicate the diaphragm in normal digestive and/or visceral fascial motility.

Psychoemotional

Interaction with pathophysiological domains of depression is a systemic phenomenon affected by and determining neuroendocrine function, neurotransmitter metabolism, neuroimmunological mechanisms, and synaptic plasticity (Eyre and Baune, 2012). Pro-inflammatory mediators are responsible, in part, for depression's pathogenesis (Littrell, 2012). Therapeutic administration of cytokine interferon alpha (IFN-α) leads to depression in a significant number of patients (Raison et al., 2006), which suggests "proinflammatory cytokines and their signaling pathways offer a unique therapeutic opportunity to treat depression and related conditions, such as fatigue, labile anger, and irritability" (Lotrich et al., 2011, p. 48).

Evidence of systemic inflammation could increase depression prevalence and risk; however, the introduction of anti-inflammatories in those with low levels of peripheral inflammation blocks the positive effects of inflammation in those with treatment-resistant depression (Raison and Miller, 2013). This finding suggests that depression treatment must be customized based on knowledge of individual risk factors for depression, not just known inflammatory levels. Environmental and personal factors that guide the WHO ICF model, as well as a person's learning preferences, sensory threshold, and level of conscious competency must factor into yogic prescription.

Respiration is perhaps the most expedient way to impact psychoneuroendocrine and physiological health. Littrell (2012) discusses multiple entry points for addressing depression in individuals, consideration of complementary and alternative methodology including: (1) yoga, (2) meditation, and (3) exercise (Pace et al., 2009; Kiecolt-Glaser et al., 2010; Greenwood and Fleshner, 2011) in order to facilitate stress resilience and reduce systemic inflammation (Littrell, 2012). Even exercise undertaken and perceived as "forced," or outside an individual's control, can still elicit positive changes in stress resistance (Greenwood et al., 2013).

Reproductive, urological, and sexual

The respiratory diaphragm and the pelvic diaphragm share intimate connections. The pelvic floor works to resist increased intra-abdominal pressure and contribute to continence of bowel and bladder. A lesser known function of the pelvic floor is to control the pressure of intra-abdominal fluid via healthy respiration (Bordoni and Zanier, 2013). In real-time magnetic resonance imaging (MRI) there is a directly proportional change in pelvic floor length/tension during use of the diaphragm, whether for breathing or coughing (Talasz et al., 2011). Symmetrical electrical activity can be found in the pelvic floor and TA and internal obliques during anticipated inhalation (Talasz et al., 2011), establishing necessity for inclusion of pelvic rehabilitation principles in yoga prescription for urological, reproductive, sexual function, and also lumbopelvic function (see next section).

Lumbopelvic

Yoga is a powerful modality for achieving lumbopelvic stabilization, prevention, and management of back pain, and management of a plethora of women's health diagnoses (Delitto et al., 2012; Fritz et al., 2012; Gellhorn et al., 2012; Hoffman and Gabel, 2013; Janssens et al., 2013), especially when the current evidence base in rehabilitation is applied to evolve yoga. The respiratory diaphragm, for example, provides a stabilizing function in the management and prevention of lumbopelvic pain (Kolar et al., 2010, 2012; Stokes, 2010). Further, early utilization of physical therapy using the BPS framework of MTY carries tremendous implications for improving patient satisfaction and outcomes (Fritz et al., 2012; Gellhorn et al., 2012), especially since worsening trends in back pain management and underutilization of conservative and noninvasive (i.e. physical therapy) treatment are well documented (Mafi et al., 2013). The distinct physiological benefits for employing respiration affect biomechanical principles of movement in the lumbopelvic region, the physiological science of lumbopelvic action, and provision of safety and clinical efficacy in lumbopelvic management (Bordoni and Zanier, 2013).

The role of the lumbopelvic spine and hip, and its surrounding soft tissue, must be considered for pelvic floor and pelvic pain interventions and vice versa (Eliasson et al., 2008; Arab et al., 2010; Bi et al., 2013; Bush et al., 2013). The integrated continence system (ICS) describes intimate interaction of three structural systems and their modifiable factors (Grewar and McLean, 2008), while Bordoni and Zanier (2013, 2015) establish the intimate fascial and neurophysiological connection between the respiratory and pelvic diaphragm (Table 3.5). The ICS includes three elements: intrinsic urethral closure, urethral support, and lumbopelvic stability systems; modifiable factors include motor control, and musculoskeletal and behavioral factors (Grewar and McLean, 2008), all of which must be evaluated during posture or breath prescription, which would affect the pelvic floor or lumbopelvic region(s).

Table 3.5
The integrated continence system

Factors that affect urinary continence	
Structural systems	**Modifiable factors**
Intrinsic urethral closure	Behavioral
	• Chronic ↑ in IAP
	• Sedentary lifestyle
	• Altered hydration or voiding patterns
	• Psychosocial comorbidities
Urethral support	Musculoskeletal
	• ↓ROM
	• ↓Strength
	• ↓Endurance
Lumbopelvic stability	Motor control
	• PFM dysfunction
	• Postural/movement dysfunction
	• LBP/pelvic pain
	• Diaphragmatic dysfunction

(Adapted from Grewar and McLean, 2008.)
IAP, intra-abdominal pressure; PFM, pelvic floor muscle; LBP, low back pain; ROM, range of motion.

Pelvic floor muscle dysfunction, postural movement and coordination, and breathing habits are *modifiable motor control factors*, while loss of ROM (Hasebe et al., 2014), strength, and endurance are *modifiable musculoskeletal factors.* Inactivity, poor psychoemotional–social health, poor nutritional habits, and poor mind–body awareness are all *modifiable behavioral factors* (Grewar and McLean, 2008).

Via the vagus nerve's anastomoses with the phrenic nerve, yogic intervention can be adapted to address all modifiable factors in order to exert a positive effect on the ICS model's three systems and to influence fascial connection(s) and ventral circuit vagal activity. Gender-specific therapeutic yoga must again be considered because women with back pain have an even greater increased risk of stress urinary incontinence (Eliasson et al., 2008; Bush et al., 2013). Patients with chronic pelvic pain in general have systemic pain which can include interstitial cystitis, irritable bowel syndrome, levator ani syndrome, pelvic floor tension myalgia, vulvar vestibulitis, and vulvodynia, all of which have an association with limbic-associated pelvic pain (Fenton, 2007). This finding has implications for yoga application because of yoga's effects on limbic deactivation, neuroendocrine and regulatory function (Streeter et al., 2012). Higher-level assessment should be performed by a licensed and experienced healthcare provider who is trained to evaluate, diagnose, and treat these conditions.

Biomechanically, use of the TA-assisted thoracodiaphragmatic (TATD) breath is a method and early entry point for systems-based and neuromuscular intervention of the lumbopelvic region. Increased intra-abdominal pressure and its psychobiological role in adequate arousal for optimizing physical performance, functional mobility and controlled flexibility via spinal unloading during activities of daily living (ADL) (Kolar et al., 2010, 2012; Stokes, 2010) are presented in Chapter 4.

Lumbopelvic fascia

Fascial interrelationships and connective tissue links between the diaphragm, the pelvic floor, and the rest of the body are well established via the unifying connecting point of the three diaphragms (Figs 3.15 and 3.16). The fascia is well endowed with

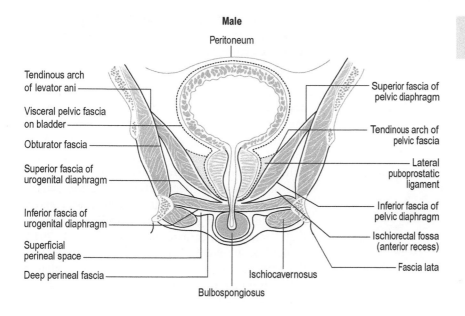

Male

Peritoneum

Tendinous arch of levator ani

Visceral pelvic fascia on bladder

Obturator fascia

Superior fascia of urogenital diaphragm

Inferior fascia of urogenital diaphragm

Superficial perineal space

Deep perineal fascia

Bulbospongiosus

Ischiocavernosus

Superior fascia of pelvic diaphragm

Tendinous arch of pelvic fascia

Lateral puboprostatic ligament

Inferior fascia of pelvic diaphragm

Ischiorectal fossa (anterior recess)

Fascia lata

Figure 3.15
Lumbopelvic fascia

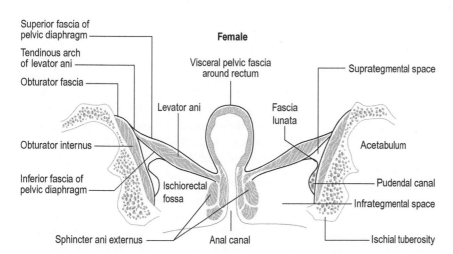

Superior fascia of pelvic diaphragm

Tendinous arch of levator ani

Obturator fascia

Obturator internus

Inferior fascia of pelvic diaphragm

Sphincter ani externus

Female

Visceral pelvic fascia around rectum

Levator ani

Ischiorectal fossa

Anal canal

Fascia lunata

Suprategmental space

Acetabulum

Pudendal canal

Infrategmental space

Ischial tuberosity

mechanoreceptors which provide invaluable proprioceptive awareness and nociceptive information, including:

- GTO and Ruffini endings, which slowly adapt and respond to tension

- Pacinian corpuscles which rapidly adapt and respond to pressure and vibration

- Meissner's corpuscles, which rapidly adapt and respond to vibration (Drake et al., 2009; Willard

et al., 2012) (see Chapter 12 for details of affecting fascial mechanoreceptors).

We can see, therefore, that problems in the diaphragmatic fascia could implicate the entire lumbopelvic region, including the rectus abdominis, internal and external obliques, cremaster, pyramidalis, transversus abdominis, psoas, quadratus lumborum, sacrospinalis, spinalis, and multifidus (Loukas et al., 2008; Stecco et al., 2011; Willard et al., 2012).

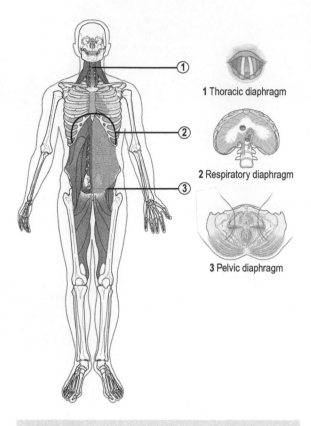

1 Thoracic diaphragm

2 Respiratory diaphragm

3 Pelvic diaphragm

Figure 3.16
Three diaphragms and fascial interrelationships

Bordoni and Zanier (2013, p. 287) posit that the tranversalis fascia, "firmly connected to the TA (Peiper et al., 2004) via the epimysium and linea alba," is a continuation of the endothoracic fascia (Skandalakis et al., 2006), which ultimately is a connecting point to the pubis via the deep cervical fascia. If the muscles within the transversalis fascia do not glide properly contractile pressures between the diaphragm, subdiaphragmatic, and perineal muscles could be affected (Bordoni and Zanier, 2013), which incriminates respiratory diaphragm dysfunction in diastasis recti abdominis management. Further, the sacroiliac joint could be affected by diaphragmatic dysfunction or force generation in the transversalis fascia secondary to the force closure that the TA, pelvic floor, and diaphragm exert as a unit (Bø and Sherburn, 2005; Paoletti, 2006; O'Sullivan and Beales, 2007). Overall, the bidirectional nature of fascia globally affects

posture prescription and could involve any area from the cervical to the sacroiliac joint region secondary to the three diaphragm connection.

The lateral raphe is also an important intersecting point demanding clinical attention in lumbopelvic integrity, stability, and mobility management. The thoracolumbar fascia, which runs posteriorly from the sacrum, thoracic, and cervical regions and is attached to the TA and internal oblique via the lateral raphe (Barker et al., 2010), can affect lumbopelvic stiffness and the latissimus dorsi, trapezii, gluteus maximus, and external oblique through its digitation-like diaphragmatic anatomical connection (Soljanik et al., 2012; Willard et al., 2012). The lateral raphe runs from the 12th rib to the iliac crest and, through shared origin and insertion from the rib to the lumbar vertebral bodies and iliac crest, involves the quadratus lumborum in lumbar stability (Schuenke, 2012). The lateral raphe, then, is an important part of the fascial system because it influences mobility and stability of the lumbopelvic region via generation of force transmission from the abdominal muscles to the lumbosacral spine (Levangie and Norkin, 2011; Schuenke, 2012). Fascia is important in lumbopelvic and respiratory health owing to its influence on optimization of muscular performance (Stecco et al., 2011; Day et al., 2012; Willard et al., 2012; Bordoni and Zanier, 2013).

Finally, it is critical to recognize that fascial research is evolving. Fascia is living and does not conform to reductionistic views that place it solely under mechanistic function (for example, fascia does not necessarily exist in lines or bands, but as a continuous network that affects the entire body in all of its movement, including yoga postures). When considering the myofascial tensile force sections under the TI (therapeutic intention) of each pose, consider these three principles: (1) the body is not hollow, (2) everything is connected, and (3) yoga is more than a physical practice.

> When considering the myofascial tensile force sections under the TI (therapeutic intention) of each pose, remember these three principles: (1)

the body is not hollow, (2) everything is connected, and (3) yoga is more than a physical practice.

Stabilization

Stabilization requires neuromuscular control. The precepts offer guidelines for creating a physiological and orthopaedic safety net in order to improve clinical efficacy and streamline clinical decision-making in yoga prescription. The purpose of finding stability in yoga postures is to encourage functional control through the cylinder concept with an eccentric contraction focus. If stability is not attended to, then many variables are at risk, including:

- Neurophysiological plasticity
- Neuromuscular (re)education – neural patterning, motor control
- Myofascial resilience
- Neurovascular integrity
- Musculoskeletal strength and endurance (power)
- Joint stability for functional ADL carryover
- Pain management
- Psychoemotional well-being
- Injury prevention and health maintenance.

Precept Four – Medical Therapeutic Yoga recommends structural alignment of postures be guided by six physiological principles and four principles of biomechanics, with a primary lumbopelvic focus and secondary scapulothoracic focus.

Primary focus: lumbopelvic

Secondary focus: scapulothoracic.

Allowing progression in posture or breath prescription is dictated by the ability to utilize TATD breath to achieve controlled flexibility in postures that require dynamic control. Breath mastery, somatosensory consciousness, emotional intelligence, and health literacy determine yoga practitioner skill. Even though a breath pattern is full, complete, and physiologically correct it does not mean a pose is biomechanically safe or even healthy to perform. Clinicians should ask critical questions prior to posture performance, such as:

- "What are my hamstrings' anatomical limit?"
- "Do the fibers of my Achilles tendon glide/slide adequately within the fascial sheath to be safe in a downward-facing dog pose?"
- "Do I have neural tension in the dura mater of the spinal cord in the morning, and if so, how does that affect my practice and the postures I choose?"
- "Should I do arm balances or warrior II pose using full hip FABER (flexion, abduction, and external rotation) if I have diagnosed excessive femoral anteversion or an anterior acetabular labral tear?"
- "How will pelvic floor tension or pelvic pain be affected by seated twists?"

Use of the breath provides only one measure of safety. Not to oversimplify the parameters, however, a practitioner is advanced only when he/she recognizes and acknowledges his/her own weaknesses and honors BPS impairments.

Posture performance is not a static or even dynamic stretch, since that would only imply flexibility as a terminal goal. Further, stability is not about amplitude of motion but rather about how well an individual can control the amount of movement they have (Lee, 2006). An advanced student works to establish stability, even in large or extreme ranges of motion outside spinal neutral, because the nervous system ultimately dictates control, dynamic mobility, and vitality of the musculoskeletal system.

Panjabi's early work (1992a, 1992b) defined stability as an exclusive task that only occurs when passive, active, and control systems work together to transfer load safely and efficiently. Lee (2005) elaborates on Panjabi's definition, saying stability is therefore dynamic and requires four components. These clinical definitions (Lee and Vleeming, 1998; Lee, 2005, 2006) dictate stability as a prerequisite for introduction of mobility. Hodges and Cholewicki (2007) discuss the importance of functional integration of research in establishing control of the spine and acquisition of movement and stability in lumbopelvic pain. Therefore, basic guiding principles for finding stability in yoga postures follow.

General joint stabilization requisites during movement (Hodges and Richardson, 1996; Richardson et al., 1999; Garner, 2001; Willson et al., 2005) require the practitioner to:

1. Initiate slow, controlled closed kinetic chain activities — The slower and more coordinated an individual's progress through a movement or motor pattern, the better the overall proprioceptive awareness, neuromuscular control and collagen remodeling (for fascial health) potential (Schleip and Muller, 2013).

2. Facilitate co-contraction of the surrounding musculature during activity rather than unidirectional strength training.

3. Follow current biomechanical theory for safe joint positioning — Knowledge of osteokinematic (ROM) and arthrokinematic (joint play) joint mechanics and open- and close-packed joint positions helps maximize safety and efficacy in posture alignment.

4. Position joints slowly and carefully — Move slowly through the ROM to assess neural tension, fascial restriction, adhesions, movement impairment, proprioceptive ability, or strength-building. Once this is established, usually with high-level athletes, then careful positioning and pre-positioning of joints can occur at high speed.

5. Introduce unstable environments judiciously to increase difficulty and implement the overload principle for strength training.

6. Foster postural alignment with precision and control — For example, individuals with low back pain can exhibit impaired postural control strategies and demonstrate errors in self-correction of seated poor posture (repositioning) that correlate with pain and disability (O'Sullivan et al., 2013).

7. Utilize low-load force levels that change postures and movement patterns to strengthen joints in varying ranges and train multijoint synergists. This is not to say yoga postures must also only include low-velocity level movement. Indeed, Schleip and Muller (2012) recommend use of both high- and low-velocity training to induce elastic storage capacity in fascia while also increasing strength and volume in muscle, a method used with anecdotal success for two decades (Garner, 2001). High-velocity work, however, must be undertaken while honoring guideline four.

These requirements are summarized in Table 3.6.

The importance of stability in developing flexibility: controlled flexibility theory

Now we return to the discussion on flexibility. Flexibility is important, but used in the absence of control or stability it can be injurious and counterproductive. Therefore, stability is the vital entry point for posture practice. The concept of developing stable mobility is described as controlled flexibility theory, a concept synthesized from the literature, comprising and being dependent on multiple variables that

Table 3.6
Stability requisites

1. Initiate	Initiate slow, controlled closed kinetic chain activities
2. Facilitate	Facilitate co-contraction
3. Follow	Follow current biomechanical theory for safe joint positioning
4. Position	Position joints slowly and carefully
5. Introduce	Introduce unstable environments judiciously
6. Foster	Foster postural alignment with precision and control
7. Utilize	Utilize low-load force levels

affect muscle extensibility, which include (Garner, 2013):

- Sarcomere length

- Mechanical deformation

- Active and passive insufficiency

- The phenomenon of creep

- Torque and angle curve and length/tension relationship (stiffness, compliance and hysteresis)

- Neuromuscular relaxation

- Muscle extensibility and sensory adaptation, which includes neurovascular, osteokinematic and arthrokinematic joint mobility, and segmental stability (Chan et al., 2001; de Weijer et al., 2003; Weppler and Magnusson, 2010).

Factors that inform controlled flexibility theory are dependent on three variables: (1) exercise, (2) disuse, and (3) age, which contribute to both muscular contractile and tendon morphology changes and are compounded by the presence of:

- Joint hypermobility (benign) syndrome

- Decreased muscle extensibility

- Recurrent musculotendinous strain/injury (Magnusson et al., 2008).

A description of controlled flexibility theory is not currently found in a review of the literature as it relates to biomechanics. It is, however, discussed in relationship to mechanical engineering, physics, and biomechanics of equipment such as ski boots and skis, the shaft of golf clubs, prostheses, and orthotics. The conclusions concerning muscle extensibility include the following:

1. It is of "to-be-determined" importance to consider use of a yogic algorithm, presented in Chapter 5. Achieving controlled flexibility can safely streamline injury prevention and rehabilitation regimens. Many strategies exist to achieve flexibility but none possesses such a lengthy list of systemic health benefits as yoga. The algorithm provides a method for assessing stability and flexibility simultaneously through yoga. It is based on provision of joint stability via proprioceptive neuromuscular facilitation when joints are in vulnerable positions (Minshull et al., 2014). Establishing a foundation for developing controlled flexibility is vital, especially since yoga is often oversimplified and misunderstood as a modality for flexibility only.

2. There are many strategies available to achieve stability. These are based on the individual's anatomical and biomechanical factors, such as connective tissue extensibility, muscle strength, body weight, joint surface shape, motor control patterns, as well as psychosocial factors and the loads they need to control. When motion control is inadequate, too much or too little compression occurs across joint surfaces; while too much compression over a long period of time can wear out the joints and lead to osteoarthritis, too little creates episodes of giving way and collapse (Lee, 2011).

3. Consider limb stiffness in generation of joint stability versus inhibition of attaining flexibility (Hoge et al., 2010). A minimum of 2 minutes stretch time is purported to facilitate a decrease in musculotendinous stiffness (Ryan et al., 2008).

4. There is a great need for synthesis of the current evidence base concerning the physiological couplings found between muscles spindles and GTOs, the need for gender-specific clinical guidelines for flexibility prescription, minimization and/or training of the MSR for improved motor response and posture control, and employment of the GTO when flexibility is desired.

5. Since stretch reflexes contribute to joint stability and the regulation of extremity stability (Shemmell et al., 2010), the mechanical execution of yoga postures must consider requisites for joint stability as they relate to gender-specific needs.

6. Gender-specificity for yoga prescription would mandate men hold stretches longer or at a higher intensity than women in order to achieve the same ROM increases as women (Hoge et al., 2010). In contrast, when joint stability and ligamentous

injury prevention is the therapeutic goal, musculotendinous stiffness is desired, which is congruent with research that supports the theory that stretching could result in compromised performance (Knudson et al., 2000). The implication for women is that due to increased flexibility, perhaps from decreased muscle stretch reflex during ovulation (Casey et al., 2014), they have increased injury risk during this phase, especially for ligamentous structures such as the anterior cruciate ligament (ACL) (injury risk is four to six times higher in females than in males) (Malone et al., 1993; Arendt and Dick, 1995; Hewett et al., 2004, 2007; Myer et al., 2004; Barber-Westin et al., 2009).

7. Frequent stretching may need to be accompanied by high-grade joint mobilizations (Jacobs and Sciascia, 2011) to affect overall osteokinematic ROM via arthrokinetmatic manual therapy, respectively. Yoga postures alone will not correct joint hypomobility if joint arthrokinematics (joint play movements recognized as rolling, spinning, or gliding, and determined by convex and concave absolutes of joint biomechanics) are impaired. Clinical success for remodeling of connective tissue depends on the total end-range time or intensity, frequency, and duration of the stretching program, which can vary from minutes (0–30 min) to days, as in the case of serial casting (Jacobs and Sciascia, 2011). Joint mobility directives that affect tissue extensibility can be found later in this chapter.

Research on reflexes can be assimilated into practice based on their relationship with proprioceptive neuromuscular facilitation (PNF). PNF employs the GTO as the basis for achieving outcomes in flexibility and increased joint ROM when arthrokinematics are not an issue. In other words, a stretch that is held for a given amount of time, ranging from 30 seconds (Bandy, 1997; Cipriani et al., 2012) to 2 minutes (Doebler, 2000; Ryan et al., 2008), is a generally accepted rule allowing the GTO to reflexively inhibit muscle contraction, thus increasing the theoretical limit for joint ROM and mobility so long as the stretching program is maintained a minimum

of twice weekly (Rancour et al., 2009) after an initial 4-week, daily stretching program is completed. However, early evidence using bioengineered tendons suggests that influencing wound healing at the morphological level via the extracellular matrix requires myofascial strain/hold times in excess of 2 minutes (Cao et al., 2015). A review of literature cites 120–300 seconds as a standard for slow, sustained pressure to restricted fascial layers (Ajimsha et al., 2015). Certain conditions, for example adhesive capsulitis or patellar hypomobility, may require combinations of high-grade joint mobilizations and home-based stretching to achieve the best results (Jacobs and Sciascia, 2011). This can be accomplished through a combination of manual therapy and proprioceptive neuromuscular facilitation in osteopathic medicine or physical therapy, combined with evidence-based yoga prescription. Table 3.7 provides examples of PNF types. See Chapter 6 (Neurophysiological rationale for the "step back") for elaboration on how PNF, MSR, GTO, and joint stability theory is applied for functional, sport-specific, and ADL training posture via a single posture, warrior I.

Historical relevance of lumbopelvic research

The "canister" or "cylinder" concept, presented by multiple researchers (Lee and Vleeming, 1998; Richardson et al., 1999) over more than 20 years of back pain research in the field of physical therapy and physiotherapy, posits a simple theory with a complex rationale: there must be a minimum competence level and integrity of the lumbopelvic region with concurrent co-activation of muscle groups in order to provide a basic level of stability for the spinal column and trunk. Spinal neutral was defined as the following (Panjabi, 1992b):

- Spinal neutral is the posture of the spine in which the overall internal stresses in the spinal column and the muscular effort needed to hold the posture are minimal.

- Furthermore, spinal neutral is the position of the spine when a vertical force exerted allows equal weight transference or distribution into the weight-bearing surface. In sitting this is the ischial tuberosities and in standing, the feet.

Table 3.7
Proprioceptive neuromuscular facilitation (PNF): tissue response and extensibility

PNF – Tissue response and extensibility	
Reciprocal inhibition	Contract–relax pattern
Reciprocal inhibition	Hold–relax pattern
Autogenic inhibition	Contract–relax pattern
Autogenic inhibition	Hold–relax pattern

Yogic lumbar stabilization including TATD breath, in a 3-year case study, was efficacious in reducing pain and increasing functional mobility (Garner Wood, 2004). Blocks, straps, walls, chairs, bolsters, and extremities can assist in external support for safe postural transition and execution until the TA regains integrity (including fascial) and neural control.

Application of mechanical stability theory to the lumbopelvic region requires consideration of two historical biomechanical findings: (1) motor control problems are identified in those patients with spinal pain, implicating the TA and lumbar mulitifidus (Richardson et al., 1999; Jull and Richardson, 2000); and (2) control of the spine is offered by the "cylinder" or "canister" and contains four elements or planes of control (Richardson et al., 1999; Lee, 2011):

Four planes of control (Fig. 3.17)

1. Superior control is provided by the respiratory diaphragm (Hodges and Gandevia, 2000; Hodges et al., 2003).

2. Transverse or global control was attributed to provision by the TA (Hodges and Richardson, 1996), with an additional but unknown degree of contribution from the psoas, quadratus lumborum, and multifidus (Jemmett et al., 2004). The TA was thought to have an anticipatory role that might contribute to "preparatory stabilization of the spine against reactive forces resulting from limb movement" (Hodges and Richardson, 1999) and

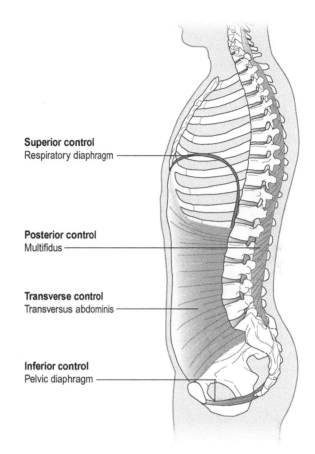

Superior control
Respiratory diaphragm

Posterior control
Multifidus

Transverse control
Transversus abdominis

Inferior control
Pelvic diaphragm

Figure 3.17
Historical planes of control

was initially implicated as the primary abdominal muscle responsible for increased intra-abdominal pressure (Cresswell et al., 1992).

3. Posterior control was attributed to the multifidus (Richardson et al., 1999; Hides et al., 2001; MacDonald et al., 2006), which does not experience automatic recovery after resolution of an acute first episode of low back pain (Hides et al., 1996). Possible stabilizing effects in the lumbopelvic region include the superficial and less able paraspinal group. They function as a spinal extensor or rotator and are theorized to provide more endurance rather than finite execution of lumbopelvic stabilization or control

Chapter 3

(Jorgensen et al., 1993; Fryer et al., 2004). The more proximal location of the multifidi have a more logical mechanical ability to control spinal segmental stability rather than distally located paraspinals.

4. Inferior control or support was attributed to the pelvic diaphragm (Sapsford et al., 2001). The lock system (Chapter 4) of the pelvic floor is described as a '*bandha*', which means lock.

This description of the cylinder/canister system is certainly not an exhaustive discussion, nor an inclusive list, of the history of lumbopelvic stabilization in rehabilitation. The concept that stability of the spine can be provided by a succinct group of "local stabilizers" is also controversial and evolving, with long-term outcomes and biomechanical theory under constant scrutiny (Standaert and Herring, 2007; Allison and Morris, 2008; Lederman, 2010; Morris et al., 2012, 2013; Wang et al., 2012). This discussion only provides a historical context for the creation of TATD breath. Chapter 4 covers contemporary support and instruction.

Scapulothoracic and glenohumeral

Scapulothoracic or periscapular stabilization follows, and is interrelated with, the primary biomechanical focus of lumbopelvic integrity via regional interdependence theory and myofascial lines. Regional interdependence theory posits remotely discovered impairments from the primary symptomatic site are instrumental in the evaluation and treatment of musculoskeletal conditions and are of particular use in manual therapy for affecting outcomes in the area of primary musculoskeletal dysfunction (Wainner et al., 2007; Bialosky et al., 2008).

Joint requisites are clearly established in the shoulder complex, implicating force coupling (Fig. 3.18) as a necessary variable in achieving healthy scapular kinesis (Kibler et al., 2013). Muscles which function in shoulder stabilization through scapulohumeral rhythm, and scapulothoracic and glenohumeral stabilization include the serratus anterior, levator scapula, rhomboids, trapezeii group, and the rotator cuff, comprising the supraspinatus, infraspinatus, teres minor, and subscapularis (Escamilla et al., 2009).

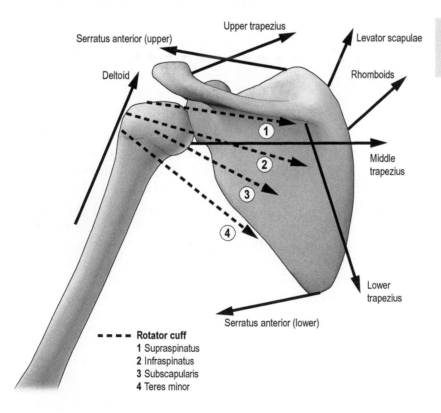

Figure 3.18
Force coupling of scapular kinesis and rotator cuff

Serratus anterior (upper)

Upper trapezius

Levator scapulae

Deltoid

Rhomboids

Middle trapezius

Lower trapezius

Serratus anterior (lower)

- - - - **Rotator cuff**
1 Supraspinatus
2 Infraspinatus
3 Subscapularis
4 Teres minor

Femoroacetabular and tibiofemoral

The contribution of hip impairment to knee pain is well established in biomedical science (Meira and Brummitt, 2011; Boling and Padua, 2013; Lee and Powers, 2013). Contributing factors to patellofemoral pain syndrome (PFPS), a common cause of knee pain, include anatomical malalignment, inadequate hip and thigh musculature strength, nonoptimal lower extremity mechanical strategy during dynamic activity (Powers, 2010; Boling and Padua, 2013). Absence of adequate motor control of the lower extremity has been associated with increases in patellofemoral joint stress due to alterations in frontal and transverse plane motion at the hip and knee leading to inadequate segmental alignment of the lower extremity during weight-bearing tasks (Boling and Padua, 2013; Lee and Powers, 2013). Reasons for this increased stress target decreased hip rotator and abductor strength, specifically eccentric control and for provision of local stability to the lower extremity (Powers, 2010; Bolgla et al., 2011; Lee and Powers, 2013), as well as poor flexion-based postural habits.

Additionally, when managing PFPS, optimal outcomes for both functional performance and pain depend on use of closed kinetic chain hip strengthening movements such as warrior I, chair, and squats, in addition to isolated hip strengthening for hip abduction and external rotation (Ismail et al., 2013). Because the hip rotators and abductors play such a critical role in lower quarter stability during weight-bearing, it is important to train and test their strength in a closed kinetic chain, or weight-bearing, position (Lee and Powers, 2013). See Fig. 3.19 for an illustration of the hip "rotator cuff," an image that mirrors, but is distinct from, scapulohumeral force coupling and scapular kinesis provided by the shoulder. Hip abductor weakness is a significant predictor for exertional medial tibial pain in women, dictating that preventive screening methods for exertional medial tibial pain should include this "proximal contributing factor" (Verrelst et al., 2014). Knee valgus cannot yet be attributed to weak hip abductors or rotators (Cashman, 2012). A systematic review concluded that inclusion of proximal (hip and lumbopelvic) exercises for strengthening are beneficial for distal joint

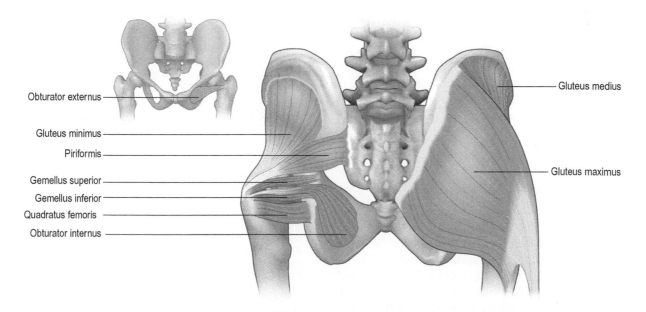

Obturator externus

Gluteus minimus

Piriformis

Gemellus superior

Gemellus inferior

Quadratus femoris

Obturator internus

Gluteus medius

Gluteus maximus

Figure 3.19

Force couple of hip kinesis and rotator cuff

pain caused by PFPS in the knee (Peters and Tyson, 2013). See Chapter 11 for a patellofemoral pain syndrome case study.

> **Tip!** See patellofemoral case example in Chapter 11.

Support

Support for yoga postures is informed by attending to lumbopelvic and scapulothoracic awareness and postural control, and comes through two different mechanisms: internal and external.

Internal/intrinsic control

Internal or intrinsic control in yoga postures is provided by multiple variables, such as fascial force transmission, connective tissue responsiveness, visceral mobility, and neural patterning, but it is directed practically via a focus on lumbopelvic and scapulohumeral rhythm and control. Co-contraction in spinal neutral is only a first step in a lengthy process of achieving control in all ranges of motion in the spine. Co-contraction is not always indicative of practical carryover to functional task completion, such as unilateral arm raising (Allison and Morris, 2008). In other words, TA function is task-specific. Therefore, contralateral contraction must be considered for establishing stability in unilateral stance or asymmetrical postures such as in tree pose (i.e. when the left leg lifts, the right leg and trunk must provide stability).

Work in spinal neutral constitutes a novice level of awareness, after which the intermediate to advanced practitioner will employ internal control throughout the entire ROM in the spine.

The locks system, a series of muscular co-contractions and osteokinematic movements of the axial or appendicular skeleton, further explains the critical internal support system of the body. Chin lock, shoulder lock (closed kinetic chain) and arm spiral (open kinetic chain), abdominal lock (abdominal contraction), anterior and posterior root lock (pelvic floor contraction), and hip lock (hip external rotator and abductor engagement) are part of the yogic locks (Chapter 4).

Use of spinal neutral with concomitant employment of TATD breath using the trunk cylinder/canister concept in standing, supine, prone, and sidelying postures can be used to establish neuromotor control and adequate psychobiological arousal in beginners. TATD breath consists of a selective abdominal lock using the TA and anterior and posterior contraction of the pelvic floor. Co-contraction or unilateral TA isolation should use a range of variable levels of MVIC (maximum voluntary isometric contraction) (from 0% to 100%) that is task-dependent. TATD breath, like yoga postures, does not always require 100% MVIC or global co-contraction to provide safety and stability. See Fig. 3.20 for an internally supported triangle pose.

External/extrinsic control

The concept of external or extrinsic support is based on creating success and safety for those who cannot maintain internal or intrinsic control, chiefly through the utilization of TATD breath and the locks system (discussed in Chapter 4). When the locks are not adequate

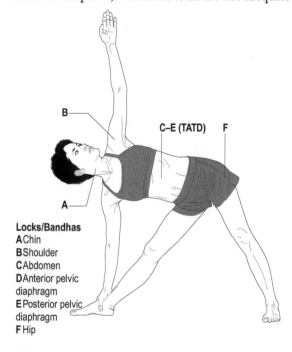

Locks/Bandhas
A Chin
B Shoulder
C Abdomen
D Anterior pelvic diaphragm
E Posterior pelvic diaphragm
F Hip

Figure 3.20

Internally supported triangle pose (TATD, transversus abdominis-assisted thoracodiaphragmatic breath)

for safe movement, external support can be provided by blocks, bolsters, wedges, blankets, straps, ropes, walls, or chairs. The therapist or partner can decrease allostatic load, facilitate abdominal–diaphragmatic breathing, and minimize sympathetic nervous system reaction. Those offering assistance maintain safe biomechanical alignment while progressing osteokinematic or arthrokinematic motion. See Fig. 3.21 for an externally supported triangle pose.

Mobilization

Addressing movement in yoga postures depends on several variables: dissection of arthrokinematics, osteokinematic absolutes, open- and close-packed joint positions, manual therapies, and self-management training, all of which affect fascial health and neural mobility. Addressing mobility also recognizes the energetic and psychoemotional contributions of behavioral organization, including sensorimotor connection,

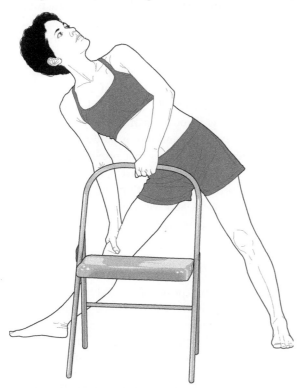

Figure 3.21
Externally supported triangle pose

mind–body interaction, and consciousness that distinguishes between the self and the ego. This means mobility is not just a mechanical phenomenon, but a psychobiological one as well.

Joint mechanics are also ultimately influenced by fascia. But fascia has value beyond the mechanical (Schleip, 2003). It is also a sensory organ (Schleip, 2009; Schleip et al., 2014; Turvey and Fonseca, 2014), together with the extracellular matrix, and is the interface for (1) connecting muscles to bone, (2) sensory integration in movement through detecting internal and external mechanical changes (proprioception), (3) fibroblast-influenced fluid exchange, and (4) autonomic nervous system regulation through visceral fascial affective input via subdiaphragmatic vagus nerve function, also implicated in interoception or "gut intelligence." See Fig. 3.22 for fascia's 12 main distinctions. A discussion of joint and spinal kinematics and fascial and neural mobilization, as it relates to general mobilization, follows.

Joint positioning

With clear knowledge of how each joint works in its subtle and gross forms (arthrokinematics and osteokinematics, respectively), the therapist is better equipped to explain the effects of a yoga posture on the joints of the body. Evaluation of a resting open-packed joint position is the position used for traction and joint mobilization. As a general rule, the extremes of joint ROM are close-packed, while the midrange positions are open-packed. Knowledge of joint positioning (open- and close-packed) provides a biomechanical safety net and platform for dissociation, downtraining, or uptraining (neuromuscular re-education) of muscle groups.

Functional joint mobility requires an understanding of several key concepts:

- Closed kinetic chain — A weight-bearing position where the upper or lower extremities are in contact with the ground or are terra firma with another immovable objects (wall, bench).

- Open kinetic chain — Positions are non-weight-bearing, where the upper or lower extremities are not in contact with the ground.

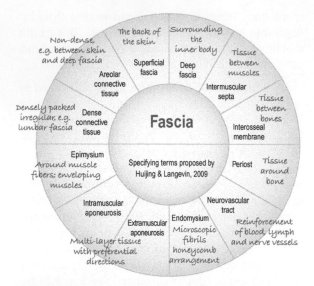

Figure 3.22

Twelve fascial distinctions (reproduced with the kind permission of Joanne Avison and Handspring Publishing)

- Open-packed joint position — The position that allows the most arthrokinematic mobility or where the joint capsule and ligaments are most relaxed and articulating surfaces are maximally separated. To increase ROM and avoid joint impingement, open-packed joint positions should be used. However, the joint is most vulnerable in this position and therefore requires following the joint requisites for stabilization and postural control. Postural progression to larger ranges of motion must sometimes include use of the open-packed position of a joint, as compared to a beginner or individual without intrinsic joint support who could use close-packed positions coupled with an inhibitory (inhalation) breath to prevent excessive joint movement. The breath can be used concomitantly with open- or close-packed joint position in a yoga pose to either progress (exhalation) or limit (inhalation) ROM. In this way joint positioning can prevent injury or manage instability via joint protection. (See Table 3.8 for a joint-by-joint review of open- and close-packed joint positions.)

- Close-packed joint position — The position that allows the least amount of arthrokinematic mobility or where joint surfaces are in maximal contact with one another. Close-packed positioning can be used to facilitate stability in those not capable of obtaining intrinsic stability, such as patients with neurodevelopmental disabilities (for example, cerebral palsy), neurovascular (for example, neuropathy), or neurological (spinal cord injury or traumatic brain injury) deficits. Spinal alignment is also influenced by use of open- and close-packed joint positioning. For example, the individual with sacroiliac joint dysfunction due to postpartum instability and deconditioning may be at risk for injury if allowed to perpetually counternutate (unlock/open-packed position) or nutate (lock/close-packed position) the sacroiliac joint during normal standing or task completion. (See Fig. 3.23 for an illustration of open- and close-packed positions of the sacrum.) She may need postural retraining, which would include assessment of neural patterning in order to facilitate proper force and form closure during functional task completion. Retraining can be accomplished through the use of yoga postures, coupled with the breath, to establish proprioceptive awareness through tactile acuity (Luomajoki and Moseley, 2011) and motor patterning encased in a series of movements that provide continuous input to the thoracolumbar fascia, which helps with sensory cortical reorganization and pain management (Luomajoki and Moseley, 2011), and collagen remodeling for fascial structure (Schleip and Muller, 2013).

Arthrokinematic joint mobility

Open-packed joint position should also be used to facilitate arthrokinematic joint mobilization. Arthrokinematic joint motion is described as joint play, or the roll, spin, and gliding that happens between joint surfaces. Osteokinematic motion, also known as ROM in flexion, extension, abduction, adduction, internal rotation, external rotation, or a combination of movements called circumduction, depends on arthrokinematic motion. In the absence

Table 3.8

Open-packed and close-packed joint positions

Joint	Open-packed position	Close-packed position
Facet (spine)	Midway between flexion and extension	Extension
Sacroiliac	Counternutation	Nutation
Temporomandibular	Mouth slightly open	Clenched teeth
Glenohumeral	55 degrees abduction, 30 degrees horizontal adduction	Abduction, lateral rotation
Acromioclavicular	Physiological position, resting	90 degrees abduction of arm
Sternoclavicular	Physiological position, resting	Maximum shoulder elevation
Ulnohumeral (elbow)	70 degrees flexion, 10 degrees supination	Extension
Radiocarpal (wrist)	Neutral with slight ulnar deviation	Extension with radial deviation
Metacarpophalangeal	Slight flexion	Full flexion
Hip	30 degrees abduction, slight lateral rotation	Full extension, medial rotation
Knee	25 degrees flexion	Full extension, lateral tibial rotation
Talocrural (ankle)	10 degrees plantarflexion	Maximum dorsiflexion
Metatarsophalangeal	Neutral	Full extension

of this joint play, altered kinematics at the joint are experienced, which can lead to loss of joint ROM, pain, and somatic dysfunction. The arthrokinematics of each joint are historically determined by the shape of the joint surfaces, known as the concave–convex rules (Kaltenborn et al., 1999), but the theory of biomechanical joint mobility is complicated by fascial integrity and response. Nonetheless, yoga posture prescription increases in complexity when considering whether to move, say, the acetabulum over the femur or the femur in the acetabulum. The two movements differ in how they affect the soft tissue and joint.

- The concave rule — When the joint surface that is moving is concave, both gliding and rolling motions occur in the same direction.

- The convex rule — When the joint surface that is moving is convex, gliding and rolling occur in opposite directions.

See Fig. 3.24 for an illustration of the concave/convex rule.

Treatment to normalize accessory motion in a joint would be warranted within a restorative, open-packed yoga posture when loss of ROM caused by capsular tightness creates asymmetry (also known as obligate translation) in joint motion that creates a firm end feel (Maitland 1977, 1986) or pain is present that creates an empty end feel. Joint mobilization can also be used to increase ROM in a joint via plastic deformation, increase mobility of shortened soft tissues, decrease pain,

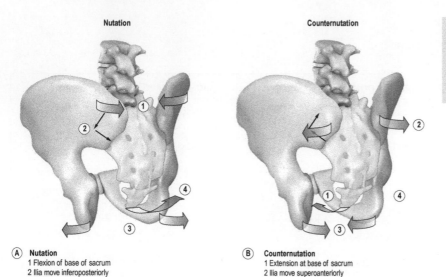

Nutation

Counternutation

A Nutation
1 Flexion of base of sacrum
2 Ilia move inferoposteriorly
3 Ischial tuberosities move anterolaterally
4 Extension at apex of sacrum

B Counternutation
1 Extension at base of sacrum
2 Ilia move superoanteriorly
3 Ischial tuberosities move posteromedially
4 Flexion at base of sacrum

Figure 3.23
(A) Close-packed sacroiliac joint position; (B) open-packed sacroiliac joint position

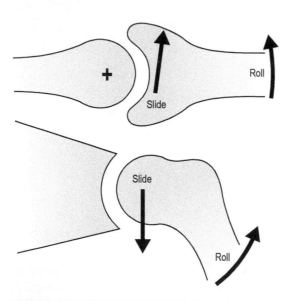

Figure 3.24
(A) Concave rule; (B) convex rule

and hypomobility. Mobilizations are graded from I to V. Mobilization grading and Kaltenborn traction levels are outside the scope of this text and should only be used as allowed by professional scope of practice.

Spinal kinematics

Finally, spinal kinematics affect yoga posture prescription and are discussed in relation to the evolution of Fryette's theoretical laws from 1957 (Parsons and Marcer, 2005) via a review of the current evidence base. Sizer (2007) posits that treating patients with spinal pain requires knowledge of three-dimensional spine coupling characteristics. To appreciate the beauty of spinal twists and flexion in yoga postures, and to teach them effectively and safely, an intimate understanding of spinal motion and what creates or impedes movement is helpful. The three-joint complex of the vertebra includes smooth, cartilage surfaces, the flexible ligament and capsule, and the synovial joint and fluid (Kapandji, 2008). In addition to the normal angles of the curvatures in the spine, defined as 30–35 degrees of lordosis in the cervical spine, 40 degrees of kyphosis in the thoracic spine, and 45 degrees of lordosis in the lumbar spine (Donatelli and Thurner, 2014), the spine undergoes coupled or uncoupled movements, depending on (1) which area of the spine is involved, (2) whether or not the movement is loaded (weighted) or performed in/outside of spinal neutral, and (3) age (Edmonston et al., 2005). An uncoupled movement is a motion that can occur independently and in the absence of another motion, while a coupled movement requires segmental vertebral movement in ipsilateral or contralateral directions (Levangie and Norkin, 2011).

Fryette's laws posit that completing motion in the spine occurs through anatomical alignment of the vertebrae and coupling of movements via multiplanar osteokinematic and arthrokinematic movements. There are three laws, which are evolving with the evidence base, making them guidelines open to clinical and investigative scrutiny.

- Type I motion — When the spine is in a neutral position, vertebral sidebending and rotation occur in opposite directions, typically found in the thoracic and lumbar spine.

- Type II motion — When the spine is outside of neutral position, vertebral sidebending and rotation occur in the same direction, found in any area of the spine.

- Type III motion — When motion is introduced in one plane, motion is naturally limited and modified in secondary and tertiary planes, respectively.

See Fig. 3.25 for an overview of spinal kinematic force coupling in the spine.

Trudelle-Jackson et al. (2011) also suggest that differing criteria should be employed, other than lumbar ROM, when determining lumbar spine impairment secondary to discrepancies in lumbar motion found between races, gender, and age groups. Chung and Wang (2009) found women have more ROM available than men in the cervical spine, upper extremities, and lower extremities, while African American women have more available lumbar extension and less available lumbar flexion than white women (Trudelle-Jackson et al., 2011). Other researchers have come to the similar conclusion that accepted normative values for lumbar ROM should be questioned based on gender, age, and race (Sullivan et al., 1994; Dvorak et al., 1995; McGregor et al., 1995; Van Herp et al., 2001; Intolo et al., 2009). These findings are of particular importance in yoga since many postures require extremes of spinal flexion or extension, which may not be available to both genders or all races and age groups. Yoga posture "norms" or the focus on achieving "normative

standards" in an end ROM of a posture should be avoided and replaced with individual prescription of yoga postures, based on gender, race, age, individual characteristics, dysfunction, and needs.

Additionally, teaching certain postures that historically exist in the yoga of India, such as extreme lumbar extension in backbends, should be reconsidered based on the evidence that the anthropometrics of the spine differ anthropologically. More research is needed on degree of spinal motion available based on gender, race, and culture.

Fascia: provision of load transfer and force generation

No longer relegated to its historical role of static mobility, the fascia is responsible for more than just passive force transmission. Hilton's law (1863) first identified the interrelationship between the joints and the overlying muscle, skin, and fascia. The evidence base clearly supports the existence of fascia as a "living" or active element in the body (Schleip, 2009).

Fascia is identified, with variations, in grossly three dimensions (Stecco et al., 2011; Findley et al., 2012): (1) superficial fascia (membranous layer of the hypodermis), (2) deep fascia (fibrous membrane enveloping joints, muscles, separating muscles, and binding structures together), and (3) epimysium, and four layers: (i) pannicular or superficial fascia, (ii) axial fascia, (iii) meningeal fascia, and (iv) visceral fascia (Willard, 2015) (Fig. 3.26). Dense, irregular connective tissue sheets of fascia are found throughout the entire human body in the form of aponeuroses, joint capsules, and muscular envelopes such as the endo-, peri-, and epimysium (Schleip et al., 2005).

Each dimension of fascia owns specific roles, which include:

- Provision of skin integrity (Stecco et al., 2011)

- Contribution of muscular contraction via smooth muscle fiber intrusion in fascia (Staubesand and Li, 1996)

- Spontaneous ligament contraction from discovery of fascia's viscoelastic properties in cadaver lumbodorsal fascia (Yahia et al., 1993)

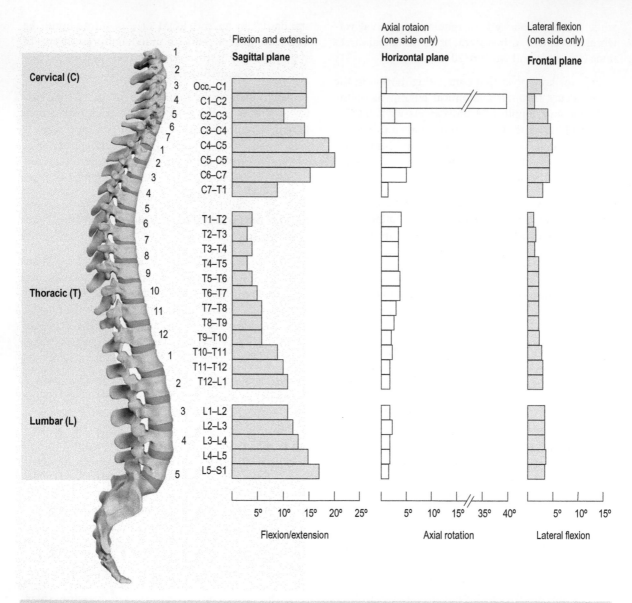

Figure 3.25

Spinal kinematics overview and segmental vertebral motion (redrawn from Sahrmann, S. et al., 2011, *Movement System Impairment Syndromes of the Extremities, Cervical and Thoracic Spines*, Elsevier/Mosby, St Louis, MO, using data from White, A.A., Panjabi, M.M. (eds), 1990, *Clinical Biomechanics of the Spine*, 2nd edn, Lipincott, Philadelphia, PA)

- Force generation and transmission in the deep layers of the thoracolumbar fascia (Barker et al., 2010; Willard et al., 2012)

- Limitation of lumbar spinal mobility (Barker et al., 2004; Schleip et al., 2005)

- Venous return (Bordoni and Zanier, 2013)

- Contribution to nociception via decreased proprioceptive awareness in involved fascia (Moseley, 2008)

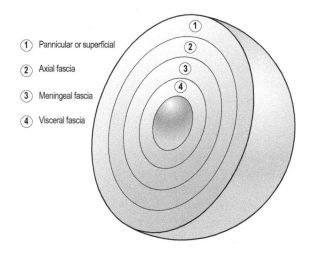

① Pannicular or superficial

② Axial fascia

③ Meningeal fascia

④ Visceral fascia

Figure 3.26
Fascial layers

- Transmission of tension between the epimysium and which validates its contribution to muscle force generation (Barker et al., 2010; Willard et al., 2012).

This is not an exhaustive list of fascia's many roles; indeed, fascia, through the theory of biotensegrity proposed by Buckminster Fuller (1975), is thought by many fascial experts (Levin, 2012; Scarr, 2014; Avison, 2015; Schleip, 2015) to provide the actual container for biomechanical and kinematic human movement through a system of compressive and tensile force akin to a geometric suspension model. It is working to expand on the compartmentalization that the body only moves via following isolated "classical mechanics and isolated lever systems" (Scarr, 2014, p. 38). Nonetheless, a systems investigation has yet to firmly establish a single unified theory that values truths in both the general relativity- and physics-based mechanical systems, and the more recent tensegrity model.

The existence of pathological fascial contractures and concomitant presence of mechanical impairment and pain underscores the active role of fascia. Schleip (2009) proposes that if myofascial manipulation can affect the local blood supply and viscosity of local tissue, then it is possible that palpable changes could be detected by the practitioner. This phenomenon was likened to "feeling with the listening hand of a sensitive practitioner" (Pischinger, 1991; Schleip, 2003).

Newer evidence confirms fascia as a force transmitter and its similar contractibility potential to smooth muscle, both of which can have serious effects on musculoskeletal dynamics (Schleip et al., 2005; Hujing, 2009; Langevin et al., 2011). Resting tone of myofascia maintains passive postural balance. Deficiency or excess of myofascial tone predisposes to pathologic muscle spindle disorders (Alfonse et al., 2010), while stimulation of Ruffini endings via lateral stretch of the fascia is posited to lower sympathetic activity (Schleip, 2003, 2009).

When tissues do not move well this may be caused by fascia that are no longer properly gliding. Microtears, dehydration, inflammation, and adhesions are thought to influence fascial layer gliding (Schleip and Muller, 2013) (Fig. 3.27). Fascial lines are described by Myers (2009, 2014) and should be considered as more than mechanical myofascial stations. See Fig. 3.28 for line illustrations.

Skin interruptions and adhesions

Interruptions in the largest organ of the body, the skin, have large potential for long-term impact on quality of life in the individual. Adhesion formation is the most common complication from abdominal or pelvic surgery (Ten Broek et al., 2013), affecting approximately 90% of postoperative patients following major abdominal surgery (Liakakosa et al., 2001; Cimen et al., 2004; Schreinemacher et al., 2010) and reducing pregnancy rates in postoperative irritable bowel patients by 50% (Ten Broek et al., 2013). The high risk of adhesions (see Fig. 3.27) should lead to improved adhesion care and prevention strategies, since adhesions can be identified as a source of bowel obstruction and chronic abdominal and/or pelvic pain (Ten Broek et al., 2013). In the abdominal area, Cimen et al. (2004) cite that myofascial restriction can contribute to chronic abdominal and or back pain and can be mistaken for internal organ dysfunction. Adhesions occur when layers of the skin are allowed to heal without some type of scar mobilization.

Laparoscopic surgery does not decrease the risk for adhesions, and overall, adhesions increase morbidity

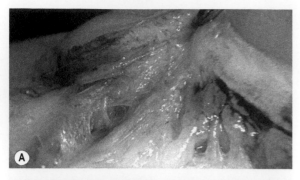

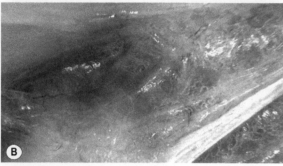

Figure 3.27

Tissue adhesion: integrity of fascia and skin layers can be interrupted by microtears, dehydration, inflammation, and/or adhesions. (A) Nature does not repair and reshape living matter exactly as it was before injury, and the results are often disappointing. This photograph shows an internal scar 1 year after the injury (×2). (B) In these scars we find reddish areas (seen as darker gray areas in this image) lined with small bunches of blood vessels, which are evidence of inflammation. Adhesions form between the scar and underlying aponeuroses (×5). Reproduced with permission from Jean-Claude Guimberteau and Colin Armstrong, *The Architecture of Human Living Fascia*, Handspring Publishing, 2015

risk and fertility treatment incidence (Ten Broek et al., 2013). Notably though, less than 10% of surgeons inform patients of adhesion risk (Parker et al., 2007; Trew et al., 2009; Schreinemacher et al., 2010).

Hernias and diastasis recti abdominis (Lee et al., 2008) also implicate the fascia, including internal organ location, via fascial generation of tension. Incisional hernias happen when organs or tissues protrude through a surgical incision, which can happen due to obesity or infection. Differential diagnosis

of myofascial restriction requires recognition of systemic issues that would include peritonitis or referred pain from internal organs and can affect respiration or vice versa. Examples of localized peritonitis that should be considered in differential diagnosis include endometriosis, hepatitis, pelvic inflammatory disease, appendicitis, peptic ulcer, colitis, abscesses, and Crohn's disease.

Fascia is innervated by smooth muscle cells and can be influenced by pain sensations. Fascial tone is influenced by the autonomic response, and because breathing is the most accessible technique for affecting the stress response, theoretically, fascia could be affected through a BPS model of intervention.

Yoga could help or harm myofascial restriction during both posture and breathing practice, and therefore must be recognized as a vital consideration in clinical prescription. Yoga prescription depends on understanding musculoskeletal pathologies that could accompany increased or decreased myofascial tonus. Doing so may offer new insights and a deeper understanding of treatments directed at fascia via use of guided imagery and manual therapies during yoga postures, including use of yogic breathing, which can impact myofascial release within yoga practice. Guidelines for myofascial release in yoga are found in Chapter 12.

Neural mobilization

Neural mobilization was born from David Butler's (1991) new frontier in manual therapy. Neural mobilization has immense therapeutic application within the context of yoga posture and breath prescription. Neural mobilization and yoga are both subtle sciences that share a common therapeutic intention; they both recognize that the nervous system is a fragile, multifaceted system capable of neural plasticity. Lorimer Moseley, however, promotes a shift in pain neuroscience nomenclature to suggest that neuroplasticity does not occur in a vacuum and affects the entire system. Therefore, bioplasticity may be a more inclusive, systems-based term (Moseley, 2014). Both yoga and neural mobilization work with a holistic approach that, through affecting neurophysiological change, aspires to facilitate allostasis in the individual.

There are two original guiding principles from Butler (1991) that inform the theory of adaptation in

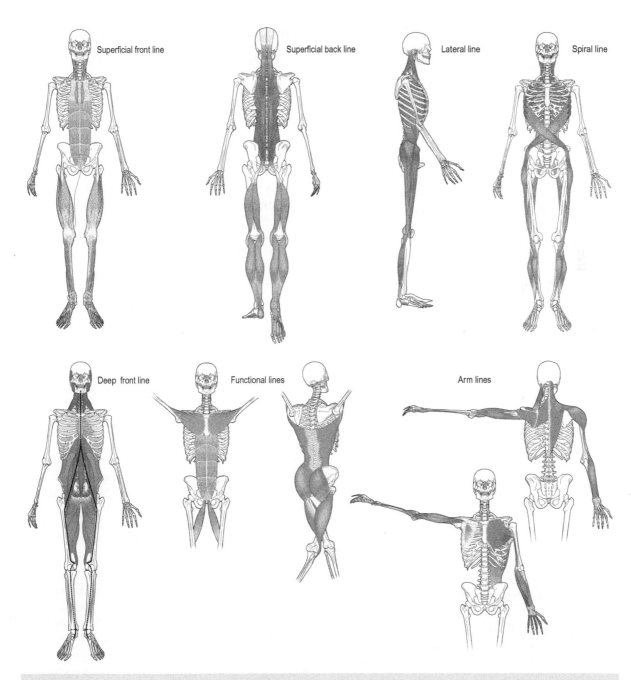

Figure 3.28
Myofascial lines

neural tissue response to intervention. First, the nervous system is susceptible to mobilization secondary to the development of tension or increased pressure within the tissue (intracranial pressure or intradural pressure). The pressure develops as a consequence of elongation and occurs in all tissues and fluids enclosed by and including the epineurium and the dura mater.

Second, movement may be considered as one of two types: (1) gross movement or movement of the system as a whole, such as a peripheral nerve sliding through the carpal tunnel in the wrist, or (2) intraneural movement between connective and neural tissues, for example the brain and spinal cord moving in relation to the surrounding cranial dura mater or the unfolding of nerve fibers that move in relation to the endoneurium. Fibrosis, edema, adhesions, or other mechanical impairment may affect both gross and intraneural movement. Guidelines for neural mobilization and assessment are found in Chapters 5 and 12.

The difference in combining yoga with neural mobilization is profound. If we consider approaching neural mobilization as not just a mechanical neurophysiological shift in tangible tissues, but also as a methodology for affecting psychoneurological change, then neural mobilization can become a more powerful modality. There is a powerful relationship between emotional response and consciousness and health status, termed "the emotional motor system" (Holstege et al., 1996). The mystery of the mind and its concrete physical and chemical characteristics is juxtaposed with its creative, spontaneous, abstract abilities and desires.

Yoga is a distinct and unique form of integrative medicine that when used in combination with other types of medicine (physical rehabilitation and conditioning, in this case), allows for treating the whole person with a preventive rather than just a pathology-based paradigm. This concept is important because presence of neural restriction should be closely monitored during all yoga prescription at all levels. Objective neurophysiological change should be guided by the sustaining principle of achieving allostasis in the individual, of discriminating between the ego, the self, and consciousness. Yoga allows for this holistic shift in intervention, unlike other movement therapies and mindfulness practices, because of its efficacy with a wide range of psychosomatic and psychiatric disorders.

Therefore, the concept of neural mobilization is not undertaken as a mechanical intervention alone, but with a compassionate attention to reorganization of behavior. Asking the question, "How can this yoga pose or breath facilitate a sensorimotor connection that allows for serious inquiry into understanding the mind–body interaction?" allows for continual advances in medicine, not just yogic prescription.

Meditation: changing the stress response

Meditation is beneficial for stress resilience and neuroendocrine regulation, a field of medicine concerned with psychoneuroendocrinology and psychoneuroimmunology (Bushell, 2009; Olivo, 2009; Kuntsevich et al., 2010, Streeter et al., 2010, 2012) and can be responsible for neural plasticity and cerebral cortex thickening (Khalsa, 2013). Meditation is purported to facilitate normal circadian rhythm via neuroendocrine regulation by reducing stress arousal and inducing positive arousal effects, including regulation of steroid hormones such as cortisol. An added benefit of neuroendocrine regulation is promotion of telomere maintenance (Epel et al., 2009), which, in short, means yoga could become a vital anti-aging, anti-cancer intervention through changing gene expression (Dusek et al., 2008; Saatcioglu, 2013).

Yogic meditation can also promote stress resilience through improving stress response and positive arousal. Improving the stress response can build resilience and develop healthy coping strategies. Stress can be your best friend, or at least your best teacher (McGonigal, 2013).

Meditation is a powerful tool to impact both psychoemotional and social health (Pace et al., 2009; Ross and Thomas, 2010) and is supported to improve mood and diminish anxiety through increasing GABA levels (Streeter et al., 2010, 2012). Mindfulness also affects emotional resilience and self-discipline through strengthening connections between the prefrontal executive zones and the amygdala (Goleman, 2013; Taren et al., 2015), with the most emotionally resilient people (those who recover most quickly after getting upset) having as much as 30 times more activation in the left prefrontal area than less resilient peers (Heller et al., 2009). See Chapter 12 for meditation guidelines.

Review

In review, use of neurophysiological principles and the interrelationship of pain neuroscience, myofascial, and neuroendocrine, and neuromuscular systems provides a framework for yoga prescription whose ultimate intention is to prevent and manage chronic disease and injury. Health promotion through the lifestyle of yoga has enormous implications to sharpen the focus of today's biomedical model, making it possible to welcome an inclusive, cross-cultural, multimodal biopsychosocial model of healthcare.

See Table 3.9 for an overview of clinical prediction guidelines and precautions.

Table 3.9
Clinical prediction guidelines and precautions*

General therapeutic intentions and clinical prediction guidelines
Cardiorespiratory – Increase heart rate variability (HRV), vital capacity, oxygen saturation, and alveolar ventilation. Inversions provide inverted diaphragmatic biofeedback wherein the inverted position could assist in deepening inhalation and metering exhalation. Inversions can provide clarity in isolation and utilization of the diaphragm, while also making exhalation easier
Cognitive – Impact movement strategy planning, executive functioning, memory recall, development of body and proprioceptive intelligence, and sensorimotor integration through scaffolded instruction and exploration
Neuroendocrine/immune – Improve autonomic stress response and inversely proportional activity that is increased in the parasympathetic and decreased in sympathetic systems; telomere maintenance and preservation, improve immunomodulation
Integumentary – Improve myofascial response and potential fascial matrix integrity
Neurovascular – Improve neural gliding in upper and lower limbs and dura sheath
Vestibular – High-level (standing, moving transitions, supine, prone lying, semi-inversion postures, and frequent transfers that involve supine-to-sit, floor-to-standing, bed transfers and/or eye/head movements) and/or low-level (seated or static postures) vestibulo-ocular reflex training
Circulatory/lymphatic – Improve vascular competency, prevention of venous insufficiency via muscle pumping action of the upper and lower extremities and in semi-inversions; prevention of orthostatic hypotension via muscle pumping action for postures which involve the lower extremities; through indirect myofascial techniques in postures, protection of vascular structures could result in diminished hypervigilance in local tissues and fascia, which could also affect global pain management of chronic orthopaedic or urogynecologic issues
Psychoemotional – Cultivate introspection (quiet) and reflection, confidence, focus, fortitude, emotional resilience, motivation, energy. Through exhalation and sound production, improve ventral vagus circuit activity to facilitate social engagement, empathic and compassion response, and regulate appropriate "fight, flight, or freeze" reactivity. Through mindfulness training via postures and breath, affect emotional resilience and self-discipline through strengthening connections between the prefrontal executive zones and the amygdala. The most emotionally resilient people have more activation in the left prefrontal area than less resilient peers
Reproductive and urologic – Focus on breath practice, meditation, visceral mobilization, and healthy movement, including weight and stress management, can potentially improve fertility, influence bladder retraining, and/or manage pelvic pain or sexual dysfunction
Pain – Influence perception and management of pain, as well as mindful attentiveness to pain source and type, and when appropriate, disengage from the faulty pain signals, which could strengthen anatomical links between periaqueductal gray (PAG), the opiate-rich area of the brain responsible for pain suppression, and the default mode network (DMN). Through polyvagal theory and potential vagus nerve stimulation via breath and sound, pain modulation can be influenced through decrease in inflammation, sympathetic nervous system activity, oxidative stress, and regulation of opioid receptors

(Continued)

Table 3.9
Clinical prediction guidelines and precautions* (*Continued*)

Gastrointestinal (GI) – Stress management and postures that include visceral mobilization (self myofascial release and manual therapy-based myofascial release) and massage effect (postures involving the force couple of twists, forward flexion, and/or inversions combined with diaphragmatic isolation) affect biochemical levels, which influence both reproductive and urological function as well as GI motility. Mobilization of GI tract can also occur within left side-lying, seated twists, myofascial release in side-lying, supine, and prone. Breathwork can also regulate functional gastrointestinal disorders (FGID) including gastroesophageal reflux disorder (GERD) and the range of signs and symptoms associated with irritable bowel syndrome (IBS). A full discussion of GI benefits is outside the scope of this text

Musculoskeletal and neuromuscular – Improve global proprioception, tactile acuity, endurance, strength, mobility; shoulder complex and pelvic and hip complex joint functioning and dynamic neuromotor balance, postural and gait training, awareness, and control, balance, bone density during weight-bearing postures combined as a dynamic sequence. Yoga locks address:

1. Spine and pelvis – Global spine and pelvic awareness, strength, tactile acuity, proprioception, reaction time, endurance, coactivation of trunk muscles at multiple joint angles and in multiple planes of motion (both unilateral and bilateral engagement); myofascial and neurovascular response and resilience in all planes

2. Lower quarter – Coactivation of lower quarter for axial and appendicular contributions to stability and controlled flexibility in both open and closed kinetic chain(s) at multiple joint angles and in multiple planes of motion; myofascial and neurovascular resilience and response in all planes

3. Upper quarter – Coactivation of upper quarter for periscapular strengthening and glenohumeral joint balance in open and closed kinetic chain(s) at multiple joint angles and in multiple planes of motion; myofascial and neurovascular resilience and response via use of arm spiral mechanism and in general postures

4. Mindful movement strategy planning via slow and fast velocity training – Yogic locks used in antigravity positions can aid in initiation of movement and muscle contraction. Yogic locks provide global trunk balance via introduction preliminary control for functional carryover into upright versions of postures (i.e. reclined tree and reclined hand to big toe can functionally carryover to their standing versions)

Elemental (*doshic*) applications

All postures affect the constitution (*doshas*): air/ether (*vata*), fire/water (*pitta*), and earth/water (*kapha*) element and are beneficial; however, a full discussion is outside the scope of this text

General precautions

General precautions are relative for all postures but as a whole include: poor body awareness, joint hypomobility or hypermobility, excessive hip anteversion (caution for poses that require external rotation since this ROM is generally limited), hip retroversion (caution for poses that require internal rotation since this ROM is generally limited), previous cartilage, labral, or meniscus injury or surgery, upper or lower quarter instability, or uncontrolled systemic illness

For postures that require trunk stability, consider:

weak or poor transversus abdominis-assisted thoracodiaphragmatic (TATD) breath endurance, which diminishes safety via lack of internal support. Substitute a static restorative approximation (SRA) or dynamic modification (DM) until internal stability makes the pose safe to perform. Orthostatic hypotension and fall risk will also require modification

*A systems-based review of therapeutic intentions, benefits, clinical prediction guidelines as well as precautions for yoga posture practice. The evidence base to support this overview is provided primarily in Chapters 1–3. Evidence-informed and evidence-based benefits specific to individual postures are found in Chapters 4–10.

This chapter provides a template assessment of the diaphragm and experience of breath techniques. Proper breath provides a basis for implementation of the functional movement assessment (FMA) presented in Chapter 5. The relationship of orofacial tonus with postural health and social engagement is also described, including a short section on orofacial phonation response exercises. This is followed by an explanation of the yogic locks system that bolsters basic postural stabilization, along with a review of pertinent special tests and screening to provide safe posture prescription. See Chapter 12 for guidelines to practice which are helpful prior to reading this chapter.

Outline

- Breath and posture therapeutic template
- Recognition of abnormal breathing patterns
- FMA: respiration – functional breathing patterns
- Orofacial assessment
- Respiratory assessment
- Orofacial phonation relaxation response
- Functional breath types
- Yogic breath types
- Yogic locks – energy anatomy for carriage maintenance
- Special tests and screening prerequisites
- Femoral version screen
- Review

Breath and posture therapeutic template

See the Glossary (p. 333) for explanations of abbreviations used in the instructional therapeutic template and definitions of terms used.

Recognition of abnormal breathing patterns

Abnormal breath patterns adversely affect human systems. These effects include psychological symptoms such as panic or anxiety, physical symptoms such as impaired trunk stability (Kolar et al., 2012), functional gastrointestinal disorders, or pelvic pain, and/or physical signs such as hypoventilation or hyperventilation. Abnormal breathing patterns include (1) thoracic breathing, chest breathing, or clavicular breathing, (2) paradoxical breathing, (3) mask breathing, and (4) open-mouthed breathing.

Abnormal patterns 1 and 2

Thoracic breath, chest breathing, and clavicular breathing are characterized by an almost silent respiratory diaphragm where the person breathes without the diaphragm and the abdomen remains still. In contrast, paradoxical breathing leaves the diaphragm unused, and it remains relaxed even as it is lifted up during inhalation. The abdominal wall is pulled superoposterior while the external intercostals lift the chest superolaterally and the ribcage expands maximally.

Abnormal respiratory patterns create an anxious, panicky, mentally degenerative or physically impaired state. They also create poor vagal response that increases allostatic load through increased sympathetic stress, inducing persistent upregulated states of "fight, flight, or shut down." According to polyvagal theory (PVT), the "shut down" response is mediated by a dorsal, unmyelinated branch of the vagus nerve (Porges, 2001, 2011). PVT is distinctly more complex than current binary theory, sympathetic versus parasympathetic response, would imply. This dorsal response is described as a vestigial reptilian response to perceived threat, characterized as an immobilizing action. In short, when an organism is threatened, it can respond by shutting down, or "freezing."

Abnormal patterns 3 and 4

Mask breathing is a form of "shut down" response characterized by a persistent recruitment of secondary muscles of respiration which includes thoracic breathing, chest breathing, or clavicular breathing, paradoxical breathing, and mask breathing. Open-mouthed breathing is less common but often found with abnormal breathing patterns 1, 2, and/or 3, in addition to comorbidities such as chronic respiratory ailments including asthma, allergies, sinus infections, chronic obstructive pulmonary disease (COPD), obesity, high stress, and allostatic load. Open-mouthed breathing is an indicator of low facial tone and myofunctional dysfunction of the orofacial complex and could correlate with sequelae that include poor proprioception in the face/mouth with possible low global tone, diminished respiratory capacity, hypermobility syndromes such as Ehlers–Danlos (DeFelice et al., 2001), and postural dysfunction (Conti et al., 2011; Olivi et al., 2012). Open-mouthed breathing is a paradoxical opposite of mask breathing. It can adversely affect dentofacial and craniofacial development in children and youth (Harari et al., 2010) that can lead to cervical, temporomandibular, and postural malalignment. The presence of low tone associated with open-mouthed breathing should also suggest consideration of airway obstruction in supine postures (i.e. sleep) that could contribute to sleep apnea, as well as any known history of bruxism, jaw clenching, or associated temporomandibular joint (TMJ) dysfunction. See Fig. 4.1 and Table 4.1 for overviews of abnormal breathing patterns.

FMA: respiration – functional breathing patterns

Two breath types, abdominodiaphragmatic (A-D) breath and transversus abdominis-assisted thoracodiaphragmatic (TATD) breath, are considered functional breathing patterns. The former is used for regular at-rest breathing and the latter for trunk stability and safety during posture practice and completion of activities of daily living (ADL). Both are prerequisites for progression and mastery of yogic breath and posture practice.

Therapeutic intention

The systemic benefits and therapeutic intentions of breath practices are discussed in Chapters 1 and 3.

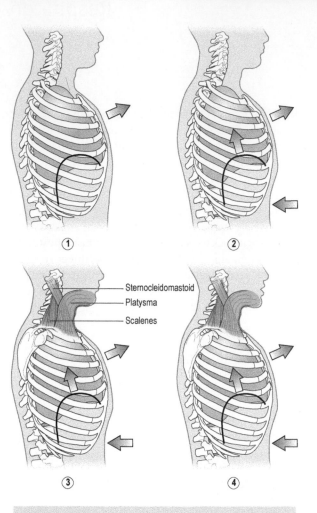

Figure 4.1

Abnormal breathing patterns. 1. Chest/clavicular/thoracic breath. 2. Paradoxical breath. 3. Mask breathing 4. Open-mouthed breathing. Note that this breathing pattern could take on characteristics of 1, 2, or 3 breath types

Additional individual therapeutic intentions are included with each breath type.

Orofacial assessment

1. Begin with history-taking. Note any history of teeth clenching, grinding, or TMJ issues. Check for point tenderness or trigger points around the mandible, TMJ, hyoid, platysma, sternocleidomastoid, and mastoid process.

Table 4.1

Characteristics of abnormal breathing patterns

Abnormal breathing pattern characteristics	
I: Thoracic breathing, chest breathing, or clavicular breathing	An almost silent respiratory diaphragm where the person breathes without the diaphragm and the abdomen remains still
II: Paradoxical breathing	Leaves the diaphragm unused, where it remains relaxed even as it is improperly lifted up during inhalation
III: Mask breathing	A persistent recruitment of secondary muscles of respiration
IV: Open-mouthed breathing	An indicator of low facial tone and myofunctional dysfunction of the orofacial complex

2. Assess for lip seal and jaw position. The lips should close, in the absence of allergies or structural abnormalities such as restricted labial frenulum or orthodontia. With an adequate lip seal, the tongue should be lifted and rest behind the front teeth, which widens the airway and opens the mandible. Any malocclusion of the mandible can adversely affect not only the neck and head, but also distal postural alignment (Sakaguchi et al., 2007).

3. If any remarkable history is noted or the lip seal and jaw position are difficult to attain, consider the following two screens:

   • Lingual frenulum length — A tethered frenulum affects the ability of the tongue to lift, which is associated with postural dysfunctions such as cervical and lumbar hyperlordosis, excessive thoracic kyphosis, abdominal ptosis, increased inguinal hernia risk, and stability during gait (Olivi et al., 2012), all of which can lead to pain related to structural alignment or myofascial

length/tension relationships. In contrast, an absent lingual frenulum is associated with states of hypermobility such as Ehlers–Danlos syndrome (DeFelice et al., 2001). *The test*: Open the mouth and place the tongue on the roof of the mouth. A positive test is an inability to touch the roof of the mouth with the tongue.

   • Mallampati score — The height of the mouth determines the amount of airway space available. *The test*: Open the mouth and stick out the tongue. The soft palate and uvula should be visible. If they are not, the test is positive and the patient should be referred out for further testing. The screen can be done with or without phonation (vocalizing a sound such as "ahh").

Respiratory assessment

Start with a supine assessment of the breath and progress to seated or functional positions such as dynamic yoga postures as each level is mastered. The root of the tongue should remain relaxed with A-D breath, and the soft palate of the mouth should remain soft (not rigid) and lift gently, along with the uvula, during postures that require TATD breath or overcoming/victorious breath.

Loss of coordination of the three diaphragms (coordinating the relaxed descent of the thoracic, respiratory, and pelvic diaphragms during regular abdominal breathing) could contribute to obstructive sleep apnea, sleep difficulties, bruxism, and insomnia and prevent proper TATD breath during functional activities and posture execution that require local and global spine stability.

Note quality and/or quantity of the following:

1. Resting body position on the yoga couch — The body should rest comfortably in spinal neutral in plumb line alignment (head to hip). Any physiological deviation from this alignment should be documented and addressed.

2. Diaphragm's position at rest — A caudally located portion of the anterior and middle diaphragmatic portions, coupled with a steeper slope in the middle to crural sections, can contribute to low back pain (Kolar et al., 2012).

3. Respiratory rate at rest — This should be under 14–18 breaths per minute without intervention to qualify as a normal (non-hyperventilating) range (Hodges et al., 1997; Hodges and Gandevia, 2000; Gandevia and McKenzie, 2008; Janssens et al., 2013). Note any abnormal breath patterns:

- Concentric (descent) and eccentric (ascent) diaphragmatic action — Is it smooth and even? Are inhale and exhale equal? Are there any fascial restrictions in the pannicular (superficial) skin layer that may indicate deeper restriction of hemi-excursion (asymmetry) in the respiratory diaphragm? See Fig. 4.2 for an illustration of the three diaphragm layers.

Differential diagnosis should rule out the following systemic impairments related to diaphragmatic dysfunction:

1. Orofacial difficulties and airway occlusion (see above)

2. Gastrointestinal motility impairment via the left descending colon's intersection with the

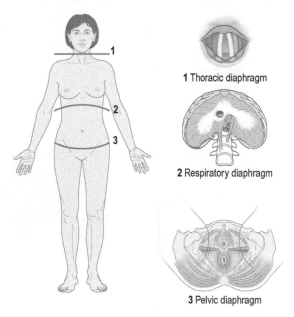

Figure 4.2
Muscular layers of the three diaphragms

1 Thoracic diaphragm

2 Respiratory diaphragm

3 Pelvic diaphragm

phrenicocolic ligament. The ligament attaches to the subdiaphragmatic peritoneal thickening, and could also affect dorsal vagus nerve activity via phrenic anastomoses. Any diaphragmatic dysfunction could create what Porges (2011) identifies as a lack of vagal brake, which downregulates sympathetic activity, prevents dorsal vagal surges (Porges, 2015), and prevents a parasympathetic "rest and digest" response, which could interfere with normal gastrointestinal motility

3. Liver or gallbladder impairment could refer pain to the diaphragm secondary to the shared phrenic nerve connection (Barrall and Mercier, 2006, 2007; Bordoni and Zanier 2013)

4. Cardiopulmonary regulation is strongly influenced by respiratory function via the vagus nerve (Porges, 2011) with diaphragmatic functioning and evaluation by physical therapy shown to correct problems related to venous drainage (Byeon et al., 2012) and venous stasis (Chiappa et al., 2008; Restrepo et al., 2008; Bordoni and Zanier 2013)

5. Lymphatic drainage and absorption depends on "rhythm and stretch" of the diaphragm to affect intraperitoneal pressure (Abu-Hijleh et al., 1995; Moriondo et al., 2008)

6. Refer to systemic effects of the diaphragm (Chapter 3).

Orofacial phonation relaxation response

A great deal of the topographical surface area of the primary somatosensory cortex is assigned to the lips, tongue, and fingers. The diagram of the cortical homunculus in Fig. 4.3 is MRI-supported as an accurate, if bizarre, representation of somatosensory function (Nakamura et al., 1998). The dominating cutaneous sensory input provision from the lips and tongue via the thalamus demands attention, especially since those areas are the entry point for healthy respiratory habits, which dictate systemic health. A short series of orofacial phonation relaxation exercises is provided to address this connection.

The focus of orofacial phonation relaxation is a three-pronged approach that considers (1) resonation,

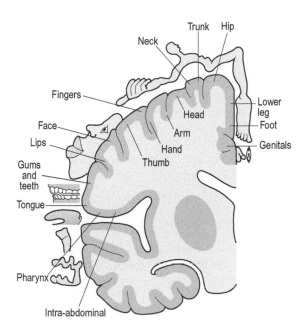

Figure 4.3
Sensory homunculus

(2) projection, and (3) yogic breathing. Resonation and projection will be emphasized through orofacial phonation relaxation while yogic breathing is prefaced by the introduction of two functional breath types. Although beyond the scope of this text, it is important to harness the powerful potential of the voice and breath as symbiotic functions through which we communicate, both intra- and interpersonally.

The voice and the breath are two key entry points for accessing the myelinated ventral vagal circuit, which functions in social engagement via the trigeminal nerve, in cardiorespiratory health through the phrenic nerve/ventral vagal anastomoses, and in visceral function through the subdiaphragmatic vagus connection. There is also a neuromuscular pelvic connection to the thoracic (voice) and respiratory diaphragms. Formally trained vocalists and brass players were found to have the best neuromuscular patterning and pelvic floor control with forced expiratory flow (Talasz et al., 2010), a skillset required to sing, to play an instrument, and also to sneeze, cough, and master yogic breath techniques such as overcoming breath.

1. Choose a comfortable, maintainable pitch that falls between the tones heard when you say the word "*uh-huh*" several times.

2. Exhale. Inhale and then, on the exhale, sustain the sound of the note as long as possible without a grip or closure-like feeling of the tongue or throat. During the sustained note hold, "chew" on the sound of the note. Keep the mouth closed and open and close the jaw in every direction possible without pain. The tongue should contact the roof of the mouth without tension at the root of the tongue and with a wide airway. Tension in the jaw, tongue, or throat will close the airway. Exhalation is most helpful for inducing a ventral vagus nerve response (Porges, 2015).

3. Recite the phrase "*The lips, the teeth, and the tongue.*" Feel the way the tip of the tongue contacts the teeth and anterior hard palate when you say the words "the" and "lips," respectively. Feel how the tongue contacts the anterior palate (first) and the teeth (second) when you articulate "teeth." Finally, feel how the tongue contacts the anterior hard palate on articulating "ton" and the posterior hard palate on "gue."

4. Repeat 2 and place a hand over the throat. The skin and fascia of the throat and the platysma, sternocleidomastoid, and scalenes should remain loose and pliable. The thoracic diaphragm should remain neutral during breathing and normal talking but may slightly lift or lower with animated speaking or singing. Tension here will adversely affect airway width, flow, and subsequently, resonance and projection, two of the three gateways to systemic health.

5. Repeat 3 and follow instructions from 4.

6. Phonate three syllables in succession: (1) *ahhh*, (2) *oooh*, and (3) *mmmm*, while chewing on the exhaled sound. "*Ahhh*" and "*oooh*" should be open mouthed with "*ahhh*" maintaining a dropped jaw position and "*oooh*" maintaining a circle shape with the lips. "*Mmmm*" is a closed mouth position. "*Ahhh*" should resonate low in the abdominal and pelvic cavity, "*oooh*" should resonate in the chest and throat, and "*mmmm*" should resonate in the sinuses and skull. The combination of these three syllables recited makes the mantram "*Om*" and allows for more

complete (1) resonation, (2) projection, and (3) yogic breathing for systemic benefit via the ventral vagus nerve motor circuit (Fig. 4.4 and Table 4.2).

Therapeutic technique

Changing pitch (higher or lower), resonation (lower lungs, chest, throat, sinuses, or skull), projection (altered through volume, conscious resonation in the cavities of the body), and conscious relaxation of the soft tissue structures of the head, throat, and inside the mouth can all improve orofacial relaxation and response.

Advanced technique

Practice orofacial phonation relaxation with the yogic locks introduced at the end of the chapter. Maintain a full breath while practicing each of the locks. Focus on maintaining a connecting point between each of the three diaphragms and the locks during a full A-D breath with no valsalva. (See Fig. 4.4 for an overview of resonation between the three diaphragms and the yogic locks.)

Functional breath types

Abdominodiaphragmatic (A-D) breath

> **Code 4.1** (free code)
> Abdominodiaphragmatic (A-D) breath with tri-diaphragmatic action

Passive descent of the respiratory diaphragm secondary to active, at-rest inhalation is critical to normal autonomic and systemic function and ultimately, stress control (Porges, 2011; Bordoni and Zanier, 2013), and is the gold standard mechanism for physiological employment of the respiratory diaphragm. A-D breath terminology was first defined by Coulter (2001) and should be expanded to include a neutral position of the thoracic diaphragm and passive descent of the respiratory and pelvic diaphragms (Fig. 4.5 and Code 4.1).

Prerequisites   Orofacial and respiratory assessment.

TI (therapeutic intention)

- Low arousal state conducive to relaxation and sleep hygiene in non-stabilization yoga postures

Table 4.2
Phonation review

Phonation of "aum" (OM)		
Syllable	Mouth position	Location
Ahhh	Open, dropped jaw	Low abdomen and pelvic cavity
Oooh	Open, circle shaped lips	Chest and throat
Mmmm	Closed	Sinuses and skull

Figure 4.4
Corollary substrate of resonation in the three diaphragms

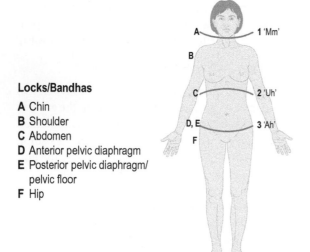

Locks/Bandhas

A Chin
B Shoulder
C Abdomen
D Anterior pelvic diaphragm
E Posterior pelvic diaphragm/ pelvic floor
F Hip

Resonation

1 Thoracic diaphragm
2 Respiratory diaphragm
3 Pelvic diaphragm

'Aum' = ' Om'

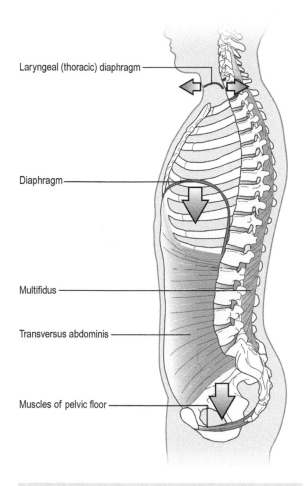

Laryngeal (thoracic) diaphragm

Diaphragm

Multifidus

Transversus abdominis

Muscles of pelvic floor

Figure 4.5
Abdominodiaphragmatic breath

- Induction of inhibitory neural impulses to baroreceptors (blood pressure and heart rate monitors) in the carotids (Jerath et al., 2006) via diaphragmatic descent which stimulates the slowly adapting stretch receptors (SARs) in order to downregulate sympathetic tone. What follows is a symphony of systemic activity in the mind–body: cardiovascular, pulmonary, immune, neuromuscular, neuroendocrine (through decreased salivary cortisol and downregulation of the hypothalamic–pituitary–adrenal axis), and gastrointestinal system function actively work toward homeostasis, thus potentially reducing overall allostatic load (Jerath et al., 2006; Kuntsevich et al., 2010; Sivakumar et al., 2011;

Tharion et al., 2012; Adhana et al., 2013; Jyotsna et al., 2013; Turankar et al., 2013)

- Foster neuroplasticity and alteration of the stress response to improve psychoemotional health, which exacts an anti-inflammatory response and affects genetic transcription, attributed to yogic breathing practice (Dusek et al., 2008; Pullen et al., 2008; Qu et al., 2013)

- Effective non-pharmacological method of GERD (gastroesophageal reflux disease) management via reduction of long-term drug dependency, increased quality of life, and improved pH-metry (Eherer et al., 2012)

- Access ventral vagal circuit via repetitious exhalation practice (for dose response) using good diaphragmatic biomechanics in yogic breathing, which via inhalation stimulates stretch receptors in the alveoli of the lungs, baroreceptors, chemoreceptors, and sensors in the respiratory anatomy. Deep breathing affects perception, cognition, emotion regulation, somatic expression, and behavior (Brown and Gerbarg, 2009; Streeter et al., 2012)

- Vocal and speech functioning, including orofacial tone and impairments related to ASD (autism spectrum disorders)

- Bowel and bladder management

- Depression, schizophrenia, ADHD (attention deficit hyperactivity disorder), sleep disorders (Balasubramaniam et al., 2013)

- Pulmonary functioning in stroke patients via neuro-re-education of the diaphragm (Jung et al., 2014)

- Effective in beginner sessions, restorative yoga, or for correction of faulty breathing habits.

SP (starting position)   Any posture, but especially corpse or child's pose.

Entry   Exhale. Inhale and allow the abdomen to expand without force. The spine is in neutral, plumb line alignment. The extremities are in anatomical position. A-D breath should eventually become involuntary and able to be performed in any posture or position.

Exit Exhale and passively allow the belly to return to a resting position.

SRAs (static restorative approximations) and DMs (dynamic modifications)

- Guided imagery or motor imagery
- Partner-assist in supine lying
- Sandbag breathing
- Perform from: (1) child's pose, (2) corpse, or (3) yoga couch.

TTCP (teaching and tactical cuing primer)

- A-D breath is taught first.
- Beginners start with a 3–4 count exhale and subsequent 3–4 count inhale, progressing to 8–15 seconds or more for each cycle.
- Deepen the breath via exhale elongation, then equalize inhale with exhale.
- Watch for abnormal breath habits defined earlier in the chapter.
- This breath requires not just "belly" expansion, but also "back body or rib" expansion.

Contraindications Use a semi-upright or upright position for asthma, chronic obstructive pulmonary disease (COPD), or second trimester pregnancy and beyond; not for postures that require postural stability.

Transversus abdominis-assisted thoracodiaphragmatic (TATD) breath

Code 4.2 (free code)

Transversus abdominis-assisted thoraco-diaphragmatic (TATD) breath

TATD breath (Fig. 4.6; Code 4.2) is a simultaneous employment of yogic locks that includes the following:

- Abdominal lock, which is specifically defined as engaging the transversus abdominis (TA). The TA is thought to be a primary stabilizer of the lumbar

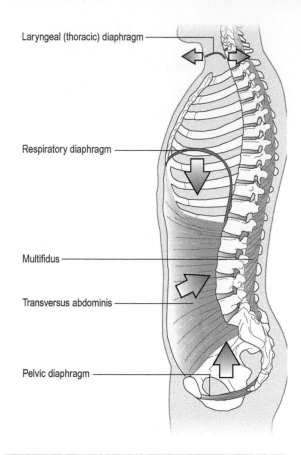

Laryngeal (thoracic) diaphragm

Respiratory diaphragm

Multifidus

Transversus abdominis

Pelvic diaphragm

Figure 4.6

Transversus abdominis-assisted thoracodiaphragmatic (TATD) breath with tri-diaphragmatic action

spine and mechanism for healthy load transfer between the trunk and lower extremity (Hodges et al., 2003; Barker et al., 2007; Hodges, 2008)

- Anterior root lock (anterior pelvic floor)
- Posterior root lock (posterior pelvic floor).

These three locks are practiced together without valsalva, known as "partial or mild" versions of the traditional full versions (historically taught with breath holds). TATD also includes multifidus action and increased recruitment of the respiratory diaphragm through the increased resistance (intra-abdominal pressure) offered through TA recruitment. TATD recruitment is variable and task-dependent based on research that shows TA activity varies with the extent of postural demand (Crommert et al., 2011). Recruitment of the TA during TATD breath may also be asymmetrical. For example, if the task includes rapid arm movements or trunk rotation, the TA does not co-contract prior to introduction of rapid postural changes (Allison and Morris, 2008; Hodges, 2008; Morris et al., 2012, 2013). Urquhart and Hodges (2005) found that the TA is active with both directions of rotation but greater on the ipsilateral side of trunk rotation. Lastly, the degree of recruitment can range from 1% to 100% maximum voluntary isometric contraction. The obliques may also be involved with TATD breath but would not dominate a spinal neutral isometric contraction strategy. In the case of rotational movement of the spine, the contralateral external oblique and ipsilateral internal oblique may contribute most to torque (Urquhart et al., 2005), with the TA having small torque potential (Urquhart and Hodges, 2005).

TATD breath differs from Coulter's (2001) early definition of thoracodiaphragmatic breath. TATD breath is a biomechanical and neural evolution that identifies the TA as a chief stabilizer of the trunk, rather than the rectus abdominis (as was previously identified in Coulter's work).

Mindful effort involving three diaphragms

TATD breath requires conscious involvement of three diaphragms – thoracic, respiratory, and pelvic – in order to facilitate adequate intra-abdominal pressure through contraction of the TA, the pelvic floor (anterior/posterior root locks), and conscious relaxation of the thoracic diaphragm (which could be associated with a chin lock).

Prerequisites

- Orofacial assessment
- Respiratory assessment
- A-D breath
- Abdominal lock (end of chapter)
- Root lock (anterior and posterior; end of chapter).

TI (therapeutic intention) In support of the use of TATD breath for posture performance, optimal

arousal state has both a neuromotor and psychobiological mechanism.

Neuromotor and physiological mechanisms

- Provide optimal arousal state for achieving a "*best fit*" motor performance for dynamic stability in postures, which can be supported by the Yerkes–Dodson law (Yerkes and Dodson, 1908) (Fig. 4.7). Optimal performance is associated with a certain level of arousal, as proposed in the Yerkes–Dodson law, and is, like TATD, task-dependent

- Dynamic postural control in and outside of neutral through provision of lumbopelvic stability and the biological plausibility provided via Kolar et al. (2010, 2012)

- Provide synergistic regional stability (via scapulothoracic stability) in order to provide functional carryover for ADL and work task performance

- Foster postural/trunk awareness and control of the diaphragm, TA, pelvic floor, multifidus (Kolar et al., 2010, 2012), and related synergists for safety and

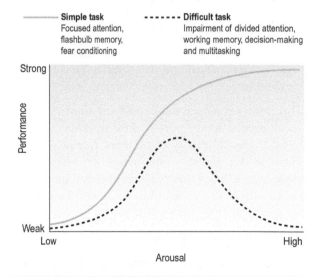

Figure 4.7

Yerkes–Dodson law. The original Yerkes and Dodson law was formulated in 1908 (https://commons.wikimedia.org/wiki/File:OriginalYerkesDodson.svg#/media/File:OriginalYerkesDodson.svg)

efficacy in dynamic yoga postures and to prevent and/or rehabilitate lumbopelvic injury, pelvic pain, respiratory impairment, or incontinence (Hung et al., 2010; Talasz et al., 2010)

- Engage the trunk cylinder/canister bilaterally or unilaterally at a level below maximum voluntary isometric contraction except during postures where maximum lumbosacral/pelvic stability is needed, when 100% maximum voluntary contraction TATD breath could feasibly be used

- Facilitate increased pelvic floor muscle strength through forced expiratory flow training via use of combined TATD breath and overcoming breath as described, but not specifically named, in Talasz et al. (2010)

- Aid in resolution of urinary incontinence via diaphragmatic retraining in concert with TA and pelvic floor muscle coordinated function (Hung et al., 2010), described by the authors as a new technique reported by Sapsford (2004) that prefers coordinated muscle strengthening in place of isolated strengthening. TATD breath was originally described in 2001 (Garner, 2001)

- Facilitate healthy load transfer via tension transmission through the transversalis fascia to the lateral raphe

- Improve segmental stability of the lumbar spine and reduce hyperlordosis through Kolar et al.'s (2012) posited theory of balanced recruitment of agonists/antagonists, essentially the respiratory diaphragm (balanced excursion of all components), pelvic floor, abdominal wall, and spinal extensors, respectively (Kolar et al., 2012).

Psychobiological perspective

The physiological and neuromotor mechanisms for TATD breath are important, but they are not the only rationale for its use:

- Provide optimal arousal state via provision of ventral vagal motor stimulation, which must be present to facilitate hypothalamic–pituitary–adrenal (HPA) axis regulation and allostasis. If arousal is too high, sympathetic input is dominant and is associated with negative stress hormone regulation, chiefly glucocorticoid regulation, which is instrumental in HPA axis regulation. Ironically, normal regulation of one of the most important glucocorticoid hormones, cortisol, shows a striking resemblance to the Yerkes–Dodson law (Fig. 4.8) (Lupien et al., 2005, 2007).

Persistent high states of glucocorticoids are correlated with memory and cognitive impairments and a smaller hippocampus. Optimal performance state, then, is both a biomechanical and a psychobiological phenomenon. This *zen zone* is also associated with maximum cognitive efficiency, which Daniel Goleman (2012) calls "*neural harmony*." In a state of lower arousal, for example, as the neural circuit of TATD breath is firmly established, task completion becomes an effortless, an almost involuntary event.

- In the case of TA function, the bank of scientific evidence that supports the importance of effortless involuntary function is substantial (Chapter 3), showing, among other findings, that the TA should fire involuntarily during ADL task completion. During injury, however, this involuntary control is frequently lost. Voluntarily training the TATD under varying states of arousal, to improve performance, while also attending to the psychobiological needs of the patient is critical for effective, safe yoga prescription that offers functional ADL completion value. Yoga is, in effect, a neural exercise that can affect vagal tone on both ends. Yoga can influence visceral afferent and diaphragmatic input to the brain, which modulates myelinated ventral vagal efferent influences. The benefits of yoga practice can be enhanced further through inclusion of vocal sound production and listening (auricular branch of the vagus) due to the influence of the vagus on the larynx, pharynx, heart, and middle ear muscles (orofacial function). The psychobiological and neurophysiological influences of TATD breath, then, are supported by the inverted U principle (Yerkes–Dodson law) because they optimize motor performance (bio) and mental health and social engagement (psychosocial) through influencing arousal level.

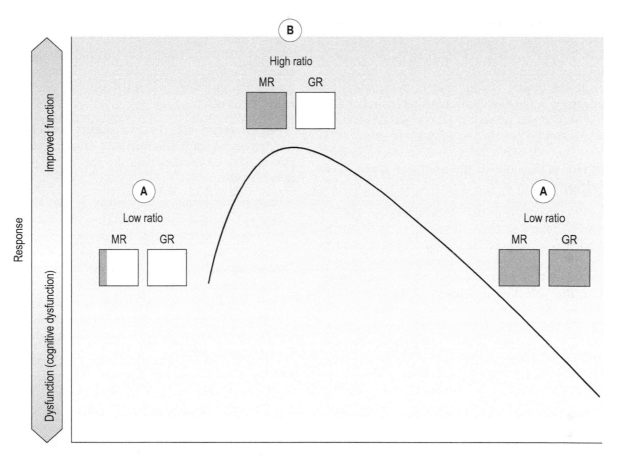

Figure 4.8

Circulating levels of glucocorticoids on human cognition (memory and learning) (adapted in part from Lupien et al., 2005). Hormesis describes the beneficial effect that a usually toxic substance can have at low doses. This figure resembles the Yerkes–Dodson inverted U-shape that simplifies the complex concept of how stress hormones, chiefly glucocorticoids (GR) and mineralocorticoids (MR), are task- or context-dependent on the type of stress incurred (eustress/arousal or distress/negative stress) and circadian rhythm (HPA (hypothalamus–pituitary–adrenal) axis response dictates cortisol release). While MR are present in the limbic system, GR are present preferentially in the prefrontal cortex and also in subcortical (paraventricular nucleus, hypothalamic nuclei, hippocampus, and parahippocampal gyrus) and cortical areas. All of these areas dictate cognitive functioning, specifically human memory and learning. While a single figure cannot represent all the variables that influence cortisol levels and divisions of human learning and memory, some general conclusions are represented in this figure. Cognitive function is optimal when most of the MR and a portion of GR are activated (B). However, if GR levels are extreme (high or low) (A), cognitive function declines (represented by extremes of the inverted U-shape). A final note that emphasizes the importance of context: emotional memory is an anomaly not represented by the Yerkes–Dodson law. High circulating levels of GR consistently (100% of reviewed studies in Lupien et al., 2005) enhance emotional memory recall, which has enormous implications for patient populations in chronic pain or distress (post-traumatic stress disorder, for example)

SP (starting position)   Perform from any dynamic yoga posture or functional movement that requires stability and control. For learning purposes, place the hands on the ribcage in a "C" grip. After mastering the breath, tactile input of the hands is not necessary. Beginners should start by learning TATD in A/P (anterior/posterior) (Fig. 4.9) and lateral spinal neutral (Fig. 4.10) and progress by using TATD breath outside of neutral and with increasingly more degrees of freedom in the axial and appendicular skeleton.

Entry   To perform the breath, engage the TA firmly enough to create a sensation of lift in the pelvic floor in a position of spinal neutral. A slight corset-like "drawing-in" or concentric shortening of the waistline and trunk should occur. Inhale, appreciate the palpable movement of the ribcage lifting laterally like bucket handles and the posterior ribs flaring. Exhale allows the ribcage diameter to diminish in size but TATD is maintained throughout respiration.

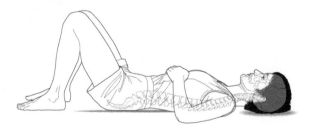

Figure 4.9
Anterior/posterior spinal neutral

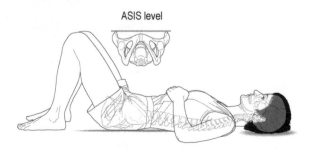

Figure 4.10
Lateral neutral

Exit   Release TATD breath and return to A-D breath when stability in postures is no longer required or TATD breath is involuntarily and/or adequately engaged via low level maximum voluntary isometric contraction such that there is safety during postures and movement.

"Cough assessment"   To test a patient's involuntary TA strategy, which is also indicative of load transfer during ADL completion, have the patient cough or clear the throat.

- Improper involuntary TA strategy — The lateral edges of the abdominals would become concave and the area of the rectus abdominis would become convex – "*rectus loaf.*" The external obliques would dominate and angularly indent soft tissue at the caudad ribcage angles, creating a downward compression of the abdominal contents and lower abdominal "pooch." Lumbar or thoracic flexion or posterior tilt would likely also occur during throat clearing or cough.

- Proper involuntary TA strategy — The abdominal muscles remain flat with no "rectus loaf." The spine could maintain neutral with no posterior shear stress in the spine due to hemidiaphragmatic or partial diaphragmatic expansion. Palpation of the TA just medial to the ASIS (anterior superior iliac spine), above the pubic symphysis, or into the inguinal region (note that the TA is not present below the iliac crest in all individuals; Urquhart and Hodges, 2005) would reveal TA activation without rectus or oblique dominance. Adequate lift of the pelvic floor during cough or throat clearing should also occur and is palpated externally just above the pubic symphysis.

SRAs (static restorative approximations) and DMs (dynamic modifications)

- Beginner — Use motor imagery to guide breath mastery:

  - feel the belly button draw in slightly and up toward the ribcage

  - feel the muscles of the TA engage like a corset around the waist and draw the waist in smaller

- feel as if the front ASIS or "hip points" draw toward one another.

- Progression — Initiate TATD breath in prone or supine hook lying first without a head lift.

- Progression — Teach in four-point position followed by upright-seated static position.

- Final progression — Move from static to dynamic postures, sequences, or ADL where contralateral and ipsilateral contraction of the TA is required.

TTCP (teaching and tactical cuing primer)

- During TATD, the perineum should never bulge, no urine or feces should be expressed (stress incontinence), and there should be no valsalva and no heavy or painful feeling in the pelvis or pelvic floor muscles.

- Maintain breath duration as in abdominal breath.

- Improper movement strategy cannot always be blamed on poor neuromuscular patterning or timing. It can also be related to poor stress response and a lack of feeling "safe" within movement, the body, or the environment. For example, external oblique and rectus abdominis dominance during the cough assessment can result in an unconscious return to a more visceral, primitive, dorsal vagal response (shut down state). See the case study recounting Eva's story.

Case study

Acute loss of TATD function: physiological or psychobiological? – Eva's story

Eva,* a highly trained athlete who previously demonstrated TA recruitment and patterning, had an injury which created psychosocial and physical stress. She then underwent surgery (not directly involving the TA muscle). After surgery, the therapist noted the athlete's almost absent TATD function, despite having demonstrated excellent TA and pelvic floor functioning and patterning just days prior to surgery. This shutdown of TATD breath, as a responsive neuromuscular phenomenon, could be possibly correlated to the diaphragm's intimate connection to the

vagus nerve's predominant afferent function, through its anastomoses with the phrenic nerve and through altered sinus node rhythm. In other words, a dorsal vagal response due to the psychoemotional trauma from surgery, chronic disability, and functional impairment, could have created a "freeze" response that elicited the primitive visceral response which resulted in loss of higher order lumbopelvic control. Another plausible explanation for the TATD shutdown was that the three diaphragms were mechanically inhibited in their recruitment as a result of intubation during surgery, as a purely myofascial phenomenon, through its common attachment with the diaphragm through the pretracheal, pericardial, endothoracic, and transversalis and related lumbopelvic fascia. Whatever the psychobiological phenomenon, Eva was only left with a predominant external oblique and rectus abdominis strategy (which strangely, and ironically, resembles the neuromuscular action of a fetal position, which a person automatically assumes when they feel threatened) that had to be retrained through neuromuscular re-education of TATD breath over several months of therapy. Future research should focus not only on the physiological etiology of impaired lumbopelvic load transfer due to acute and unexplained external oblique and/or rectus abdominis dominance, but perhaps more importantly on the psychobiological influence of the dorsal vagal circuit on TATD function in orthopaedic rehabilitation.

*Please note that the patient's name has been changed to protect her privacy.

Contraindications None, since TATD breath can be performed with the smallest maximum voluntary isometric contraction, or even guided imagery.

Yogic breath types

Prerequisites

- Orofacial and respiratory assessment

- A-D breath (beginner to intermediate practice)

- TATD breath (advanced practice – progress by performing the yogic breath types with TATD breath).

Three-part breath; **Dirga [der-guh] pranayama [prah-nuh-yahm]***; supine three-part breath with/without sandbag breathing* (Fig. 4.11)

> **Code 4.3** (free code)
> Three-part breath
>

TI (therapeutic intention)

- Meter or pace the breath to achieve optimum respiration rates for improving heart rate variability, which is thought to be at or near 6 breaths per minute (Vaschillo et al., 2006) with a range of 4–6 breaths per minute, although the optimum respiratory rate for improving self-regulation and stress response via affecting heart rate variability and respiratory sinus arrhythmia (systemic autonomic coherence) should ideally be determined via resonance frequency analysis

- Paced breathing can improve insomnia and vagal activity (Tsai et al., 2015)

- Elongate breath

- Equalize inhale and exhale.

SP (starting position) Any posture.

Teach three-part breath in supine lying using the yoga couch and guided imagery of inhaling two counts into three sections of the torso – the lower abdomen, the lower ribcage, and the upper ribcage. For chest/clavicular/scalene/sternocleidomastoid breathers, avoid using the upper ribcage as a point for breath manifestation. The upper ribcage is reserved for four-part breath, which is an advanced technique.

Entry and exit

1. Exhale.

2. Using A-D breath, inhale and on this breath inhale 2–3 counts into the lower abdomen and pelvis.

3. Continue inhalation and inhale 2–3 counts into the ribcage.

4. Continue inhalation and inhale the final 2–3 counts into the upper lobes of the lungs under the clavicles and ribcage. Do this without using secondary muscles of respiration in the neck, such as the scalenes or sternocleidomastoid (SCM), and without chest breathing.

5. Exhale in the exact reverse order. Empty the glass of the lungs from the top – exhale from the upper lobes of the lungs for 2–3 counts, followed by the middle lungs or ribcage and abdomen for 2–3 counts, followed by the lower lobes of the lungs in the lumbar spine for 2–3 counts.

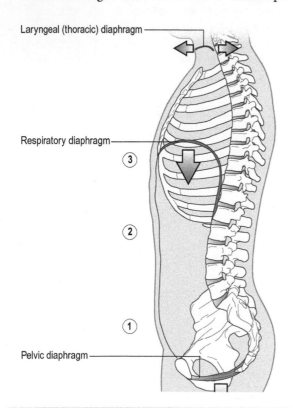

Laryngeal (thoracic) diaphragm

Respiratory diaphragm

③

②

①

Pelvic diaphragm

Figure 4.11
Three-part breath

6. Repeat for at least 3–5 breaths and then return to a normal full breath. Notice any changes.

7. Progress by performing the same breath using TATD breath.

Alignment Follow abdominal breath unless in a dynamic yoga posture, then follow TATD breathing alignment.

SRAs (static restorative approximations) Guided or motor imagery using "*filling the glass*" of the lungs (from the bottom up on the inhale and the top down on the exhale).

DMs (dynamic modifications)

• Novices may inhale/exhale 1 count in each of the three parts of the body, rather than the 2–3 count in each part, making for a 3-count inhale and 3-count exhale. Experienced practitioners can move to the 4-count breath, taking a 4-count inhale at each part of the body, making for a 12-count inhale and a 12-count exhale, or approximately 2 breaths per minute.

• If the patient has difficulty with three-part breath, attempt a lightweight (under 10 pounds) version of sandbag breathing. The patient's interlaced fingers or a book weighing less than a regular sandbag can be placed on the abdomen above the pelvis and below the ribcage, in order to identify functional impairment in the breath, such as noted staccato-like moments in the breath, clipped or non-linear patterns that deviate from a smooth and equalized inhalation and exhalation.

• Alternately, a progression to a four-part breath is optional.

Four-part breath (Fig. 4.12)

Code 4.4 (free code)
Four-part breath

1. Exhale.

2. Inhale and take 2–3 counts of inhale into the lower pelvis.

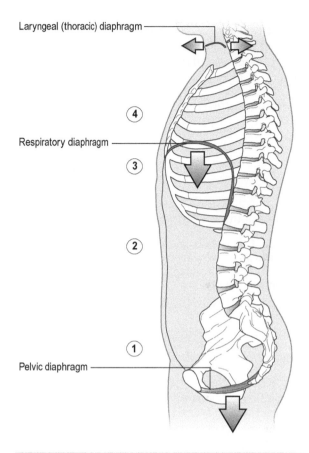

Figure 4.12
Four-part breath

3. The next 2–3 inhale counts go into the lower abdomen.

4. The next 2–3 counts go into the ribcage and clavicles/upper lung lobes.

5. The remaining 2–3 counts overflow into the upper lobes of the lungs and the skull, behind the eyes, and crown of the head.

6. Reverse the breath by exhaling out of the skull, then clavicles, then ribcage, then abdomen, then pelvis.

TTCP (teaching and tactical cuing primer) Make the breath smooth and seamless. Do not differentiate between "levels" of the body or breath by making the breath a staccato (detached) motion.

Contraindications No breath-holding during this pose but especially for those with hypertension, pregnancy, cardiovascular or cerebrovascular disease, anxiety, or anyone prone to panic disorder.

Sandbag breath (Fig. 4.13)

Code 4.5 (free code)
Sandbag breath

TI (therapeutic intention)

- Teach A-D breath and/or combine with overcoming breath.
- Elongate the breath.
- Improve alveolar ventilation.
- Meter or pace breath (see TI of three-part breath).
- Equalize inhale and exhale.
- In quadriplegics, weighted supine abdominal breathing re-establishes CO_2 and O_2 levels (hyperventilation) measured via electromyography (EMG) of inspiratory muscles, mouth pressure, inspiratory flow, and inspiratory volume (Kwan-Hwa Lin et al., 1999).

SP (starting position) Corpse.

Props needed Sandbag (typical weight is 10 lb but weight should be determined based on ability to perform without anxiety and with good form); 2–4 blankets, as needed.

Entry Place the sandbag over the lower abdomen, on and below the navel, below the ribs and above the pelvis, approximately. Breathe steadily and slowly, feeling the rise of the sandbag on inhalation and its steady descent on exhalation.

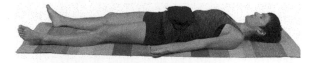

Figure 4.13
Sandbag breath

Exit Remove the sandbag by dragging it off the belly to the left side. Remain here and notice any changes. After several breath cycles, transition to right sidelying, then to seated meditation. Spend several breath cycles in seated meditation to center and notice any changes.

Alignment Honor the curves of the spine (plumb line alignment), while in corpse.

SRAs (static restorative approximations)

1. Manual cuing — Use the hands to provide weight instead of a sandbag.
2. Pose adaptation — Start with a heavy book instead of a sandbag.
3. Pose adaptation — Incline the pose for those who cannot remain supine secondary to musculoskeletal, cardiopulmonary, or other complications.

DMs (dynamic modifications)

1. Support the lumbar spine with a rolled blanket under the knees.
2. Rest in yoga couch for pregnancy, respiratory difficulties or impairment, or vestibular impairment that causes vertigo or dizziness with supine lying.

TTCP (teaching and tactical cuing primer) Cue for careful observation of the breath before having the student change anything about the breath.

Contraindications Pregnancy or postpartum do not use a sandbag but instead rest the hands on the abdomen for biofeedback. Those with abdominal surgeries, hernias, anxiety, ulcers, GERD, or a history of panic attacks should refrain from sandbag use until comfortable with weighted breathing.

Victorious/overcoming breath (Ujyaii pranayama [ooo-ja-ee prah-nahyuhm]) (Fig. 4.14)

Code 4.6 (free code)
Victorious/overcoming breath

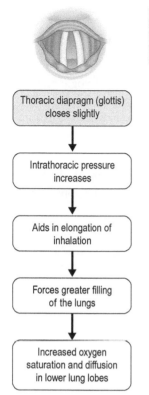

Figure 4.14
Victorious/overcoming breath

Thoracic diaphragm (glottis) closes slightly

↓

Intrathoracic pressure increases

↓

Aids in elongation of inhalation

↓

Forces greater filling of the lungs

↓

Increased oxygen saturation and diffusion in lower lung lobes

TI (therapeutic intention)

- Eccentric strength and conditioning for the respiratory diaphragm

- Methodology for vocal preservation and throat clearing without cough, including establishing sub-threshold phonation for accessing vagus tone via its auricular branch and through the trigeminal nerve, both of which can also employ throat widening through lifting of the soft palate and uvula. This action teaches orofacial relaxation and could potentially improve circadian rhythm through affecting sleep quality via improved cardiorespiratory function

- Widen or relax the airway and orofacial area with a slowed respiratory rate

- Through common connections of the diaphragm with pericardial (attaches to central tendon of diaphragm), endothoracic, pretracheal, and transversalis fascia, slow, controlled victorious breath affects visceral fascial functioning and related recruitment

of local trunk stabilizers as well as the global stress response through target of the ventral vagus circuit. This breath technique could be an effective form of both dynamic myofascial release through slow, controlled concentric and eccentric employment of the respiratory diaphragm via increasing resistance to airflow through the glottis/thoracic diaphragm

- This technique, through the same mechanical mechanism, can also more adequately clear air from the distal alveoli, as it is commonly "trapped" in patients with COPD (chronic obstructive pulmonary disease) or asthma

- Similar benefits to deep abdominal or diaphragmatic breathing in systemic measures of cardiac, pulmonary, and biochemical functioning via replacing pursed lip breathing to increase cardiac–vagal baroreflex sensitivity to improve oxygen saturation, lower blood pressure, reduce anxiety, increase parasympathetic activation, influence vagus nerve stimulation, increase oxygen absorption, and increase tidal volume (Mason et al., 2013).

SP (starting position)   Supine, seated, or in any yoga posture. A slight chin lock may prevent chest breathing by increasing sensory input to the required slight closure of the glottis.

Entry   With quiet, feel openness at the back of soft palate and throat. Let the tongue drop away from the roof of the mouth. Facilitate a relaxed breath in supine lying supported with blankets. Once mastered, lengthen inhalation and exhalation. Once a steady, inaudible, long inhale and exhale are mastered, perform in seated. Breathe with the mouth open. Next, slightly close the back of the throat or glottis on the inhale. Listen to the sound of inhalation, to the sighing quality of it. Adjust the cadence, sound, and speed to improve breath control. Slow the breath and listen to it resonate inside the body. Pause briefly between inhalation and exhalation. Note the lift of the soft palate and uvula, and a corresponding wider airway as the air flows past the vocal cords with increased resistance due to the slightly closed glottis/thoracic diaphragm.

Exit   Exhale and pretend to "fog a window." Maintain the slight closing of the glottis. To perform full "*ujyaii*," close the mouth and breathe only through the nose. The sound of the breath should now be likened to hearing the distant ocean surf or someone in deep sleep.

SRAs (static restorative approximations) and DMs (dynamic modifications)

1. Guided or motor imagery — "*Filling the glass*" (fill and empty lungs like a glass of water) or "*massage the trunk*" with the entire breath.

2. Begin with an open-mouthed "fog" breath where the inhale occurs through the nose and exhales through the open mouth.

3. Progress to a closed mouth "fog" breath where inhale and exhale occur through the nose.

4. Breathe less vigorously (for less heat) and more vigorously (for more heat) as desired.

5. In an SRA, use A-D and/or three-part breath in combination with victorious breath. If upright or in any posture that requires stability, perform in combination with TATD breath.

TTCP (teaching and tactical cuing primer)

- Be observant. The slight contraction or closure of the glottis creates breath resistance, making success dependent on increased intrathoracic pressure, which requires greater effort than normal slow breathing.

- The sound on the inhale should be "ssss."

- The sound on the exhale should be "hhhh."

Contraindications Any condition where increasing internal body temperature is contraindicated, for example in pregnancy; also not for those who cannot master good principles of breathing at rest or those who cannot breathe without tension in the eyes, ears, face, or neck.

Alternate nostril breath (Nadi shodana [nah-dee show-dah-nuh])

> **Code 4.7** (free code)
> Alternate nostril breath
>
>

Additional prerequisite Overcoming/victorious breath.

TI (therapeutic intention)

- Alternate nostril breath and general yogic breathing affect mental health, cortical control, cognition and decision-making, as well as blood pressure and heart rate variability (Ghiya and Lee, 2012; Telles et al., 2012a, 2012b, 2013a, 2013b)

- Improve attention, language, spatial abilities, depression, and anxiety in post-stroke populations (Marshall et al., 2014)

- Improve parasympathetic activity and cardiac autonomic function, found in young adults who practice alternate nostril breath (Upadhyay et al., 2008).

SP (starting position) Any posture suited for meditation.

Entry

1. The right hand is held, palm facing the body, with the first two fingers closed into the palm, and the thumb, ring finger, and little finger held extended (Fig. 4.15).

2. Place the thumb on the skin of the right nostril and the edge of the ring finger on the skin of the left nostril (Fig. 4.16).

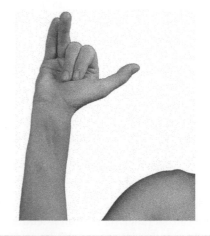

Figure 4.15
Alternate nostril breath, hand posture

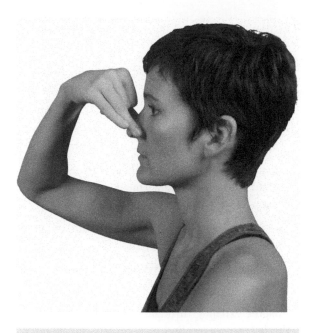

Figure 4.16
Alternate nostril breath, hand position on face

3. Exhale completely without nostril blocking.

4. Block the right nostril and inhale through the left, inhale steadily and slowly until the lungs are full.

5. Block the left nostril. Observe the silence between inhale and exhale as both nostrils are blocked.

6. Release the right nostril. Exhale through the right nostril until the lungs are empty.

7. Inhale through the right nostril.

8. Block the right nostril and release the left nostril to exhale through it.

9. Begin the cycle again from step 4.

SRAs (static restorative approximations)   Guided or motor imagery.

DMs (dynamic modifications)

• Alternate nostril breath can be performed with A-D breath (for relaxation) or with TATD breath (for seated version where trunk support is needed). To induce a relaxation response, inhale through the left nostril and exhale through the right only in a

circular pattern, known as Moon breath (*chandra bedhana*).

• For mental clarity, inhale through the right nostril and exhale through the left in a circular pattern, known as Sun breath (*surya bedhana*).

• If the fingers cannot conform to the mudra, use imaginary digital palpation.

TTCP (teaching and tactical cuing primer)

• Requires delicate adjustments with fingertips.

• Keep the wrist out of the way of the taking in of breath. Lift the wrist out of the way of the airway of the nostrils.

• Bring the head down and the chest up, which silences the frontal brain and activates the contemplative back brain.

Contraindications   Loss of sensory awareness or motor control in the fingertips to digital palpation and dexterity/coordination to hold the right hand posture (*mudra*) is only a relative contraindication and does not preclude the use of imagery (imagining digital palpation) or other modification.

Bee breath (Bhramari pranayama [bruh-mah-ree prah-nuh-yahm])

Code 4.8 (free code)
Bee breath

Additional   prerequisite   Overcoming/victorious breath.

TI (therapeutic intention)

• Mimics the sound of a buzzing bee or sighing exhale sound. The therapeutic benefits for bee breath are similar but potentially more effective than A-D breath, for its induction of a relaxation response, ventral vagus nerve circuit stimulation, pain management, and HPA axis regulation via the combined benefits of breath and sound production

- Paced sigh or spontaneous augmented breath, which is a neural exercise that affects cardiac vagal tone by acting as a psychophysiological reset to improve respiratory stability, heart rate variability (beat-to-beat interval variation), emotional coping and stress, and allostasis (Vleminx et al., 2013; Ramirez, 2014; Vaschillo et al., 2015). Much like heart rate variability, which is intimately connected to respiration, healthy breathing is not a metronome-like event (Ramirez, 2014)

- Use of phonation or subphonation can further increase the positive effects of ventral vagus nerve response due to the psychobiological benefits of vocalization discussed earlier

- Paced sighing (one sigh every 50 seconds interspersed with normal abdominal breathing or 0.02 or even 0.01 Hz, a low frequency range which equates to less than 6 breaths per minute) may improve vascular tone (Vaschillo et al., 2015), while spontaneous sighing is posited to provide optimal recovery from mental stress over instructed sighing (Vlemnicx et al., 2010). Differentiate the controlled bee breath or sighing breath from excessive sighing, the latter of which is implicated in prevention of homeostasis and is indicative of persistent panic, pain, irregular or maladaptive breathing patterns (Vleminx et al., 2013).

SP (starting position) Any posture, but especially corpse or child's pose.

Entry Exhale. Inhale with A-D, TATD, or overcoming breath, and exhale with a light vocalization that sounds like a buzzing bee. The exhale can also take on a sighing quality, which is defined as a deep but quick inspiratory phase that is 50% longer than the preceding respiratory cycle (Cherniack et al., 1981).

Exit Return to A-D, TATD, or overcoming breath.

SRAs (static restorative approximations) and DMs (dynamic modifications)

- Breathe without vocalization (subthreshhold phonation); practicing a light sigh, like a heavy sleep.

- Phonation may be preferred to augment ventral vagus circuit response through:

- stimulation of the auricular branch (hearing sound)

- increasing eccentric diaphragmatic function through metered slowing of the breath (exhalation), and/or

- augmentation of vocal fold laryngeal nerve stimulation (vocalization).

- Phonation can be light or heavy, depending on desired pain, stress management, or social engagement needs (see Fig. 4.17 for an illustration).

- The breath can also be combined with sandbag, three-part, or four-part breath.

TTCP (teaching and tactical cuing primer) Guided imagery:

- Imagine exhaling through an instrument, such as the harmonica or flute, which requires metered, slow, controlled breathing and will assist with performance of bee breath.

- Imagine exhaling slowly enough to make a pinwheel turn.

- Imagine exhalation that sounds like a gentle wind.

Contraindications None. Bee breath can be adapted for any population.

Yogic locks – energy anatomy for carriage maintenance

The word *bandha* (Sanskrit) means lock or seal. The locks in prevention and rehabilitation of lumbopelvic and orthopaedic injury serve as musculoskeletal and neuromuscular re-education and awareness and to facilitate neural patterning for form closure, force closure, and load transfer across joint surfaces. The locks are different from traditional yogic locks in that they are based on the following musculoskeletal and neuromuscular concepts:

1. Limit degrees of movement based on available controlled flexibility

2. No valsalva at any time

3. Use a graded range (1–100%) of maximum voluntary isometric (and sometimes isotonic)

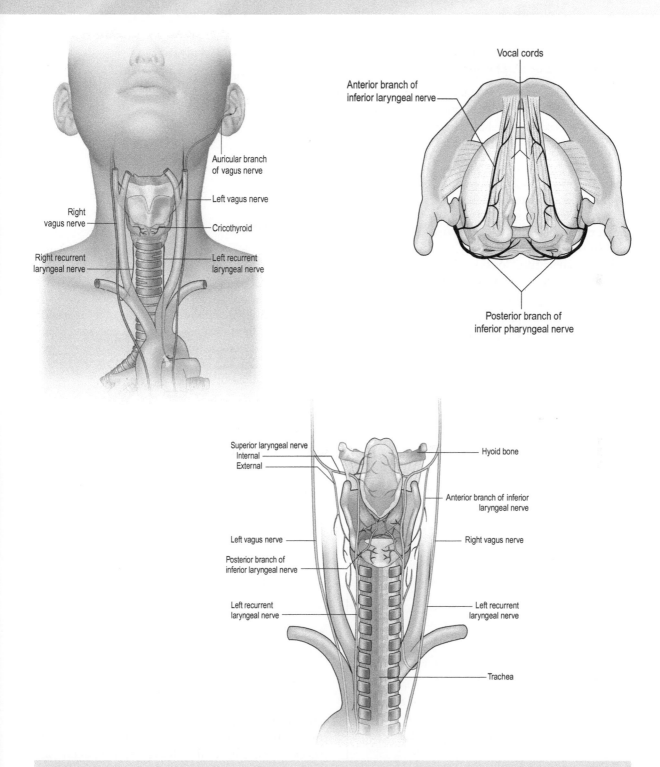

Figure 4.17
Phonation physiology and ventral vagus circuit relationship

contraction to facilitate safety in functional task (yoga posture or ADL) completion

4. Choose a voluntary isometric and/or isotonic contraction that is the minimum needed to elicit controlled flexibility (stability through form closure, force closure, and safe load transfer) through a joint.

Use of these guidelines modernizes use of yogic locks for today's patient populations, especially for those people with cardiovascular disease, pregnancy, glaucoma, metabolic syndrome, or any type of chronic pain, for whom breath-holding or unmitigated movement (movement with stability) is contraindicated. The energy anatomy of locks use is not negated in this text; however, their use has scant evidence base and is outside the scope of this text.

All traditional yogic locks are redefined and evolved according to the evidence base and are "mild" forms of their traditional (full) counterparts. This nomenclature is used in order to avoid confusion with traditional teachings that use breath holds, valsalva, or unmitigated flexibility. There are seven locks used in this text (Table 4.3):

Table 4.3
Yogic locks

Lock	Figure
1. Chin (*jalandhara bandha*)	Figure 4.18 Figure 4.19
2. Abdominal (*uddiyanda bandha*)	Figure 4.20
3. Root anterior (*mula bandha*)	Figure 4.23
4. Root posterior (*ashwini mudra*)	Figure 4.23
5. Shoulder (*anjali*)	Figure 4.21
6. Hip	Figure 4.22
7. Great seal pose (*maha mudra*)	Figure 4.24

1. Chin (*jalandhara bandha*)

2. Abdominal (*uddiyanda bandha*)

3. Root anterior (*mula bandha*)

4. Root posterior (*ashwini mudra*)

5. Shoulder

6. Hip

7. Great seal pose (*maha mudra*).

Lock assessment

Locks should be assessed first inside the spinal neutral zone in the following postures: (1) hook lying, (2) prone, (3) seated, (4) mountain, (5) sidelying, (6) four point (hands and knees). Once lock performance in spinal neutral has been mastered, yoga postures and movements that introduce planes of spinal motion can be introduced. Begin with the anterior/posterior plane of motion and progress to lateral planes. Locks should assess the following:

- Quality of bony alignment (form closure)

- Muscle contraction (force closure)

- Coordination and timing (neural patterning), all of which will be completed through the FMA

- Performance of the lock without valsalva.

Chin lock (Jalandhara bandha)

Prerequisites

- Orofacial assessment

- Respiratory assessment

- A-D breath

- TATD breath

- Overcoming breath – aid locks performance.

Partial The mild chin lock employs a posterior glide of the occipital condyles over C1 of approximately 10 degrees. A gentle cervical retraction (not sheer) is made up of the gliding of the cranium on C1 in the absence of cervical flexion. It is used often for postural retraining, minimizing greater occipital nerve tension, and improving "overcoming breath" (*ujyaii pranayama*) efficiency (Fig. 4.18).

Full   A "full" chin lock employs cervical retraction and flexion of C2–C7 within safe osteokinematic ROM allowed per the individual. It can be used to facilitate healthy cervical flexion ROM and in proprioception training for overcoming breath, in order to assist in partial glottis (thoracic diaphragm) closure (Fig. 4.19).

Abdominal lock (Uddiyanda bandha) (Fig. 4.20)

Prerequisites   Same as chin lock.

Partial   The partial abdominal lock is not synonymous with TATD breath because it does not employ the force couple of pelvic floor or root lock recruitment. However, it does employ less than a 100%

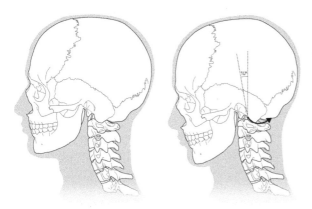

Figure 4.18
Partial chin lock

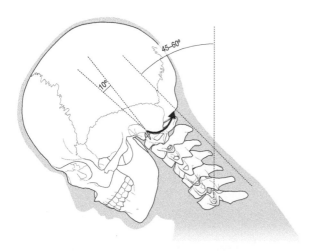

Figure 4.19
Full chin lock

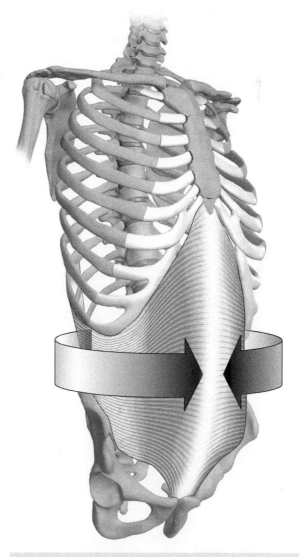

Figure 4.20
Abdominal lock

maximum voluntary isometric contraction and does not use a valsalva. The mild abdominal lock should be perfected in a small spinal neutral zone before attempting to teach the lock outside of spinal neutral in order to avoid compensatory patterns such as gluteal gripping, paraspinal tonic contraction, breath-holding, or use of the external oblique or rectus abdominis muscles in place of the TA. Excessive recruitment of the external oblique during attempted TATD breath is considered a nonoptimal strategy and can negatively affect load transfer to the pelvis as well as increasing pelvic floor descent/pressure.

Full   The full abdominal lock represents a non-breath-holding TATD breath with a 100% maximum voluntary isometric contraction while maintaining spinal neutral and a full breath. It can be used in short bouts for high level strength training or advanced

yoga posture completion, such as arm balances, headstands, or shoulderstands. Hip synergists (those muscles which contribute to spinal stability and are located in the hip, such as the hip external rotators) can also be employed as a part of abdominal lock in the mild or full versions, which constitutes addition of the hip lock.

Shoulder lock (Anjali mudra *plus*) (Fig. 4.21)

Prerequisites   Same as chin lock plus three- or four-part breath helpful but not required.

Prayer hands (*anjali mudra*) is a classic hand posture in yoga. However, using prayer hands alone without the shoulder lock mechanism cannot address scapulothoracic stabilization and awareness. Shoulder lock is akin to a "prayer hands plus," and is used for the following:

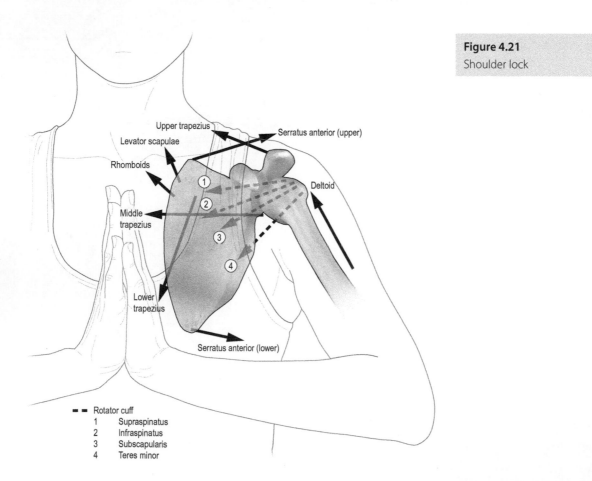

Figure 4.21
Shoulder lock

Upper trapezius
Levator scapulae
Rhomboids
Serratus anterior (upper)
Deltoid
Middle trapezius
1
2
3
4
Lower trapezius
Serratus anterior (lower)

Rotator cuff
1   Supraspinatus
2   Infraspinatus
3   Subscapularis
4   Teres minor

- Assessment of A-D breath quality — A-D breath should occur with proper diaphragmatic descent and without the use of secondary muscles of respiration. It should also occur with chest heaving or lifting, and without strain of the rigidity of the root of the tongue and soft palate

- Therapeutic intervention through co-activation of the upper extremity and periscapular musculature

- Inhibition of flexion synergy pattern through prolonged static elongation in tonic forearm muscles of hemiparetic side of the body through simulation of closed kinetic chain (weight-bearing) activity (Eng and Chu, 2002)

- Prevention or minimization of chest breathing through a kind of "locking-out" mechanism that offers resistance to chest expansion via creation of a natural loop of biofeedback through co-contraction recruitment

- Assessment of scapulothoracic stabilization and scapulohumeral rhythm

- Therapeutic intervention via simulation of a closed kinetic chain position and using proprioceptive neuromuscular facilitation and motor imagery through facilitating proper form closure, force closure, and load transfer through the four joints of the shoulder complex, the shoulder rotator cuff and the periscapular stabilizers.

Hip lock (Fig. 4.22)

Prerequisites Same as chin lock but overcoming breath not requisite.

The hip lock provides dynamic lower quarter stability and is chiefly influence by the hip rotator cuff and gluteals. Just as a house must have a sturdy foundation, building a yoga posture requires the same approach. Foot, ankle, and knee alignment can intimately affect

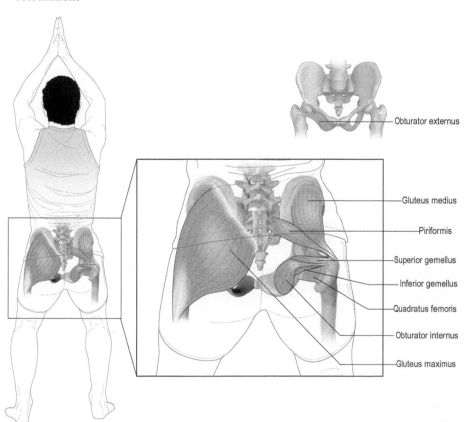

Figure 4.22
Hip lock

Obturator externus

Gluteus medius

Piriformis

Superior gemellus

Inferior gemellus

Quadratus femoris

Obturator internus

Gluteus maximus

the health of and ability to proximally stabilize joints, and vice-versa (Earl, 2011). Co-activation and synergistic contraction that contribute to musculoskeletal balance and health in the lower quarter are heavily influenced by proximal stability, especially in the lumbopelvic region (Earl, 2011). This means that the hip lock contributes, by synergy and in conjunction with TATD breath, to lumbopelvic integrity.

The hip external rotators (local) and gluteus maximus (global) function as synergists in lumbopelvic, hip, and sacroiliac joint (SIJ) stabilization, while the gluteus medius provides primary lateral hip stability (Reiman et al., 2012). The hip external rotators include the piriformis, gemellus superior and inferior, obturator externus and internus, and quadratus femoris. The hip lock is used in yoga postures through isotonic and isometric contraction via both open and closed kinetic chain movements. Teaching high-level dissociation of the gluteals from the hamstrings, pelvic floor, hip abductors, and hip external rotators is a chief neuromuscular retraining and neural patterning goal of hip lock. Force closure and healthy load transfer through the lumbosacral and lumbopelvic complex can be accomplished, in part, through identification and use of the hip lock in yoga postures.

Femoroacetabular impingement, a recently discovered structural deformity of the hip joint, is implicated in yoga prescription owing to its etiology, which is attributed to adverse mechanical forces at the acetabulum and related labrum due to various processes including osteoarthritis of the hip, congenital or developmental dysplasia, traumatic malformation, or thickening of the acetabular labrum (Beaule et al., 2009; Grant et al., 2012a). The implication is those patients who demonstrate hip muscle weakness, specifically hip adduction, flexion, external rotation, and abduction, are at increased risk for symptomatic and potentially pathomechanical femoroacetabular impingement (Casartelli et al., 2011).

Differences in hip torque generation from left to right in the same individual can influence development of knee injuries. Internal rotation torque is greatest at 90 degrees of hip flexion, less at 40 degrees, and least at 10 degrees. External rotation torque does not vary based on degree of hip flexion (Johnson and Hoffman, 2010).

Root lock, anterior (Mula bandha) and posterior (Ashwini mudra) (Fig. 4.23)

Prerequisites Same as chin lock plus bee breath helpful but not required.

Use of the pelvic floor includes the three lower diaphragms of the pelvic floor and the anterior/posterior root lock. Superficial muscles are the superficial transverse perineal muscle, the bulbocavernosus, and the ischiocavernosus. The muscles of the urogenital diaphragm are the sphincter urethrae membranaceae, and the deep transverse perineal muscles. The pubococcygeus, puborectalis, and iliococcygeus form the deepest layer.

Internal assessment should only be used in accordance with a healthcare professional's Practice Act. Referral to a pelvic floor specialist, such as a pelvic physical therapist or physiotherapist, is warranted for internal assessment. Use of root locks should include assessing whether the pelvic floor is capable of both a peak, sustained contraction and a baseline resting non-contraction state.

Finally, the anatomic connection of the respiratory diaphragm to the pelvic floor makes assessment of forced expiration (Talasz et al., 2010) and concomitant pelvic floor integrity and force closure important in prevention and management of diastasis recti abdominis and stress urinary incontinence.

Great seal lock (Maha mudra) (Fig. 4.24)

Prerequisites

- Orofacial assessment

- Respiratory assessment

- All previous six locks.

The great seal lock employs all six previous locks in one final seventh lock, performed in a seated, head-to-knee (*janu sirsasana*), gravity-dependent position. Feeling the contact of the perineum on the floor or on a blanketed surface or chair can provide biofeedback while facilitating adductor length, pelvic outlet

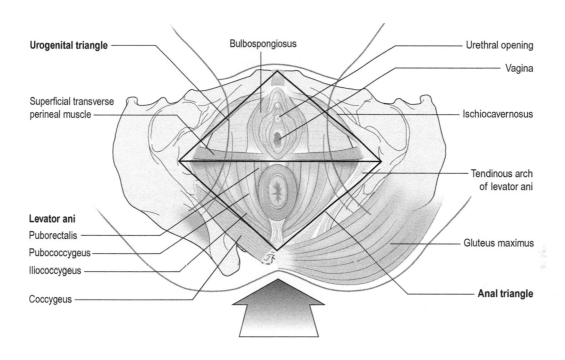

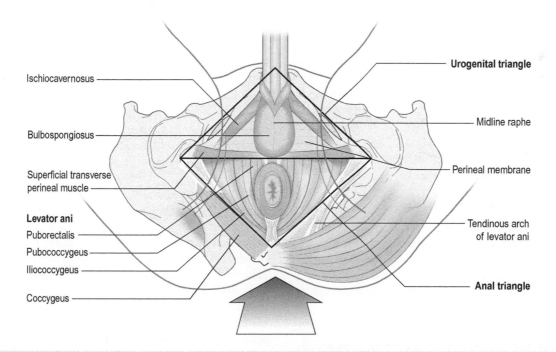

Figure 4.23
Anterior root lock and posterior root lock (top illustration: female; bottom illustration: male)

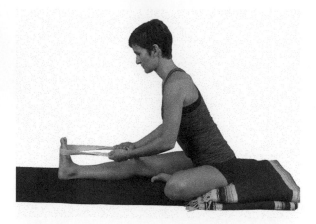

Figure 4.24
Great seal lock

opening, myofascial mobilization via deep respiration, hamstring length, neural mobilization for the sciatic nerve, pelvic awareness, postural and trunk control and awareness, and neural patterning via a proprioceptive neuromuscular facilitation (PNF) hold/relax pattern.

Special tests and screening prerequisites

Before beginning the FMA (Chapter 5), the femoral version test should be completed. Other tests will be specifically performed via the FMA (Chapter 5), including: (1) the scapular repositioning test and the scapular assistance test (performed during standing or seated arm floats/upstretched mountain), as well as upper or lower limb neural tension tests, SIJ screening, and multifidus screening.

Femoral version screen

Screen for abnormal pelvic bony development by identifying hip excessive anteversion or hip retroversion. The presence of excessive femoral anteversion, greater than 12–15 degrees, increased risk and incidence of labral tears by 2.2 times in an investigation of 204 hips (Ejnisman et al., 2013).

Femoral anteversion is defined as the angle between the proximal femoral neck axis and the distal femoral condylar axis (Yoon et al., 2014). Femoral retroversion is present if the angle is less than 12–15 degrees of anteversion (Yoon et al., 2014).

Because hip torque rotation production varies according to flexion angle, leg, and sex, individual measurement should occur prior to prescription in order to prevent or manage hip or knee pain. Additionally, measurement of 64 subjects where hip muscle strength was measured at zero degrees and mid-range hip joint positions found that "differences in muscle strength are dependent on the position that the hip rotator muscle is tested and the type of hip rotation symmetry or asymmetry present" (Cibulka et al., 2010). This finding further underscores the need to measure hip ROM and identify unilateral asymmetry in hip ROM, including screening for acetabular orientation via manual hip joint version (anteversion and retroversion) measurement, prior to yogic prescription. The implication is especially important prior to prescription of yoga postures which require hip joint internal or external rotation, since excessive hip anteversion is associated with limited hip joint external rotation and subsequent premature aging in the joint (Ejnisman et al., 2013); while hip retroversion is associated with increased hip external rotation, decreased hip internal rotation, and similar hip joint instability, leading to early degenerative osteoarthritis or femoroacetabular impingement, especially in the pediatric population and those with developmental delays (Friend and Kelly, 2009). For example, adults with cerebral palsy who are ambulatory and demonstrate hip dysplasia, which could stem from excessive femoral anteversion, often develop severe degenerative osteoarthritis and/or arthrodesis (Murphy, 2009). The same could be true with any adult with congenital or acquired malformation of the hip. As a result the global concern for healthcare providers using yoga should be hip and spine preservation in anyone with or without disability, but especially for those with functional impairment. Premature aging secondary to adverse load transfer from faulty mechanics or failure to recognize faulty mechanics should be prevented wherever possible, which begins with a firm foundation of hip and spine mechanics and requirements for neural patterning to facilitate functionally appropriate movement patterns.

Limitations in hip ROM, combined with any evidence of hip instability or lack of control, such as in the case of an orthopaedic injury, postpartum deconditioning, or cerebral palsy affecting gait, put the anterior acetabular labrum at risk via increasing hip extension without stability; and due to its anatomical and physiological function of improving hip stability, pressurizing the hip joint to prevent consolidation and decreasing contact forces, an individual would be put at even greater risk for premature degeneration and arthritis (Grant et al., 2012b). As a result, increases in hip ROM would have to be executed in a protected, controlled manner in order to avoid risk of labral degeneration or subsequent chondral lesions.

Measuring hip version angle (Fig. 4.25)

Code 4.9 (free code)

Femoral version screen/Craig test

There are two methods for the Craig test measurement described by Yoon et al. (2014): (1) the trochanteric prominence angle test (TPAT) and (2) the transcondylar angle test (TCAT). Both tests are performed from prone lying and utilize a digital inclinometer or smartphone Tiltmeter application (Yoon et al., 2014). Of 19 hips, the TCAT demonstrated superior intra- and inter-rater (ICC = 0.94, 0.89, respectively) reliability (Yoon et al., 2014).

Trochanteric prominence angle test (TPAT)

From prone lying with the knee flexed 90 degrees, the clinician internally and externally rotates the hip until the greater trochanter is palpated as being most prominent at the lateral hip joint. The angle is measured by placing the measurement tool (inclinometer or appropriate smartphone application) at mid-shaft of the tibia (Yoon et al., 2014).

Transcondylar angle test (TCAT)

Follow the same directions as the TPAT, but instead measure version via palpation of bilateral femoral condyles. Draw a horizontal line between the condyles. The angle is measured by aligning the measurement device on the transcondylar line, providing the femoral version angle (Yoon et al., 2014).

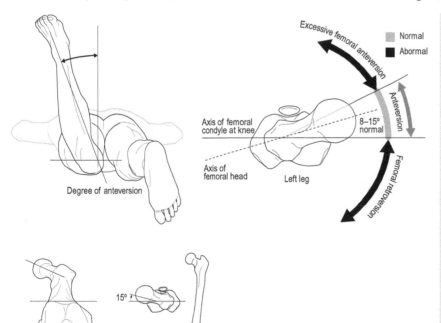

Figure 4.25

Femoral version screen option 1: trochanteric prominence angle test. An angle is determined by quantifying the angle from the vertical (line perpendicular to the earth) to the tibia with a manual, digital or smartphone goniometer. The lower picture depicts the optimal range of femoral anteversion. Femoral version screen option 2: transcondylar angle test is taken by capturing the same angle as shown, but taking the measurement by drawing a line between the femoral condyles (top left horizontal line) and measuring the angle with a smartphone goniometer. Adapted from Yoon et al. (2014).

Normal clinical external or internal rotation is not typically found in excessively anteverted and retroverted hips, respectively. External rotation is typically lacking in excessive anteversion, and internal rotation is lacking in retroverted femoral necks. However, someone with hypermobility syndrome or a long history of yoga, dance, or gymnastics practice could have forced "normal" internal or external rotation by aggressively moving the hip past its normal range. In these cases, risk for hip labral injury is even higher.

Yoga prescription implication for those with excessive femoral anteversion should avoid forcing end-range hip external rotation (i.e. lotus, half-lotus, or warrior II), while those with hip retroversion should avoid forcing end-range hip internal rotation (i.e. hero or the back leg in pigeon). However, due to inherent capsular and/or ligamentous laxity that accompanies excessive ROM in a joint, end-ranges in either extreme of rotation should be avoided because of excessive loads being placed on either the anterior or posterior labrum, and an emphasis on high level femoroacetabular and lumbopelvic stability should be pursued.

Review

Orofacial relaxation, vagus nerve response, respiratory techniques, and yogic lock mastery should be attended to prior to yoga posture prescription or FMA use. Special testing is also critical for clinical efficacy and safety in posture prescription.

Medical Therapeutic Yoga (MTY) expands on the idea that yoga can and does evolve via scientific inquiry and creative innovation by offering an evidence-based approach for therapeutic alignment of postures. The discussion is incomplete without offering a methodology for ordering the postures in a logical psychobiological fashion. This algorithmic ordering offers options for progression via a series of preliminary yoga breath techniques and postures. The method is not without exceptions and, as a result, is not offered as an absolute, but rather as a clinical guideline for fluid qualitative and quantitative musculoskeletal systems-based assessment. Refer to Chapter 12 for verbal and manual cuing and patient monitoring guidelines to practice.

Outline

- Defining the algorithm and its use

- The functional movement assessment (FMA) algorithm

- Safety in the algorithms: guidelines to posture prescription

- The vector analysis

- The FMA algorithms

- Other biomechanical considerations

- FMA – the primary diagnostic algorithm

- FMA: adult form

- FMA: geriatric form

- Review

Defining the algorithm and its use
(Fig. 5.1)

An algorithm is a type of decision tree to help streamline clinical decision-making. The algorithms are designed to provide a framework for clinical decision-making while affording the clinician autonomy to modify as needed, based on the unique needs of the patient and the clinician's professional expertise. For example, IF the individual can master a breath type or posture type, THEN they should have some measure of safety and competency in order to progress to the next step (yoga posture or breath type).

The algorithm(s) also allows for a large body of information to be organized into succinct substructures that indicate to the learner a level of difficulty and thus, help determine the application or use of the variable. A medical algorithm is typically set up in a flow chart format and is recognized as a method to assist in medical assessment and inform decision-making. The intention of the algorithms in this chapter is to improve and streamline decision-making in the delivery of yoga as medicine, realizing that algorithms are working theories that evolve as the evidence base matures.

Two catalysts have driven development of the algorithms. First, there is no current agreement on how yoga postures or breath should be biomechanically aligned or executed (Garner, 2011). Yoga postures have historically been taught based on verbal knowledge, handed down from guru to student, rather than on scientific evidence and rationale (Garner, 2011). The algorithms do not attempt to replace the rich heritage and wisdom of this experiential knowledge. What they do provide is an evidence-informed method for biomechanically safe and effective application of yoga postures based on biological plausibility, the evidence base in rehabilitation, and clinical expertise.

Second, the algorithms can allow for application and prescription of yoga in complex patient populations. The current research in yoga is limited in its ability to address complex medical histories. The algorithms make provision for establishment of inter-rater and intra-rater reliability during future research through a baseline standard for biomechanical alignment of postures, which allows for further scrutiny of yoga's ability to address complex patient populations.

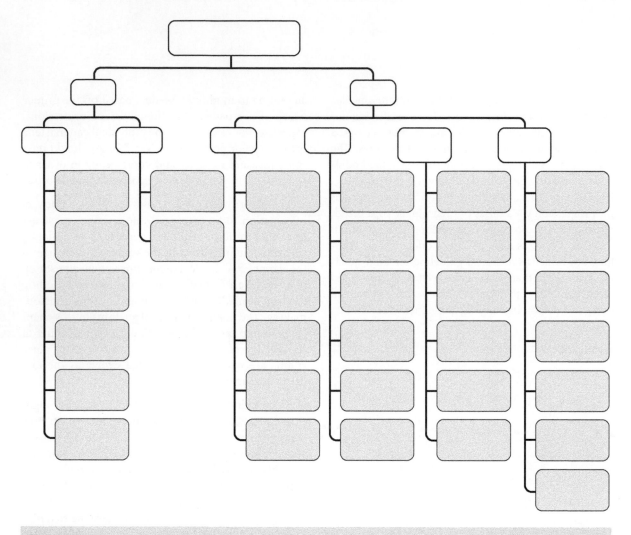

Figure 5.1
Algorithm skeleton

The functional movement assessment (FMA) algorithm

The existence of a functional movement evaluation is not new (Onate et al., 2012; Tehyen et al., 2012; Smith et al., 2013). The functional movement screen (FMS) is a qualitative tool developed to screen movement patterns in athletics to quantify risk for injury via identification of compensatory patterns within these movement patterns (Smith et al., 2013). This development is an important step in identifying dyskinesis and predicting injury risk, thereby improving injury prevention measures and, ultimately, improving decision-making in rehabilitation.

The future of FMA in yoga, as used in this text, is to establish reliability as it is beginning to be established with the FMS (Onate et al., 2012; Teyhen et al., 2012; Smith et al., 2013). An additional use for the FMA is to allow for a wider range of application for patient and wellness populations through incorporation of a yogic model. The FMA is a prototype that allows for objective quantitative and qualitative assessment of yoga postures for orthopaedic benefit. And, encased in the biopsychosocial (BPS) model, it is distinctly different from the sports medicine-based FMS.

Safety in algorithm use: guidelines to posture prescription

Safety in the algorithm is guided by returning to the 10 precepts (Chapter 1). The algorithms should be used in the context of an interdisciplinary, individualized, culturally sensitive, holistic plan of care, and not as a physical practice only.

Biomechanical assessment: safe posture prescription depends on "vector analysis" (Garner, 2001) and is additionally informed by McCreary et al. (2005), Reese and Bandy (2002), and Sahrmann (2002):

Yoga prescription for prevention or pathophysiology requires careful biomechanical analyses within the yoga posture or breath and depends on a two-step process:

1. *Centering through breath mastery* — The concept of centering is based on precepts one, two, and three, which support the theory that breath dictates health (Gandevia and McKenzie, 2008); therefore, monitoring of respiration and mastery of a basic skillset in respiration is a prerequisite for yoga posture performance. Centering is a deliberate action the individual initiates to create mind–body connectedness throughout each of the five facets of the BPS model. Since each of the pentagons is interrelated, the most effective way to affect centering is to teach breath awareness first (found in Chapter 4).

2. *Addressing six subsystems of movement for proximal to distal control* — Yoga is a complementary therapy capable of addressing all six subsystems of movement (Fig. 5.2) due to its mind–body component (Deutsch and Anderson, 2008; Hoffman and Gabel, 2013). BPS stability should be addressed before mobility. Stability begins with lumbopelvic evaluation, followed by shoulder complex/upper quarter assessment and lower quarter assessment as stated in the precepts. Stability assessment is found in this chapter and in Chapters 6–10.

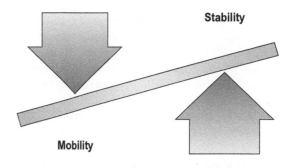

Figure 5.2

A finer balance: the mind–body ground substance of yoga includes six subsystems of movement classified into two categories: stability and mobility. Hoffman and Gabel (2013) posit that each category demonstrates passive, neural, and active components which, together, complete the six subsystems. Therefore, stability and mobility depend on a finer balance of achieving passive, neural, and active equilibrium

The vector analysis

A "ground-up and inside-out" approach should be taken by performing a "vector analysis." This is an assessment of the yoga posture or breath in all planes of motion: (1) coronal or frontal (lateral), (2) sagittal (anterior-posterior), and (3) transverse (horizontal) (Fig. 5.3).

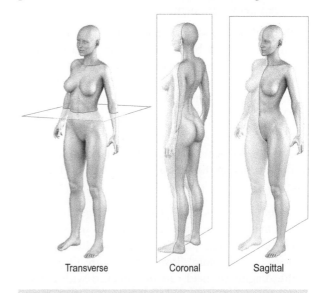

Transverse   Coronal   Sagittal

Figure 5.3
Planes of analysis

For example, in standing postures the entire kinetic chain includes the toe tips to fingertips and soles of the feet to the cranial crown, recognizing that fascia also plays a major role in postural performance (Alfonse et al., 2010), breath, and alignment via variables including, but not limited to, muscle contractility through force generation (Schleip et al., 2005; Sakuma et al., 2012), force transmission (Barker et al., 2004; Hujing, 2009; Langevin et al., 2011; Findley et al., 2015), viscoelasticity and plastic deformation (Schleip, 2003; Chaudry et al., 2007), and tensile force capability (Chaudry, 2011), which includes proprioception via mechanoreceptors, as well as nociception (Stecco et al., 2016). In standing postures, the yoga posture is constructed from the ground up and from the inside out, given that fascia is "malleable, coordinates components of motor units in the myofascial unit and connects element between body joints by means of retinacula. The fascia and the muscles act as rigging that guarantees verticality of our body" (Stecco, 2004., p. 11; Findley et al., 2012).

When aligning a posture from an orthopaedic perspective, work proximally to distally. For example, in extended side angle, if the glenohumeral or tibiofemoral joints appear compromised or unsafe, check proximal joint alignment before attempting to change distal segment alignment.

Through postural assessment, the FMA identifies anomalies such as, but not limited to, dysfunctional neuromuscular, myofascial response, or recruitment patterns, since these variables are instrumental in pain management, increasing range of motion (ROM), and facilitating tissue healing (Hoffman and Gabel, 2013).

The four critical domains for evaluating postures and breath using the vector analysis method include (Table 5.1):

1. *Optimal kinematics* (OK) — To properly assess kinematic control and load transfer in postures, introduce single planar movements, limiting the degrees of freedom allowed in a posture. Otherwise the diagnostic field can be muddied with excess variables for proper differential diagnosis. Note presence or absence of reasonably normal spinal curves and extremity positioning.

Table 5.1
The vector analysis

Critical components	Description
Optimal kinematics	Assess kinematic control and load transfer in postures, limiting degrees of freedom for diagnostic accuracy and safety
Efficient motor patterns	Note initiation or isolation of individual muscles or muscle groups, range of motion, and control
Ability to adapt to imposed stresses	Note the psychobiological response to imposed stress(es) via polyvagal theory assessment
Tissue extensibility and sensorimotor integration	Deeper attention is given to neurovascular, myofascial, and/or soft tissue resilience and response, as well as sensorimotor integration

2. *Efficient motor patterns* (MP) — Note initiation or isolation of an individual muscle or muscle group (including the three diaphragms) to facilitate stability, indicative of adequate load transfer and optimal movement strategy. Note if ROM is completed in a smooth, coordinated fashion with both concentric and eccentric control. Note if momentum, rather than control, is used to complete a movement pattern, which is considered a nonoptimal movement strategy.

3. *Ability to adapt to imposed stresses* — In all postures, note the psychobiological response to imposed stress. Document subdiaphragmatic (visceral "fight or flight" or dorsal vagal "shut down" response) phenomena versus supradiaphragmatic (ventral vagal response with psychobiological "centering," e.g. calm disposition, even, smooth breathing at 12 or fewer respirations per minute, and where applicable, maintenance of transversus abdominis-assisted thoracodiaphragmatic (TATD) breath for provision of safety in

yoga posture performance) response. Note any changes derivative of a dorsal vagal or "shut down" response (Porges, 2011), such as breath shortening or holding, emotional dissociation or lack of social engagement, changes in the voice, skin, or fascial expression, or alternately, sympathetic nervous system (flight or fight) response.

4. *Tissue extensibility and sensorimotor integration* (TESMI) — Deeper attention is given to neurovascular, myofascial, and/or soft tissue resilience and response, in addition to sensorimotor integration. Postures in the FMA can be used to assess ability to follow instructions, body awareness, attention to task performance, attitude, cooperation, need for tactile prompting or other form of learning. All fascia is relevant because it has the capability of being on tension in order to maintain a posture, especially if the theory of biotensegrity is considered. However, if a linear approach is desired, which could be reductionist, then corresponding myofasical lines (Myers, 2014) are provided for theoretical but not myopic or isolated application (found in Chapters 5–10). Myofascial restriction and identification of diaphragmatic impairment or contribution of other soft tissue or neural factors (hamstring or posterior fascia limitation, sciatic nerve tension) should be identified by observation or by the clinician's "listening hand," as described in the work of Robert Schleip (2003). See Chapter 3 for a myofascial lines overview. The entry point for this assessment is to complete real-time assessment of ROM (osteokinematic motion) during posture performance. Loss of osteokinematic ROM is a red flag that necessitates evaluation of arthrokinematic ROM (accessory motion or joint play). Sensorimotor integration also considers contributing mechanical factors such as joint hyper- or hypomobility of the spine and extremities, how the individual responds to his/her environment through movement and breath, and the capacity of the individual to learn and move mindfully.

The FMA algorithms

There are two FMAs introduced in this text: the adult form (Fig. 5.4) and the geriatric form (Fig. 5.5). Both use postures and breath to evaluate overall functional mobility and stability. The algorithms evaluate general neuromuscular fitness including strength, flexibility, endurance, cardiorespiratory function, myofasical and neurovascular health, and emotional resilience, under the auspices of a systems-based categorical yoga posture progression(s). The second version of the FMA, the geriatric form, is appropriate for those who cannot successfully transfer from floor to standing or where floor to standing transfers are not functionally necessary.

Other biomechanical considerations

Rationale for excluding some postures in the algorithm (Table 5.2)

Functional carryover is a rationale which can be used to order the neural patterning and motor control algorithm differently or to exclude certain postures in the algorithm altogether. For example, if a stroke patient does not need to get on their hands and knees for a functional task, then it may be unnecessary to prescribe the prone position. However, in geriatric rehabilitation and fitness, safety often requires successful floor to standing transfer, which necessitates the prone series.

Exceptions to following the stabilization precept four

Reversing the proximal to distal focus

Constraint-induced movement therapy (CIMT) is another rationale that can be used to order this algorithm. The MTY precepts support proximal to distal stability in creating healthy functional movement patterns. However, in the neurological population, using stroke as an example, CIMT proponents advocate for functional development of skills in the hand for completion of activities of daily living (ADL), regardless of whether or not stability is addressed proximally. This is where algorithm operationalization is open to clinical interpretation. If working with an orthopaedic population, one may use the proximal to distal stability precept to create scapulohumeral rhythm via scapulothoracic stabilization in order to protect and optimize rotator cuff (RTC) integrity and function. However, if proximal stability is not possible due to stroke, CIMT theory may dictate a focus on

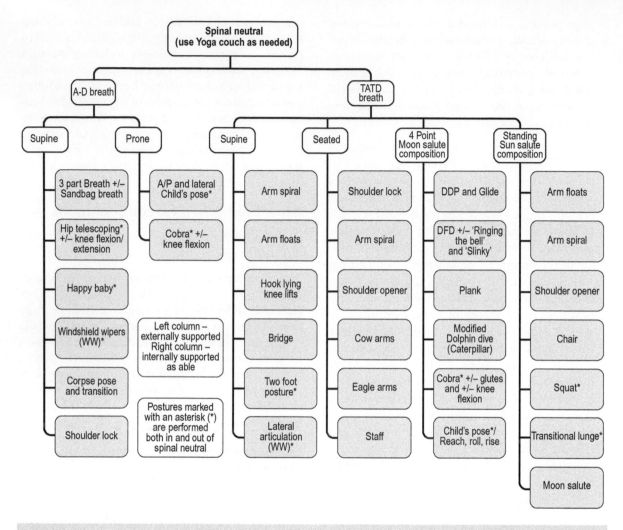

Figure 5.4
Primary functional movement assessment: adult

functional task completion and motor training in the hand. Clinicians can, through differential diagnosis, integrate the FMAs into regular practice because of their non-deterministic interpretive capacity. The algorithms become less of an "if, then" flowchart and more of a categorical guideline of yoga postures to address on an open continuum, depending on person-centered needs analysis and functional goals.

The stability–mobility paradox

There may be instances where mobility must be addressed, whether proximal or distal, before stability.

However, depending on the way mobility is defined and addressed, pursuing mobility first could still fall under the domain of achieving stability first, albeit through seeking psychoemotional stability (as a primary intention) via first affecting change in physiological mobility (as a secondary intention). A common clinical case would be the need for gentle mobilization of fascial structures prior to addressing stability due to fascia-induced neuromuscular inhibition, pain, or patient-driven fear of movement.

The pelvic floor is an ideal example of the stability–mobility paradox. There is a fine balance between

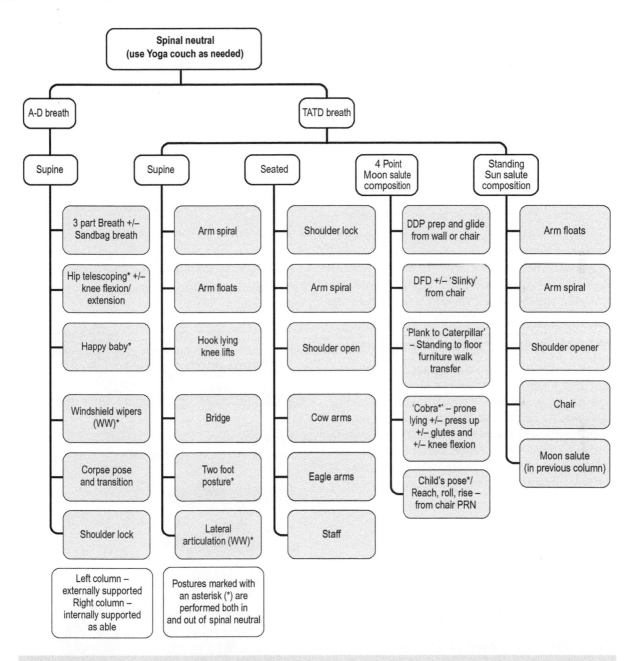

Figure 5.5

Primary functional movement assessment: geriatric

stability and mobility of the pelvic floor system. Oftentimes, pelvic floor release (mobility, resilience, and response) dictates strength and endurance capability (stability). However, the person with pelvic pain may register any movement or input as nociceptive, perhaps due to autonomic or neuroendocrine dysregulation. In this case, it would be necessary to build a sense of safety (stability) first. Safety in the therapeutic landscape and in rehabilitation intervention(s) can improve ventral vagus circuit function and effectively employ the vagal brake,

Table 5.2
Exceptions to precept four

Precept four – The Professional Yoga Therapy Institute advocates for biopsychosocial (BPS) stability as a primary focus, with mobility as a secondary focus, guided by principles of neurophysiology and biomechanics	
Exceptions to stability precept four	• Functional carryover • Constraint-induced movement therapy

which has both a supra- and a subdiaphragmatic effect. This means, although mobility via pelvic fascial manual therapies may be addressed first, which are technically categorized as mobilization, the therapies would be delivered under the biopsychosocial umbrella of seeking stability, in this case psychobiological stability, first.

FMA – the primary diagnostic algorithm

This section covers a step-by-step explanation of the adult and geriatric FMA. Pre-postures serve as prerequisites to performance of, or assessment in, any yoga postures and include breath assessment in yoga couch, hip telescoping, anterior/posterior articulation and lateral articulation, lateral child's pose, arm spiral, arm floats, shoulder opener and lock, downward-facing dog preparation, and windshield wipers.

Using the FMA

- For FMA breathwork instructions, see Chapter 4.

- For prerequisite posture instructions and assessment, see this chapter.

- For postures that only include assessment, instructions are found in their respective chapters (6–10).

Supine prerequisite postures (Table 5.3)

Instructions in Chapter 8.

1. Three-tier approach – "yoga couch" (Fig. 5.6).

Code 5.1 (free code)
Three-tier approach – "yoga couch"

Table 5.3
Supine prerequisite postures

Supine prerequisite postures	Figure	QR code
Three-tier approach – "yoga couch"	Fig. 5.6	Code 5.1
Corpse and transfers from supine to sit	Fig. 5.7	

2. Corpse and supine-to-sit transfer (Fig. 5.7).*

This pose is assessed in supine lying unless the patient is unable to lie supine or supine lying is contraindicated, in which case, use the yoga couch with a 30 degree trunk incline.

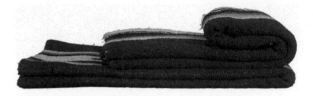

Figure 5.6
Three-tier approach – "yoga couch"

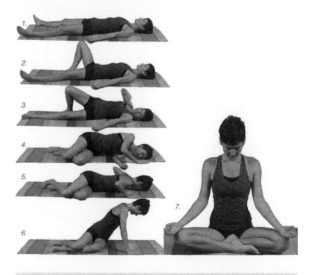

Figure 5.7
Corpse and supine-to-sit transfer

Assess and document:

OK (optimal kinematics) Plumb line alignment from crown to pelvis with spinal neutral (yoga couch) or from crown to toe (corpse). Excessive thoracic spine kyphosis creates a cervical spine extension moment, compromises postural alignment, and is indicative of loss of cervical spine osteo/arthrokinematic motion and/or vestibular impairment if dizziness or vision changes are present. Inability to lie supine or in hook lying requires differential diagnosis of orientation of bony landmarks:

1. Lumbopelvic and/or lumbosacral impairment — Anterior superior iliac spine (ASIS), pubic symphysis, and medial ilia functional symmetry

2. Shoulder complex — Anterior translation of humeral head that prevents the posterior shoulder from resting on the floor (document the distance in centimeters (cm) from posterior acromion to the floor). This finding may be due to pectoralis minor or short head of the biceps tendon inflexibility, posterior capsule restriction (Kibler et al., 2013), or related myofasical restriction

3. Hip and pelvis — Angle of anterior/posterior inclination or tilt. Femoral head positioning in acetabulum. If the psoas or other related fascia or tissue is limiting pelvic neutral alignment, excessive anterior tilt (unilateral or bilateral) of the pelvis is present. Ability of the hip joints and pelvis to rest in neutral position without myofascial restriction, visceral, abdominal, or psoas fascia tethering, back or pelvic pain, or scar adhesions. Degree and quality of resting anatomical position of hips (external rotation) via a capsule test.

Code 5.2 (free code)

Capsule test

MP (motor pattern) Transition quality entering and exiting corpse. Oftentimes injury in the workplace, recreational activity, or sport occurs not during the pose or movement itself but in the entry or exit from a movement, making assessment of transition

even more important. Assess ability to move from sit to supine through sidelying and log-rolling into position without valsalva. Leaning straight back or sitting straight up, unless there is ideal TATD control and strength, is considered a nonoptimal strategy. Abdominodiaphragmatic (A-D) breath should be mastered with full, symmetrical diaphragmatic excursion (concentric and eccentric) at all three diaphragms, either through observation or palpation.

TESMI (tissue extensibility and sensorimotor integration)

- Myofascial tension — Superficial front, superficial back, and deep front lines/bands, but consider all lines if these are unaffected

- Neural tension — Median nerve with and without arm spiral with arms positioned at 45 degrees; if there is no neural tension at 45 degrees, test at 90 degrees.

Supine A-D breath postures (Table 5.4)

Instructions in Chapter 8.

1. Knee-to-chest (*apanasana*)

2. Hip telescoping with/without knee flexion and extension (self-guided or clinician-guided scour test)

3. Happy baby

4. Windshield wipers

5. Shoulder lock.

Table 5.4

Supine abdominodiaphragmatic (A-D) breath postures

Posture	Figure	QR code
Knee-to-chest	Figs 5.8–5.9	
Hip telescoping	Figs 5.10–5.14	
Happy baby	Figs 5.15–5.18	
Windshield wipers	Figs 5.19–5.24	Code 5.3
Shoulder lock	Fig. 4.21	

Hip telescoping is a self-guided or clinician-assisted version of a scour test that includes knee-to-chest pose without compressive axial loading of the hip joint. It is a three-step assessment that includes: (1) finding spinal neutral using A-D breath; (2) performing knee-to-chest with and without loss of spinal neutral (TATD breath required on latter test); (3) telescoping the hip (flexion, abduction, external rotation (FABER) and/or flexion, adduction, internal rotation (FADDIR)) without spinal neutral and with or without knee flexion and/or extension.

Happy baby is an optional variation to include only after successful knee-to-chest and hip telescoping.

> Hip telescoping, happy baby, and windshield wipers can be identified as a *"sensory diet"* therapeutic trifecta

Hip telescoping, happy baby, and windshield wipers provide posturing, pressure, and rocking that can be beneficial for sensory integration in those with sensory processing disorders. Deep-pressure proprioception through brushing followed by joint compressions may also be of benefit in pediatric populations (May-Benson, 2007). Thus, hip telescoping, happy baby, and windshield wipers can be identified as a *"sensory diet"* therapeutic trifecta. There is also biological plausibility for these postures to affect cerebrospinal fluid (CSF) flow via postural changes, in this case spinal flexion when the postures above are performed outside of spinal neutral. While only a theory, CSF movement via sacral rocking, also known as *"the rocker"* in the Brain Gym program used in pediatric occupational therapy practice in schools, is thought to affect posture, focus, and breathing through autonomic regulation via the mechanism of promoting healthy CSF flow (identified by Cushing in 1927 as the *"third circulation"*) (Cushing, 1927; Whedon and Glassey, 2009).

Knee-to-chest, hip telescoping, and happy baby (Figs 5.8–5.18)

Assess and document:

OK (optimal kinematics)

- Unilateral and bilateral functioning and synergistic patterns of the hips and lumbopelvic area, including bilateral hip ROM comparisons and breath quality when the more complex movement patterns of bilateral hip and trunk flexion, hip abduction and external rotation, knee flexion, and ankle dorsiflexion, are introduced. Hip joint surface integrity (a non-compressive scour test in hip telescoping), smooth spinning, gliding, and rolling (arthrokinematic or joint play motions) in the hip, limitations in hip joint ROM that affect the lumbopelvic or lumbosacral spine. Shoulder complex ROM and functional mobility

- Response of the spine and extremities to movement in and outside of spinal neutral, focusing on ilia response. A sagittal anterior pelvic plane interrupts the vertical alignment of the anterior pelvic plane (APP) and pubic symphysis (the APP is the line joining the ASIS and the pubic symphysis) and is associated with acetabular malalignment that results in femoroacetabular impingement (FAI) (Legaye, 2009; Banerjee and McLean, 2011). Pain, pinching, or referred pain into the groin during FABER or FADDIR movements, which could be indicative of FAI (cam or pincer type), sacroiliac joint (SIJ) pain, or other intra-articular hip lesion, such as chondral damage, articular cartilage degeneration, acetabular undercoverage, overcoverage, or labral tear, and warrants further investigation.

MP (motor pattern)

- Upper quarter — Resting position of the scapulae. They should not leave the chest wall prematurely, since doing so limits shoulder elevation and creates impingement due to absence of scapular stabilizer or RTC involvement. Note excessive upper trapezius recruitment, along with local changes in myofascial quality or neurovascular sensory output. Quality of periscapular strength and/or any combined lack of mobility in the hip joints or loss of periscapular strength may affect the torso and

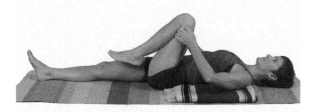

Figure 5.8
Knee-to-chest unilateral

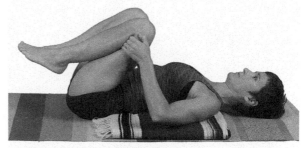

Figure 5.9
Knee-to-chest bilateral

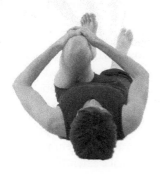

Figure 5.10
Hip telescoping step 1

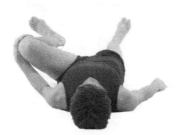

Figure 5.11
Hip telescoping step 2

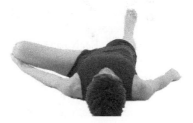

Figure 5.12
Hip telescoping step 3

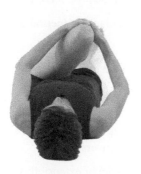

Figure 5.13
Hip telescoping step 4

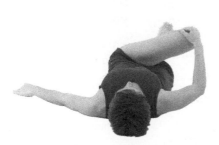

Figure 5.14
Hip telescoping step 5

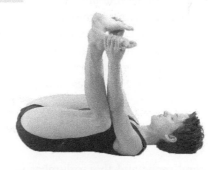

Figure 5.15
Happy baby with floating sacral apex in full posterior pelvic tilt

shoulder complex (sternoclavicular, glenohumeral, acromioclavicular, and scapulothoracic joints). Loss of functional mobility and/or appropriate movement strategy in this pose may be extrapolated to functional impairment in ADL.

- Lower quarter — Degree of implication that knee flexion versus knee extension affects the spine (hamstring length), the quality of the breath with introduction of movement, and the quality of the meditative or introspective mind with introduction

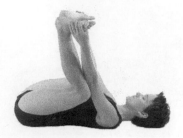

Figure 5.16

Happy baby with grounded base of sacrum and decreased posterior pelvic tilt

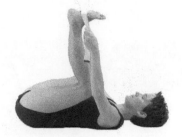

Figure 5.17

Happy baby with strap in arm spiral

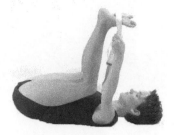

Figure 5.18

Happy baby with strap in arm spiral with floating sacral apex

of movement (*Meditation With Movement*). Note ischial tuberosity glide with single and bilateral knee to chest. Each ischial tuberosity should glide inferiorly with the ilium during hip and knee flexion, free from groin impingement, SIJ pain, and with concomitant ASIS posterior innominate rotation (knee to chest outside of neutral). Knee extension is introduced after assessment of all of the previous facets, in order to determine the degree of hamstring involvement in limitation of hip and spine functional mobility. Immediate loss of spinal neutral is indicative of impaired load transfer to the spine as a result of loss of normal sensory modulation or tissue response (posterior muscle or associated fascia, nerve, or vascular supply), which is approximately 90 degrees of hip flexion without loss of spinal neutral.

TESMI (tissue extensibility and sensorimotor integration)

- Lateral raphe and thoracolumbar fascia response, which can implicate low back, cervical and suboccipital regions and/or the pelvic floor; the transversalis fascia, owing to its connection of the cervical fascia to the pubis and inguinal regions, involving the posterior diaphragm via the retroperitoneal level (Bordoni and Zanier, 2013). Myofascial restriction rules out and/or complicates the presence of diaphragmatic dysfunction via abnormal breathing habits or through bidirectional phenomena that could cause pelvic pain, sacroiliac joint

(SIJ) dysfunction (Bordoni and Zanier, 2013), or "*fight, flight, or shut down*" response due to dorsal vagal stimulation from subdiaphragmatic vagal afferent input (Porges 1995, 2007, 2011).

- Neural tension — Assessment of single planes of motion allows for consideration of neural tension in the sciatic nerve during knee extension and spinal neutral, with the introduction of foot dorsiflexion and plantarflexion to fully complete testing for sciatic nerve neural tension. Knee-to-chest with knee extension or hand-to-big toe pose screens for:

- Straight leg raise test for radicular pain/neural tension (Butler, 1991):

  - dura mater tension (ankle dorsiflexion plus chin nod)

  - sciatic (flexion)

  - peroneal lateral variation (hip flexion plus medial rotation, plantarflexion and inversion

  - hamstring contralateral hip flexor extensibility

  - spinal integrity (neuromusuclar awareness/proprioception; gross stability (contralateral oblique and transversus abdominis control)).

- Positive test — Reproduction of lower extremity radiating/radicular pain with passive lower extremity hip flexion and knee extension

  - inability to reach 90 degrees hip flexion/knee extension without signs or symptoms.

Windshield wipers (Figs 5.19–5.24)

> **Code 5.3** (free code)
> Windshield wipers

Assess and document:

OK (optimal kinematics)

- Unilateral hip ROM in contralateral hips simultaneously (FABER and FADDIR)

- Resting postural alignment and moving postural strategy using A-D breath during descent into FABER and FADDIR

- Hip ROM using digital goniometer or inclinometer or the distance in cm of the knees from the tibiofemoral joint line to the floor

- Hip mobility restriction — Is hip ROM is within normal limits? If it is not functionally equal bilaterally, screen hypermobility of the lumbar spine, iliolumbar ligaments, or premature innominate anterior and/or medial translation. If ROM is missing in the hip joint, the typical presentation could be (1) excessive rotation through the lumbar spine and iliolumbar area with extension of the thoracolumbar area and lifting of the contralateral shoulder, (2) hypomobility of the ipsilateral or hypermobility of the contralateral SIJ, which could be identified by monitoring the ASIS and/or ischial tuberosity translation(s), or (3) knee instability or pain from a torque/rotational moment induced by loss of proximal mobility

- Also see knee-to-chest.

MP (motor pattern)   Postural control strategy using A-D breath during entry and exit.

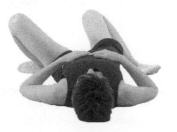

Figure 5.19
Start in hook lying (not shown).
Windshield wipers step 1

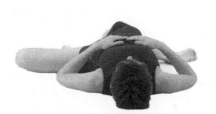

Figure 5.20
Windshield wipers step 2

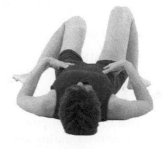

Figure 5.21
Windshield wipers step 3

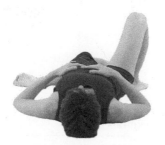

Figure 5.22
Windshield wipers step 4

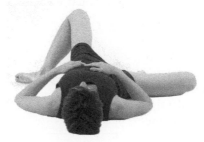

Figure 5.23
Windshield wipers step 5

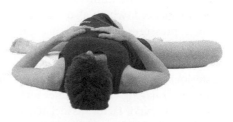

Figure 5.24
Windshield wipers step 6. Return to hook lying (not shown)

TESMI (tissue extensibility and sensorimotor integration)

- Lateral line, spiral line, functional, arm, superficial back line (on contralateral side of rotation) or deep front line restriction may diminish FADDIR while FABER may be diminished due to superficial or deep front line involvement.

- Seated version option — A seated version of windshield wipers can screen for presence of hip impingement due to bony obstruction, adhesions, thoracolumbar segmental or sacroiliac joint impairment, or myofascial restriction, or pelvic pain with orthopaedic etiology.

- Neural tension or compression is possible in the sensory distribution of the lateral femoral cutaneous nerve, which could be influenced by obesity, tight clothing or other apparatus, pregnancy, and/or scar tissue in the inguinal or thigh area.

Shoulder lock (supine) Refer to Fig. 4.21.

Assess and document:

OK (optimal kinematics) Scapular dyskinesis is present in the majority of shoulder injuries (Kibler et al., 2012, 2013) and includes altered scapular positioning and motion, including: winging/anterior tilt, tipping/internal rotation, or protraction of the scapula at rest or prematurely during arm elevation, in addition to diminished scapular external rotation and excessive upper trapezius recruitment (Huang et al., 2015; Lopes et al., 2015). In cadaver models, diminished upward rotation and increased internal rotation increase the contact area of the humeral head with the posterior superior glenoid, which also increases glenohumeral contact pressures (Kibler et al., 2013). Addressing scapular dyskinesis is correlated with successful non-operative treatment of SLAP (superior labral anterior posterior) tears (Edwards et al., 2010), while magnetic resonance imaging (MRI) studies reveal scapular dyskinesis as a "major factor" associated with loss of functional mobility (Kibler et al., 2013).

MP (motor pattern)

- Force coupling — Ability to elevate the shoulder with balanced upper trapezius, serratus anterior, and lower trapezius action without upper trapezius movement strategy domination and without neck, head, or facial pain

- Tonic contraction of the upper trapezius could be related to RTC deficiency, tendonitis, stress-induced or tension-related upper trapezius holding, or scapular dyskinesis.

TESMI (tissue extensibility and sensorimotor integration)

- Shortening of the pectoralis major or minor, which could contribute to shoulder sloping, altered humeral head contact with the glenoid, scapular dyskinesis, and RTC impairment

- Myofascial tension of all lines/bands

- Reverse Phalen's test (wrist extension using prayer hands or shoulder lock (prayer hands plus active scapulothoracic stabilization) held for 60 seconds). There should be no presence of carpal tunnel syndrome symptoms, such as numbness or tingling in the median nerve distribution. End range wrist extension, flexion, or grip can cause increased carpal tunnel pressure. The test, reproduced by a simple shoulder lock, demonstrates sensitivity ranging from 37% to 97% and a specificity of 71–93% (Cook and Hegedus, 2013).

Prone A-D breath postures (Table 5.5)

Instructions in Chapter 9.

1. Anterior/posterior (A/P) and lateral child's pose

2. Cobra +/– knee flexion.

Table 5.5
Prone abdominodiaphragmatic (A-D) breath postures

Posture	Figure
Anterior/posterior child	Fig. 5.25
Lateral child	Fig. 5.26
Cobra ± knee flexion	Figs 5.27–5.28

Child's pose and lateral child's pose (Figs 5.25 and 5.26)

The most natural position for evaluating breath in populations without contraindication is child's pose. It is a human instinct to assume the fetal position, or child's pose, when seeking physical safety or psychological preservation.

Assess and document:

OK (optimal kinematics)

- Unilateral (lateral child's) or bilateral impairment (child's pose) of the shoulder complex ROM or posterior capsule flexibility, ribcage, or segmental "thoracic ring shift" (defined by Lee, 2012, as the functional unit of the thorax which includes the bilateral ribs, its two adjacent vertebrae and disc, and the anterior attachment to the sternum) as primary drivers of impairment elsewhere in the kinetic chain

- Scoliosis of the spine, including flexion-based derangements that could include vertebral rotation or lateral shifting in the cervical, thoracic, or lumbar areas

- Sacroiliac dysfunction, which could include rotation around a vertical axis, horizontal axis, or torsion (a combination of flexion and rotation or extension and rotation, which equates to four possible torsion directions) could contribute to anterior hip impingement, creating groin, back, lateral hip, gluteal, or pelvic pain. Monitor posterior landmarks, including the SIJ, inferior lateral angle, posterior superior iliac spine (PSIS), and ischial tuberosities, which should grossly move with functional symmetry, ease, and fascial resilience

- Quality of hip flexion or FABER position and presence of any impingement symptoms, which can be indicative of intra-articular hip pathology if groin pain is present during child's/lateral child's pose, which could affect the acetabular labrum, FAI, low back, and SIJ

- Ankle ROM in plantarflexion and inversion

- Asymmetry which could be a red flag for loss of SIJ, hip, or lumbar arthrokinematic mobility, lack of knee or ankle mobility, or myofascial restriction in the thoracolumbar fascia.

MP (motor pattern)

- Proper descent of diaphragm during A-D breath should appear as a thoracolumbar and integumentary expansion as well as posterior and lateral ribcage expansion, rather than a lifting of the upper trunk due to inappropriate chest expansion. This position also allows for manual and tactile cuing or assessment of the thoracolumbar fascia and ability of the patient to breathe into the posterior ribcage, facilitating the "bucket-handle" or lateral and posterior lifting of the ribcage that is desirable for progression to TATD breath.

TESMI (tissue extensibility and sensorimotor integration)

- Myofascial response from the suboccipital region to thoracolumbar fascia, which could be driven by diaphragmatic dysfunction, scar adhesions from

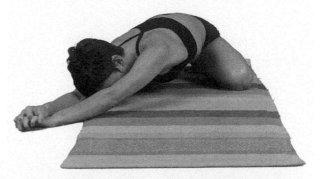

Figure 5.26
Lateral child's pose

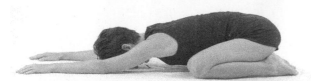

Figure 5.25
Child's pose

surgery to the abdomen or torso, chronic pain, loss of hip joint FABER, visceral fascial impairment, or loss of glenohumeral joint flexion or posterior capsule restriction. Note unilateral myofascial impairment in the lateral raphe during lateral child's pose

- Pelvic length/tension relationship could prevent proper diaphragmatic descent and/or could place excessive downward force on the pelvic floor musculature. Influential variables could include loss of hip FABER ROM, myofascial restriction in the trunk or visceral fascia, tonic recruitment or spasm of the obturator internus or pelvic floor

- Differential diagnosis of calf pliability or proximal muscle belly pain (deep vein thrombosis, gastrointestinal motility issues, edema, or electrolyte imbalance)

- Lateral child's pose — Neurovascular impairment indicative of potential thoracic outlet syndrome in more severe cases where glenohumeral horizontal abduction is not possible.

Cobra (A-D breath only) (Figs 5.27 and 5.28)

Assess and document:

OK (optimal kinematics)

- Segmental vertebral form closure during spinal extension, especially at C7–T1, T8–T12 and L4–S1, where the majority of spinal extension takes place (Neumann, 2010)

- Ribcage form closure during thoracolumbar extension (no presence of any ring (ribcage) shifts, which includes thoracic vertebral rotation)

- Humeral head form closure during shoulder extension (no presence of anterior translation, scapular protraction, pectoralis shortening)

- Presence of abnormal shear extension moment or lateral shifting of the lumbar spine

- SIJ form closure — Appropriate nutation with reciprocal posterior glide of ilia at inferior lateral angle; no presence of excessive nutation (rotation around horizontal axis), rotation around vertical axis, or a torsion moment (combination of two types of rotation can create four possible torsion moments). Lack of form closure is indicative of extension-based SIJ disorder.

MP (motor pattern)

- Cobra with only A-D breath uses the arms to extend the spine, rather than dynamic stabilization. Watch for force closure of the shoulder complex (no shoulder shrugging, loss of humeral head force closure)

- Cobra with TATD breath (dynamic stabilization) follows in the next section.

TESMI (tissue extensibility and sensorimotor integration)

- Myofascial response over superficial and deep front lines, as well as spiral, functional, and arm lines, and the response of the anterior soft tissue and fascia during knees bent position. If the psoas or rectus femoris are restricted, or any associated fascia, the pelvis will improperly rise from the floor

- How the patient responds to being asked to lie prone. This could cause anxiety in older populations, those with significant orthopaedic or neuromuscular

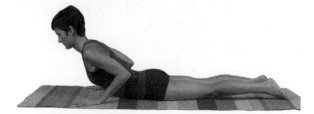

Figure 5.27
Cobra without knee flexion

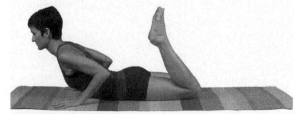

Figure 5.28
Cobra with knee flexion

impairments, or those with anxiety or history of past trauma.

Supine TATD breath postures (Table 5.6)

Instructions in Chapter 8.

Pre-posture prerequisites include:

1. Arm spiral

2. Arm floats

3. Hook lying knee lifts

4. A/P spinal non-articulation (bridge)

5. A/P spinal segmental articulation (two-foot)

6. Lateral segmental spinal articulation (TATD wind-shield wipers).

Arm spiral and arm floats – supine, seated, and/or standing (Fig. 5.29 and Fig. 5.30)

Code 5.4 (free code)	
Arm spiral	

Table 5.6

Supine transversus abdominis-assisted thoracodiaphragmatic (TATD) breath postures

Posture	Figure	QR code
Arm spiral	Figs 5.29–5.30	Code 5.4
Arm floats	Figs 5.31–5.33	
Hook lying knee lifts	Figs 5.34–5.35	Code 5.7
Anterior/posterior non-articulation (bridge)	Fig. 5.36	
Anterior/posterior articulation (two-foot)	Figs 5.37–5.42	
Lateral segmental spinal articulation	Figs 5.19–5.24	Code 5.9 Code 5.3

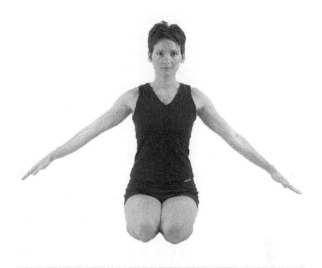

Figure 5.29
Arm spiral at 45 degrees

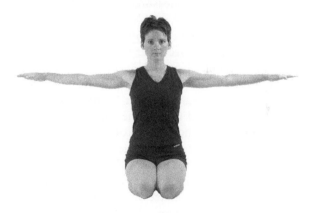

Figure 5.30
Arm spiral at 90 degrees

Supine arm spiral and arm floats are given as an option when RTC deficiency, lack of postural awareness and/or control, adverse neural tension, or shoulder injury precludes seated/against gravity shoulder functional assessment. Scapular repositioning can be performed in seated and standing arm spiral and arm floats.

Repositioning has been supported to diminish open kinetic chain-related pain with shoulder elevation (overhead motion) in diagnosed scapular dyskinesis patients who are symptomatic (Kibler et al.,

2013; Pluim, 2013). Arm spiral can be used for patient education and autogenic biofeedback for cultivation of postural awareness, proper respiration, and healthy upper extremity movement strategies that use glenohumeral joint abduction, external rotation, forearm supination and pronation, and wrist extension.

Arm floats are performed in supine and standing with a yoga apparatus such as a bamboo cane (active assistive ROM (AAROM)) or belt (higher-level AAROM) to provide tactile feedback for motor planning strategy that involves concomitant upper quarter and trunk stability. Arm floats are used as an initial measure of glenohumeral joint flexion and periscapular control and should first be assessed in supine hook lying and in full supine lying (to minimize degrees of freedom) if possible, with progression to standing assessment second. Supine hook lying offers a measure without the influence of the psoas while full supine lying measures shoulder flexion considering the secondary variable of psoas length. If the iliopsoas is shortened and impacts myofascial resilience or is impaired secondary to scarring or adhesions in the trunk placed when on full stretch, then glenohumeral flexion will be implicated in full-supine lying. If iliopsoas is not a factor in shoulder flexion, then hook lying and full supine lying will yield the same goniometric shoulder flexion ROM measurement. The upper psoas, if implicated, can cause the upper lumbar segments to flex, while the lower psoas could create a lumbar extension moment, which ultimately impairs maintenance of spinal neutral and full glenohumeral joint flexion.

Optional measures include the following:

Scapular repositioning test (SRT)

Code 5.5 (free code)
Scapular repositioning test

The SRT was validated in a study of 98 athletes with positive subacromial impingement (SAI), matched with 44 athletes with SAI. Using the SRT, approximately half had reduced pain, with half of those with reduced pain experiencing increased strength (Tate et al., 2008).

The SRT is performed during shoulder elevation via assisting the patient with scapular positioning by applying posterior tilt and external rotation motion to the scapula. A positive test is one where the patient complaining of SAI symptoms experiences decreased pain and/or increased strength with the SRT.

Scapular assistance test (SAT)

Code 5.6 (free code)
Scapular assistance test

The SAT is posited to improve scapular orientation in those with SAI symptoms (Seitz et al., 2012a, 2012b). In a study of 42 subjects, use of the SAT increased scapular posterior tilt, upward rotation, and acromiohumeral distance in various positions (rest, 45 degrees, and 90 degrees elevation) (Seitz et al., 2012a, 2012b). The SAT is performed by assisting movement of the scapula to increase subacromial space via provision of manual assistance for scapular mobility during arm elevation. This assisted action eliminates the impingement mid-arc pain in patients with dynamic/secondary impingement and implies scapula rehabilitation exercises are required. See Codes 5.5 and 5.6 for demonstration of both open and closed kinetic chain versions of the SRT and SAT.

Arm spiral and arm floats (Figs 5.31–5.33)

The entire pose is introduced here in full instructional format, rather than "assess and document" only.

TI (therapeutic intention)

- Gateway postures in the FMA. Arm spiral is a foundation for all yoga postures that involve arm movement or placement and is used in almost all open and closed kinetic chain positions during yoga posture performance. Arm floats are used during transitions in yoga postures.

- Arm spiral is necessary for stabilization of the upper extremity for writing, fine motor, visual motor, and self-care tasks. Specifically for the pediatric population with handwriting, visual motor, and fine motor difficulties, shoulder stabilization

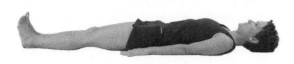

Figure 5.31
Arm floats step 1

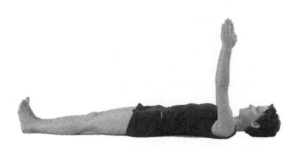

Figure 5.32
Arm floats step 2

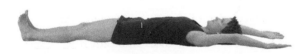

Figure 5.33
Arm floats step 3. Repeat steps 1–3 in reverse order to assess return quality of movement

is needed for distal control of the arm, wrists, and fingers (Wilson and Trombly, 1984; Jover et al., 2010).

- Arm floats can be used to quantitatively and qualitatively measure the level of ADL (e.g. removing shirt, drying hair, independent ADL such as housework, grocery shopping), work (e.g. construction worker, caregiver), or leisure activities that require overhead reaching, in particular repetitive reaching, throwing or reaching with a balance component, or lifting objects above 90 degrees of shoulder flexion.

- Identify RTC impairment — The RTC's role in abduction of the arm is important, but its role in preventing humeral head translation is paramount (Escamilla et al., 2009). Decreased RTC activity via cadaver dissection/removal of the RTC and subsequent electromyographic (EMG) analysis reveals deltoid contribution to humeral head superior translation during early abduction, leading to impingement (Page, 2011).

SP (starting position) Supine lying, hook lying (supine version), seated, or standing.

Arm spiral action

Entry Abduct the glenohumeral joint to 45 degrees. If scapular dyskinesis, RTC impingement, or neurovascular impairment is not present, abduct to 90 degrees. The elbows are in anatomical position at 45 or 90 degrees of glenohumeral abduction, while the forearm is supinated. Externally rotate the glenohumeral joints. Co-activate the biceps/triceps concomitantly with shoulder depression and medial scapular rotation. Then add forearm pronation. Scapular stability is provided from this action, predominantly by the force couple of the serratus anterior, lower trapezius, and minimal recruitment of the upper trapezius (to facilitate the force couple). The scapulae should be within functional limits for symmetry in dynamic movement without scapular internal rotation (winging) or anterior rotation (tipping), or excessive upper trapezius recruitment.

Exit Bring the arms to the side.

SRAs (static restorative approximations) Supine lying "snow angels" — Resting in supine or hook lying, assume arm spiral with the arms resting on the floor.

DMs (dynamic modifications)

- Supine "snow angels" — After performing the SRA version, actively abduct the glenohumeral joints from 0 to 90 degrees, using the arm spiral action instructions. Note impairments in musculoskeletal, neuromuscular, neurovascular, pulmonary, or myofascial function.

- Standing modification — Leave the arms in true *"anatomical position,"* described as 45 degrees or less of glenohumeral abduction, with forearm supination, if there is an active RTC or labrum lesion or remarkable dyskinesis.

TTCP (teaching and tactical cuing primer)

- Arm spiral is not a scapular retraction effort. It is a multisystem effort involving isotonic scapular depression with isometric serratus anterior action to secure the scapula to the chest wall, with the lower trapezius stabilizing the scapula and thoracic spine, as well as the preceding movements.

- Oppositional movement — The arms reach in opposition, away from one another. The biceps eccentrically co-activate while the triceps act concentrically.

- Shoulder complex autogenic biofeedback and proprioceptive training for correction of scapular dyskinesis and related abnormal breath habits.

- Concomitant co-activation — Lengthen over the anterior surface of the arm while concomitantly shortening or strengthening the posterior arm.

Contraindications   Acute RTC or glenoid labrum lesion.

Arm floats

SP (starting position)   Supine (to eliminate degrees of freedom) or standing (to progress).

Entry   With the thumbs pointing superiorly and the wrist in neutral midway between forearm supination and pronation, inhale and lift the arms to 90 degrees shoulder flexion while screening for adequate scapulohumeral rhythm and compensatory patterns such as shoulder elevation, thoracic extension or lumbar extension instead of shoulder flexion. Exhale and progress from 90 degrees flexion up to 180 degrees flexion. The point just before any compensatory patterns are noticed represents the accurate measure of glenohumeral joint flexion. Substitution of spine movement (loss of spinal neutral) can indicate glenohumeral joint restriction, lack of postural control, or myofascial restriction that inappropriately transfers load to the spine. Measure glenohumeral joint flexion with and without hip and knee flexion (hook lying) in order to differentiate regional contribution of the iliopsoas and associated fascia to glenohumeral joint ROM.

Exit   Inhale and return to 90 degrees flexion. Exhale and return to zero degrees flexion or neutral in the shoulder. Repeat 3–5 times to obtain an accurate measure and also note any deterioration of movement strategy.

SRAs (static restorative approximations)   Guided imagery.

DMs (dynamic modifications)   Limit shoulder and hip joint ROM to what can safely be completed with good technique (no compensatory patterns, breath-holding, lower quarter involvement, myofascial restriction, or neural tension). If the hip contributes to loss of shoulder ROM, perform the pose from hook lying.

TTCP (teaching and tactical cuing primer)

- Keep thumbs-up (neutral forearm) position for open coracoacromial arch space.

- Measure each upper extremity individually. The majority of individuals will not display bilaterally symmetrical shoulder flexion.

- Documentation of glenohumeral joint flexion:

  - in hook lying/bent knees and feet flat _____

    straight knees and legs flat in supine _____.

Contraindications   Conditions where AROM or AAROM of the glenohumeral joint is contraindicated, such as post-surgical RTC repair or tear.

Assess and document:

OK (optimal kinematics)

- Open (when arms are in space) and closed (when arms are in contact with the ground or other surface) kinetic chain FMA for scapular dyskinesis, should assess and document:

  - scapular winging (spinal border lifting of the scapula during shoulder abduction or internal rotation of scapula), or

  - tipping (inferior angle lifting of the scapula away from the chest wall during shoulder abduction)

- Arm spiral (screen during humeral elevation to 90 degrees) and arm floats (screen during humeral elevation to 180 degrees) — With humeral elevation, early or excessive scapular protraction decreases subacromial space and supraspinatus force abduction (Escamilla et al., 2009). Dyskinesis severely alters optimal mechanics of the shoulder complex and is associated with increased glenohumeral horizontal abduction and RTC strength imbalance and weakness or general fatigue, as well as decreased available coracoacromial arch space for clearance of the RTC due to chronically altered postural mechanics such as posterior capsular contracture and altered scapular orientation (Mihata et al., 2008), pain avoidance patterns, and local inflammation or fraying of the RTC tendon(s) (Kibler et al., 2013)

- Arthrokinematic and osteokinematic (shoulder elevation) shoulder complex assessment — Lack of arthrokinematic mobility prevents full ROM in shoulder elevation and is a red flag that warrants differential diagnosis and an arthrokinematic shoulder mobility screen

- Dissociation of spinal extension strategy from shoulder elevation, which may be seen in supine and/or standing version(s)

- Any excessive thoracic kyphosis (signified by the posterior shoulder and scapular spine not resting on the floor).

MP (motor pattern)

- Upper quarter isometric and isotonic neuromuscular patterning integrity — Motor patterning screening for contributions to scapular dyskinesis etiology including: limited glenohumeral joint internal rotation, alterations in periscapular neural patterning or weakness involving the serratus anterior's role of medial border and inferior angle scapular stabilization (preventing scapular winging and anterior tilt) (Escamilla et al., 2009) and upper or lower trapezius force coupling or delayed onset (Kibler et al., 2012)

- Postural control can be a likely culprit of scapular dyskinesis from seated or standing arm spiral or arm floats/upstretched mountain, including poor yoga execution such as allowing scapular sloping or protraction, reversal of spinal curves, excessive thoracic kyphosis or glenohumeral joint hyperflexion, otherwise known as the SICK position (scapular malposition, inferior medial border prominence, coracoid pain and malposition, and dyskinesis of scapular movement) (Kibler et al., 2012). Labral tears and directional or multidirectional stability can also be implicated as a result of, or in combination with, scapular dyskinesis.

TESMI (tissue extensibility and sensorimotor integration)

Arm spiral

- Dynamic upper limb neural tension test (median and ulnar nerves):

  - median nerve — An active version of the upper limb neural tension test can be achieved via arm spiral. The test is positive when evidence of numbness, tingling, loss of or change in sensation is felt in the first three fingers and corresponding palm of either hand

  - ulnar nerve — Ulnar nerve tension is found by adding wrist and finger extension while maintaining arm spiral and is positive when evidence of numbness, tingling, loss of or change of sensation is felt in the last two fingers and/or ulnar side of either hand. *To progress*: add elbow flexion. Note that there are often neural signs and symptoms in absence of other deficits indicative of pathological neural tension or impingement. In these cases, arm spiral can be used as a neural mobilization to address the neural tension.

- Notice trophic/skin changes and/or myofascial presentation which may commonly be found in, but are not limited to, the functional, arm, or superficial or deep front lines/bands.

- Pectoralis major and/or minor length. Soft tissue etiology of scapular dyskinesis includes pectoralis shortening and biceps (short head) muscle shortening (Escamilla et al., 2009).

Arm floats

Superficial front or back, and/or deep front line fascia resilience to glenohumeral joint mobility in hook lying versus full supine lying. In standing, all myofascial planes become relevant for screening.

Arm floats in supine

Differentiate between upper quarter (glenohumeral joint or supradiaphragmatic fascia) versus lower quarter (hip joint or subdiaphragmatic and visceral deep front line fascia) contribution/inhibition of glenohumeral joint ROM capability.

Hook lying knee lifts (Figs 5.34 and 5.35)

Code 5.7 (free code)
Hook lying knee lifts

TI (therapeutic intention)

- Assessment of postural control and lumbopelvic strength and motor planning, including pelvic floor functioning

- Foundational position for completing ADL such as ambulation, stair-climbing, or floor-to-standing (or vice versa) transfers.

SP (starting position) Lying on the back with the knees bent and feet resting flat on the mat about hip width apart.

Action

1. Place the hands with the thumbs on the distal ribcage and the middle fingers on the ASIS.

2. Find the anterior/posterior neutral spine (plumb line alignment from the ear to the knee region maintaining lumbar lordosis).

3. Find lateral neutral (position which maintains the ASIS and pubic symphysis in roughly the same plane, with ASIS grossly symmetrical in alignment in the sagittal plane).

4. Engage TATD breath.

5. Unload a single extremity (lift the heel 1–3 inches) without allowing the pelvis to translate (rock or see-saw) in space while maintaining TATD breath. If the heel can be lifted with pelvic translation, progress to lifting the entire foot (advanced).

6. Repeat for 5–10 TATD breaths while reciprocally marching.

Assess and document:

OK (optimal kinematics) Gross objective measure of pelvic translation observed during action. Movement strategy and how lifting the unilateral extremity affects load transfer to the pelvis and spine.

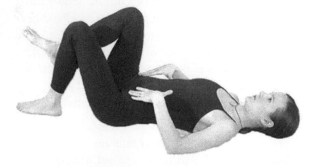

Figure 5.34
Hook lying knee lifts 1

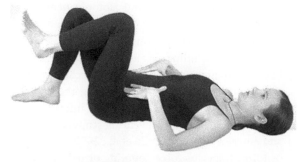

Figure 5.35
Hook lying knee lifts 2

MP (motor pattern)

- Quality and endurance of TATD contraction. All four components (transversus abdominis, respiratory and pelvic diaphragm, and multifidus) should be employed

- Compensatory patterns (use of external oblique or rectus abdominis as a dominant strategy, lack of pelvic or respiratory diaphragm engagement, downward pressure on the pelvic diaphragm, or paradoxical or absent use of the respiratory diaphragm).

TESMI (tissue extensibility and sensorimotor integration)   Pain, breath-holding, or presence of any neurovascular (pelvic area) or myofascial contribution (superficial front and back line or deep front line) could inhibit TATD breath and execution of the pre-posture. Functional and spiral lines could be implicated if any abdominal, pelvic, or hip scars are present, or if there is history of past trauma.

Bridge (A/P non-articulation) (Fig. 5.36)

Two-foot (A/P articulation) (Figs 5.37–5.42)

> **Code 5.8** (free code)
> Anterior/posterior non-articulation and segmental spinal articulation
>

SP (starting position)   Hook lying knee lift position (in neutral spine for bridge and in posterior tilt for two-foot).

Bridge does not allow for spinal segmental articulation but assesses pelvic lift quality in neutral spine and TATD to a point where a line drawn connects the pelvis to the shoulder. Two-foot allows for spinal segmental articulation and mobilization.

Assess and document:

OK (optimal kinematics)

- Bridge — Ability to maintain spinal neutral (cervical lordosis, thoracic kyphosis, and lumbar lordosis)

- Two-foot — Quality of segmental articulation in a distal to proximal fashion (lumbar to thoracic)

of each vertebral segment while maintaining TATD breath

- Identify segments that are not articulating, ones that give rise to signs or symptoms of back pain, neural tension, myofascial release, or breath alteration.

MP (motor pattern)

- The patient should be able to dissociate:

  - TATD breath from gluteal contraction as a primary movement strategy

  - gluteal contraction from hamstring action

  - hip external rotator contraction from gluteal contraction

  - anterior tibialis and quadriceps from iliopsoas dominance and hamstring contraction (which assists in iliopsoas tendonitis rehabilitation) (Edelstein, 2009), all while maintaining TATD breath.

- Once these dissociation patterns have been established, and SIJ has been ruled out, the gluteus maximus (GMAX) can be recruited again as a joint movement strategy.

TESMI (tissue extensibility and sensorimotor integration)   See previous posture for assessment recommendations.

Watch for five levels of cervical spine involvement:

1. Skin and/or trophic changes in the neck and surrounding area

2. Fascial restriction in the superficial or deep front lines/bands that could implicate other lines

3. Muscular involuntary or voluntary tonic contraction of the cervical paraspinals with or without cervical lordosis reversal

4. Nuchal ligament tension may impair diaphragmatic descent via fascial connections

5. Periodontal pain related to fascial connections via the diaphragm and the relationship of the phrenic nerve to the trigeminal nerve (Bordoni and Zanier, 2013).

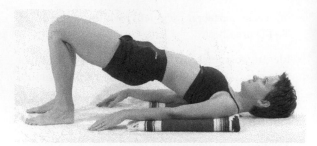

Figure 5.36
Supported bridge

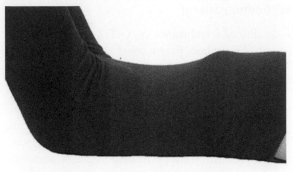

Figure 5.37
Anterior/posterior articulation (two-foot) posterior pelvic tilt

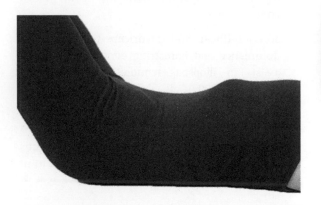

Figure 5.38
Anterior/posterior articulation (two-foot) posterior pelvic tilt with sacral apex flexion and lift

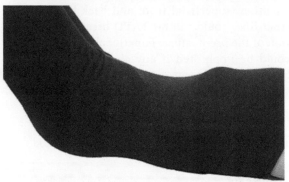

Figure 5.39
Anterior/posterior articulation (two-foot) posterior pelvic tilt with lumbar flexion and lift

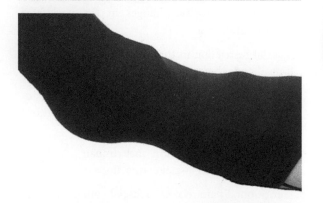

Figure 5.40
Anterior/posterior articulation (two-foot) mild posterior pelvic tilt with thoracic flexion and lift

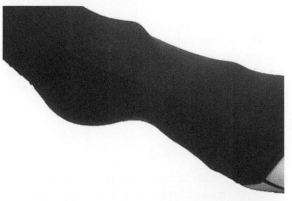

Figure 5.41
Anterior/posterior articulation (two-foot) arrive at spinal neutral (bridge)

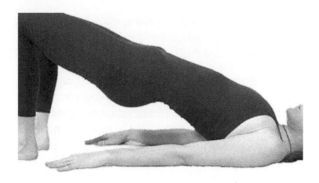

Figure 5.42
Anterior/posterior articulation (two-foot) slight glenohumeral joint external rotation and chest expansion with minimal reversal of thoracic kyphosis

Lateral articulation (windshield wipers with TATD breath)

> **Code 5.9** (free code)
> Lateral segmental spinal articulation

The theory of the lateral articulation maneuver is to assess which multifidus segments may not be firing and which vertebral segments may lack normal kinematic segmental mobility based on which vertebral segments are skipped (via palpation) during return to hook lying. Unilateral recruitment, motor patterning, fascial integrity, strength, endurance of the transversus abdominis and obliques can also be assessed using lateral articulation.

SP (starting position) Windshield wipers, which is hook lying knee lift position outside of neutral (posterior tilt). The ipsilateral hand (same hand as the direction of rotation) rests on the abdomen and the contralateral hand palpates the spine, beginning in the upper thoracic region and progressing to the lumbar region and sacrum.

1. The action of the posture allows the knees to drop independently in the same direction. Place a block or bolster under the knees to avoid terminal rotation as necessary if there is pain, excessive lumbar or limited thoracolumbar rotation, or other contraindication.

2. Exhale and engage TATD breath to segmentally return to hook lying moving from proximal to distal segments (beginning with upper thoracic spine first). The knees should follow kinetically as a consequence of, not as a primary initiator of, spinal movement.

Assess and document:

OK (optimal kinematics)

- Vertebral segments that do not articulate

- Location of spinal rotation. The majority of rotation should come from T1–T8 with a small contribution from L1–S1 (Neumann, 2010)

- Loss or delay of hip or sacroiliac joint ROM that creates functional impairment or hip impingement.

MP (motor pattern)

- Improper movement patterns such as primary recruitment of the external obliques, rectus abdominis *"loafing,"* upper trapezius, secondary muscles of respiration, mask of the face, increased pressure through the pelvic floor seen through bulging of the lower abdominal wall, valsalva, and/or failure to engage TATD breath

- Use of the hamstrings to draw the heels (isometrically) toward the body, to remove pressure from the neck and also working synergistic muscles of trunk stabilization (versus using a knee extension moment, which increases cervical spine load).

TESMI (tissue extensibility and sensorimotor integration) See windshield wipers.

Contraindication for two-foot posture and lateral articulation Osteoporosis, spondylolisthesis, anterior disc derangements, acute degenerative joint disease or degenerative disc disease, osteophyte formation or compression fractures, and possibly those with spondylosis.

Seated TATD postures (Table 5.7)

See instructions in Chapter 7 for cow arms and staff pose; Chapter 6 for eagle arms.

1. Shoulder lock (see previous section)

2. Arm spiral (see previous section)

3. Shoulder opener

4. Cow arms

5. Eagle arms

6. Staff pose.

Shoulder opener – seated and standing
(Figs 5.43–5.50)

TI (therapeutic intention)   Shoulder opener is an FMA posture and gateway pre-posture for all postures using upper extremity elevation greater than 45 degrees. It can be performed in seated and/or standing, but supine lying is also an option if arm floats do not provide adequate biofeedback for safe performance or patient self-correction. The difference between shoulder opener and arm floats is the former is performed in scaption and the latter is performed with glenohumeral flexion. In addition to arm spiral and arm float benefits therapeutic intentions include assessing the endurance and strength (power) of the upper quarter to perform repetitive motion with isometric (yoga belt) or variable isotonic (Theraband™) resistance training. The SRT or SAT can diminish subacromial

Table 5.7
Seated transversus abdominis-assisted thoracodiaphragmatic (TATD) breath postures

Postures	Figure
Shoulder opener	Figs 5.43–5.50
Cow arms	Figs 5.51–5.54
Eagle arms	Figs 5.55–5.59
Staff pose	Figs 5.60–5.62

impingement, provide periscapular biofeedback, and decrease periscapular muscle inhibition in this posture.

SP (starting position)   Supine lying or supported version over yoga couch; to increase degrees of freedom, use a seated version (thunderbolt, backless chair, or stool). Standing could be used to progress the pose for advanced practitioners who need all degrees of freedom to improve functional performance.

Entry   Use a yoga belt made of cotton or a high-resistance Theraband to maintain active horizontal abduction moment. With the arms in scaption (90 degrees flexion plus 45 degrees horizontal abduction), maintain horizontal abduction and scapular depression via strap grasp with the thumbs facing skyward. Flex the shoulder on inhale, following one of the options in DM. Maintain plumb line alignment and spinal neutral. The elbow remains in neutral (no hyperextension or flexion). Only move through a ROM that maintains proximal trunk and shoulder control.

Exit   Exhale to return to the starting position. If circumducted, inhale and return to 180 flexion.

SRAs (static restorative approximations)   Supine arm floats or guided imagery.

DMs (dynamic modifications)

- Novice — Supine shoulder opener (arm floats in scaption with strap). Use partial ROM or AAROM with a cane

- Intermediate — Seated (eliminates lower quarter degrees of freedom) with partial to full ROM

- Advanced — Standing (full version introduces all degrees of freedom in upper and lower quarter and trunk) with full ROM.

TTCP (teaching and tactical cuing primer)

- Students' bodies tend to take the path of least resistance in this pose either from ego, musculoskeletal restriction, or ignorance (*avidya*), such as lack of postural awareness or control.

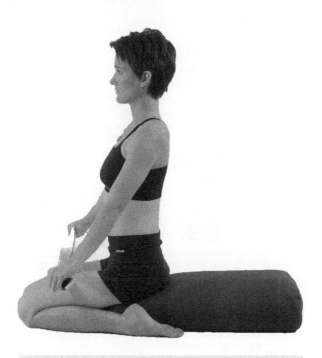

Figure 5.43
Shoulder opener step 1

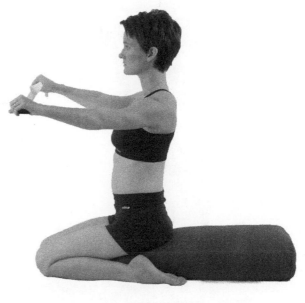

Figure 5.44
Shoulder opener step 2

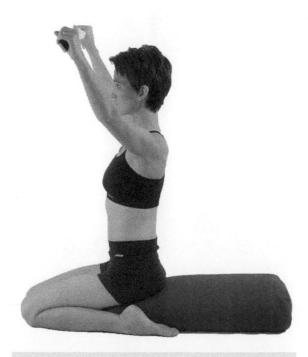

Figure 5.45
Shoulder opener step 3

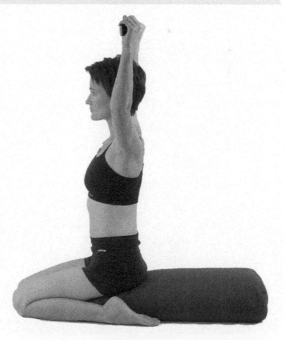

Figure 5.46
Shoulder opener step 4 (advanced). Most people will finish at step 3 and may need therapy to achieve full shoulder flexion (180 degrees) if needed for functional task completion and activities of daily living

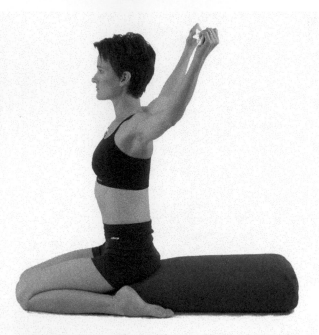

Figure 5.47
Shoulder opener step 5 (advanced)

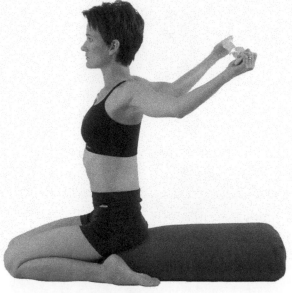

Figure 5.48
Shoulder opener step 6 (advanced)

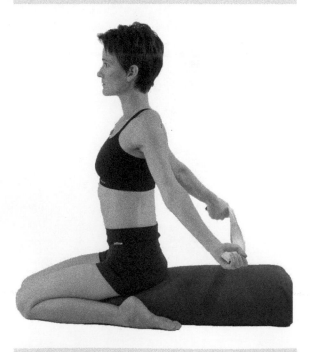

Figure 5.49
Shoulder opener step 7 (advanced)

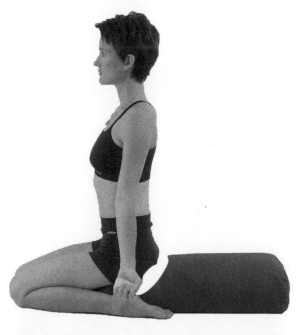

Figure 5.50
Shoulder opener step 8 (advanced)

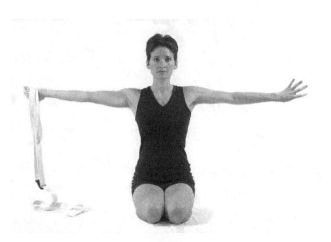

Figure 5.51
Cow arms with strap anterior sagittal view

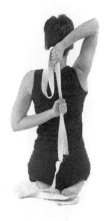

Figure 5.52
Cow arms with strap
posterior sagittal view

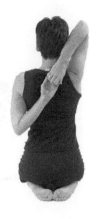

Figure 5.53
Cow arms full
posterior sagittal view

- Give tactile feedback for spinal alignment and glenohumeral and scapulothoracic positioning (hand placement on anterior glenohumeral joint for approximation and biofeedback as well as opposite hand on the inferior angle of the scapula for approximation).

Contraindications Glenohumeral instability; stubbornness; painful arc of motion, active RTC lesion, or impingement preventing pain-free shoulder elevation greater than 45–60 degrees; pregnancy should limit full circumduction.

Assess and document:

Follow recommendations for arm floats.

Cow arms (Figs 5.51–5.54)

Cow arms assess Apley's functional reach test for measuring glenohumeral external and internal rotation with simultaneous functional measurement of the following measures.

Assess and document:

OK (optimal kinematics)

- Externally rotated arm: glenohumeral abduction to 90 degrees with forearm supination, then full external rotation followed by shoulder scaption and elbow flexion

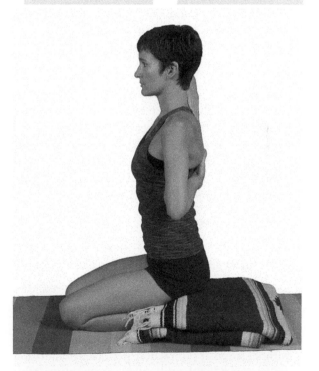

Figure 5.54
Cow arms full lateral frontal view

- Internally rotated arm: glenohumeral abduction to 90 degrees then full internal rotation followed by horizontal adduction, some shoulder extension,

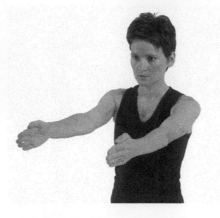

Figure 5.55
Eagle arms step 1

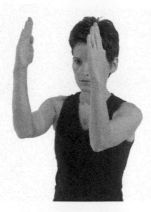

Figure 5.56
Eagle arms step 2

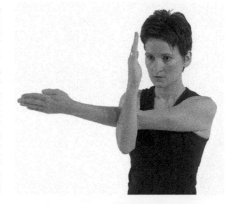

Figure 5.57
Eagle arms step 3

elbow flexion, and forearm pronation. Monitor for form closure of humerus especially on internal rotation arm. Use the "two-finger" approach

- Maintenance of spinal neutral and TATD breath

- Measure the distance between the hands (when placed behind the back) in cm or the spinal or pelvic level to which the patient can reach – for example, 5 cm distance between the hands on right cow arms (right arm in shoulder flexion/external rotation) or internal rotation – able to reach to iliac crest level; external rotation – able to reach to T2 level.

MP (motor pattern)

- Abduction to 90 degrees — Note upper trapezius recruitment and/or lack of periscapular strength

- External or internal rotation — The patient should be able to externally rotate humerus without compensatory action at the trunk (extension). The patient should be able to internally rotate the humerus without scapular protraction, pectoralis domination or "*peccing it*," or shoulder sloping without excessive arthrokinematic anterior humeral glide.

TESMI (tissue extensibility and sensorimotor integration)

- Pectoralis major/minor extensibility

- Superficial and deep front, spiral, arm (anterior for front arm and posterior for back arm), and

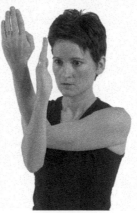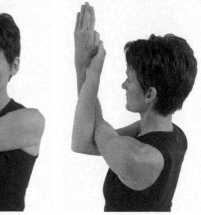

Figure 5.58
Eagle arms step 4

Figure 5.59
Eagle arms step 5

functional myofascial lines/bands may be primarily implicated

- Addition of contralateral cervical rotation away from upper arm can add myofascial tension over the face and scalene and subclavius area.

Eagle arms (Figs 5.55–5.59)

The majority of the population will not have the proprioceptive ability, postural support, and/or posterior cuff/capsule flexibility to complete the full arm position. This is inconsequential, however, because the full pose does not need to be performed. Use a dose–response ROM that provides the target therapeutic intention, which is posterior cuff and capsule stretch with concomitant periscapular strengthening to facilitate healthy glenohumeral joint ROM and correct any scapular dyskinesis. Limit degrees of freedom by not wrapping the arms, only crossing the arms, and/or eliminating elbow flexion.

Assess and document:

OK (optimal kinematics)

- Hawkins–Kennedy test for subacromial impingement (horizontal adduction coupled with 90–110 degrees shoulder flexion with neutral rotation or internal rotation), which has moderate sensitivity and specificity (Cook and Hegedus, 2013)

- ROM — Coupled shoulder flexion to 90 degrees with full horizontal adduction and external rotation

- Maintenance of spinal neutral during a hip flexion moment.

MP (motor pattern)

- Eagle arms is not a scapular protraction pose. It is a periscapular strengthener in a small zone of motion that, through scapulothoracic stabilization, isolates the posterior RTC of the shoulder. The action of eagle arms is isotonic scapular depression and medial rotation with isometric horizontal abduction once the arms are intertwined.

- Periscapular strength in scapular depression and medial rotation. Nonoperative treatment of SLAP tears has been successful with inclusion of periscapular and RTC strengthening and posterior capsule mobility and stretching, with a majority of athletes returning to sport within 6 months or less (Edwards et al., 2010).

TESMI (tissue extensibility and sensorimotor integration)

- Posterior RTC and capsule extensibility (threading the needle is the only other yoga posture that offers posterior cuff tensile force)

- Superficial back line, posterior functional, arm, and spiral myofascial lines/bands may be primarily implicated

- Presence of any neurovascular impairment in the brachial plexus.

Staff pose (Figs 5.60–5.62)

Staff pose provides the opportunity to test postural awareness and control, hamstring length, sciatic nerve and associated vascular integrity, myofascial response, and movement strategy in long-sitting.

Assess and document:

OK (optimal kinematics) Presence of abnormal load transfer from posterior pelvic tilt or SIJ dysfunction (palpate PSIS and inferior lateral angle to identify rotation or torsion moments) which would indicate a flexion-based SIJ disorder.

MP (motor pattern) Ability to long sit without iliopsoas gripping and with appropriate percentage of maximum voluntary isometric contraction (MVIC) TATD recruitment.

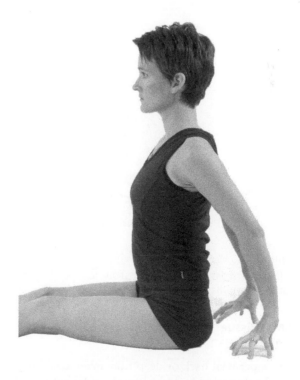

Figure 5.60
Staff pose, full with *"spider legs"* fingers

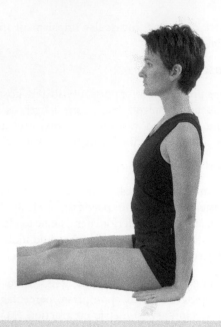

Figure 5.61
Staff pose, full with flat palm support

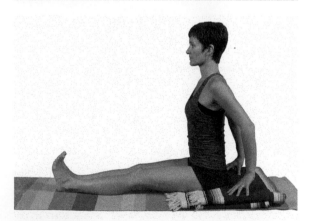

Figure 5.62
Staff pose, modified with scaffolded quarter-fold blanket support and *"spider legs"* fingers

TESMI (tissue extensibility and sensorimotor integration)

- The superficial back or deep front myofascial lines via diaphragmatic connections may be primarily implicated

- Shortening of the abdominal musculature from long-term posterior pelvic tilting, poor posture, guarding, gripping of the gluteals, or deep front or superficial back line or band restriction

- Excessive pelvic floor tension due to any of the above impairments or birth trauma or lack of post-partum rehabilitation that could contribute to or exacerbate pelvic pain

- Evidence of neural tension in the sciatic nerve (peripheral nerves) or spinal meninges, especially with knee extension and ankle dorsiflexion.

Sequenced TATD compositions (Table 5.8)

Instructions in Chapters 10 (semi-inversions) and 11 (salutations).

1. Moon salutation

2. Sun salutation.

Prone components to compositions

Instructions in Chapter 9 with exceptions as noted.

1. Cat/cow (optional)

2. Downward-facing dog preparation

3. Downward-facing dog (Chapter 10)

4. Plank

5. Modified dolphin dive (caterpillar) (Chapter 10)

6. Cobra

7. Sphinx

8. Child's pose and "reach, roll, and rise"

9. Transitional lunge (Chapter 6).

Moon salutation composition (Fig. 5.63)

Code 5.10 (free code)
Moon salute composition

Table 5.8

Sequenced transversus abdominis-assisted thoracodia-phragmatic (TATD) compositions

Posture	Figure	QR code
Moon salutation	Fig. 5.63	5.10
Sun salutation	Fig. 5.77	
Prone components to compositions		
Cat/cow	Figs 5.64–5.65 and 9.11–9.16	
Downward-facing dog preparation	Figs 5.66 and 9.17–9.18	
Downward-facing dog	Figs 5.67–5.68	
Plank	Figs 5.69 and 9.19–9.20	
Modified dolphin dive (caterpillar)	Figs 5.70–5.72	
Cobra	Figs 5.27–5.28	
Sphinx	Fig. 5.73	
Child's pose	Figs 5.25, 9.2 and 5.74–5.76	
Standing components to compositions		
Mountain	Figs 5.78 and 6.4	
Upstretched mountain	Fig. 5.79	
Chair	Fig. 5.80	
Squat	Fig. 5.81 or Fig. 6.39	
Transitional lunge	Figs 5.82 and 6.14–6.17	
Moon salutation	Fig. 5.63	

Downward-facing dog preparation posture and "glide"

Downward-facing dog preparation includes the postures four-point position, cat/cow (optional), as well as downward-facing dog preparation itself. Downward-facing dog preparation is a pre-posture designed to identify movement impairments and neuromechanical precursors for injury, for example, scapular stabilizer insufficiency or scapular dyskinesis, nonoptimal movement strategies such as trunk flexion and extreme lumbar extension, or primary recruitment of the upper trapezius to stabilize the shoulder complex during the knee lift portion of downward-facing dog preparation. Hands and knees or four-point position is required prior to performance of downward-facing dog preparation.

Assess and document:

OK (optimal kinematics)   Ability to find arm spiral and spinal neutral position from the four-point position with knees placed under the hips and wrists under the shoulders.

MP (motor pattern)   Use of TATD breath in spinal neutral without spinal motion.

TESMI (tissue extensibility and sensorimotor integration)

- Use of the force couple of periscpaular stabilizers, including serratus anterior and the upper and lower trapezius bilaterally, in order to prevent scapular protraction, winging, or tipping. The upper trapezius should not be the primary stabilizer, and should be pliable and not tonically contracted during four-point and downward-facing dog preparation position

- Nonoptimal movement strategy such as posterior gluteal clenching causing posterior pelvic tilt or obliteration of lumbar lordosis or back gripping (i.e. use of superficial paraspinals over deeper multifidus) (Lee, 2011)

- All myofascial lines are critical for identifying movement impairment in this composition.

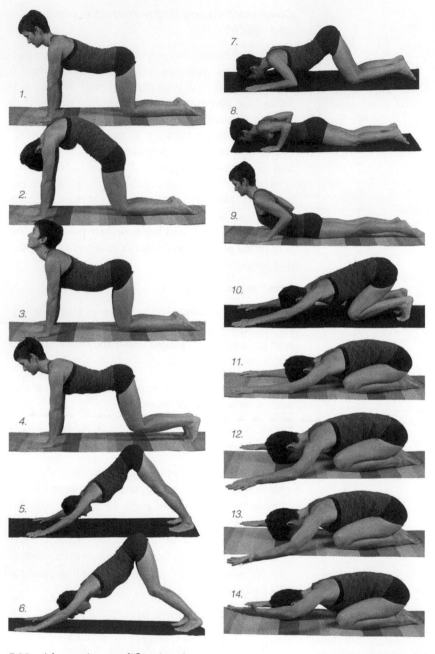

Figure 5.63
Moon salutation composition

DMs (dynamic modifications) Four-point pose can be completed in/from the following:

- Seated with hands against a wall or holding the back of a chair

- The forearms with forearm supination, eliminating elbow and wrist extension.

Cat/cow (optional) (Figs 5.64 and 5.65)

Cat/cow serves as an optional additional general screen for identifying spinal segmental and general movement (osteokinematic) impairments which could be caused by arthrokinematic deficits, musculoskeletal imbalance, pain, myofascial restriction, diaphragmatic dysfunction or poor breathing habits,

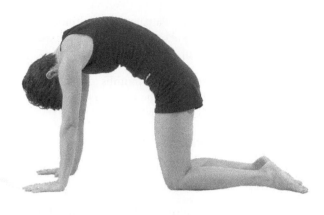

Figure 5.64
Cat

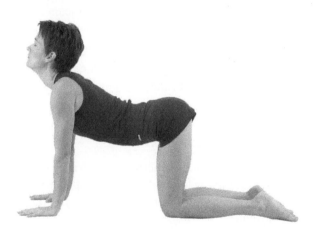

Figure 5.65
Cow

including individual or clusters of segments that do not move within the kinetic chain or that are immobile or rotated due to scoliosis (structural) or movement (functional) impairment in either spinal flexion (cat) or spinal extension (cow).

MP (motor pattern) Closed kinetic chain SAT or SRT for the scapula during entry into cat position and return to cow. The scapulae should move grossly symmetrically bilaterally. Note any premature or delayed scapular lateral rotation (transverse plane) and upward rotation/elevation (frontal plane).

TESMI (tissue extensibility and sensorimotor integration)

- Ability to marry the breath to the movement, using exhale for cat and inhale for cow that are equal in length and at least 5 seconds in duration for each posture

- Dura mater tension or superficial back or deep front myofascial lines may be primarily implicated.

Downward-facing dog preparation (Fig. 5.66)

Assess and document:

OK (optimal kinematics)

- Maintenance of spinal neutral and TATD breath for 5–10 breaths without compensatory strategies or movement in the spine indicative of lack of trunk stabilization strength or control

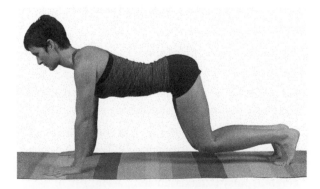

Figure 5.66
Downward-facing dog preparation

or neuromuscular patterning deficits. Although not on the FMA, cat/cow naturally occurs between four-point and downward-facing dog preparation.

Assess and document:

OK (optimal kinematics)

- Ability to begin with lumbosacral movement first rather than leading the movement at the reverse end of the kinetic chain (cervical spine)

- Sacroiliac, lumbar, ribcage, thoracic, or cervical impairment during rest and dynamic movement,

- ROM — Hip flexion, shoulder flexion, wrist extension, shoulder external rotation, forearm pronation, ankle dorsiflexion and plantarflexion, toe flexion and extension, and with cat/cow, global spinal flexion and extension respectively

- Scapular dyskinesis — Scapular winging or tipping or early, delayed, or excessive scapular protraction

- Downward-facing dog preparation "glide" — Ability to glide forward and back (not up and down) while maintaining the 1–2 inch distance of the knees from the floor in downward-facing dog preparation. Continually assess for degradation of movement strategy, structural and functional alignment.

MP (motor pattern)

- Multifidus function screen (see multifidus assessment, below)

- Segmental spinal stability and endurance

- Scapulothoracic stability and endurance

- Progress the pose (lateral weight shift) by having the patient weight shift from left to right hand. Monitor scapular and spinal response

- Progress the pose by having the patient (A/P weight shift) weight shift from the hands to the feet. Monitor for maintenance of spinal neutral or evidence of degradation of the pose (due to lack of endurance, functional scoliosis, multifidus weakness or inhibition, or fascial restriction).

TESMI (tissue extensibility and sensorimotor integration)

- Resting position of global fascia and response during downward-facing dog preparation

- Response of the three diaphragms during the holding phase of downward-facing dog preparation

- Response of forearm flexors and composite extension in four-point position for children with delayed fine motor skills, general developmental delays, or cerebral palsy (Chakerian and Larson, 1993).

Modifications can include supine hook lying TATD or supine hook lying knee lift.

Multifidus assessment Palpate the multifidus to screen for synergistic co-activation with the transversus abdominis for postural control.

Position of therapist Use the thumbs to palpate for multifidus function between the transverse processes of the lumbar spine at each level.

SP (starting position) Four-point or prone.

Action On exhale, engage TATD and breathe while maintaining the contraction.

Negative test The multifidus should be palpable as gradually rising under the thumbs to maintain a tonic contraction. The contraction should release under voluntary action of the student/patient.

The clinician should be able to palpate the multifidus rising under their thumbs and note the following:

- The multifidus "swells" slowly under the thumbs, and should not "pop" up with a quick contraction. "Popping up" is usually the paraspinals substituting for proper multifidus function

- Differences when asking the patient to engage the pelvic floor simultaneously

- Unilateral strength deficits or differences in strength at varying levels of the lumbar spine which may correlate to functional deficits or asymmetry in movement.

Positive test (weak or absent multifidus contribution to postural control) The therapist will feel a quick contraction of the paraspinals that try to compensate for the absence of multifidus function, no multifidus contraction, or a fasciculation or muscle tremor that quickly fades.

Revisit multifidus palpation every 4–6 weeks for changes in contraction quality and quantity. Note the following:

- Length of time contraction is maintained

- Quality of contraction

- Left versus right side comparison

- Varying lumbar level comparison

- Posterior or anterior pelvic tilt
- Gluteal contraction or gripping
- Lumbar flexion
- Thoracic flexion
- Valsalva.

Downward-facing dog posture with and without "ringing the bell" and "slinky"
(Figs 5.67 and 5.68)

Downward-facing dog is an advanced posture because its full form requires full glenohumeral joint flexion in partial arm spiral and full, untethered neuromuscular, myofascial, or neurovascular posterior tissue integrity and upper and lower quarter form and force closure. Use of downward-facing dog as a neuromuscular and musculoskeletal screen requires enough myofasical and neurovascular integrity not to implicate the sciatic nerve or thoracolumbar fascia.

Assess and document:

OK (optimal kinematics)

- Maintenance of spinal curves (avoid reversal of thoracic kyphosis, especially upper thoracic segments, which commonly happens in experienced yoga practitioners; reversal of lumbar lordosis), and shoulder complex (avoid subacromial impingement) integrity
- Performance of downward-facing dog with knees bent and knees straight (if spinal curves can be

maintained) in order to address both the soleus and gastrocnemius length/tension relationship, respectively

- Ability to maintain cervical positioning in the presence of full glenohumeral joint flexion (180 degrees), which the patient can self-evaluate using the "*ringing the bell*" maneuver. This maneuver can be achieved only with 180 degrees of shoulder flexion so that if the cervical spine is sidebent in each direction alternately, the ears touch the medial portion of the proximal humerus bilaterally. Hence, the name "*ringing the bell*," since the head mimics a striker (head) contacting the insides of a bell (shaped bilaterally by each humerus).

MP (motor pattern)

- Maintenance of TATD breath
- Ability to segmentally stabilize and mobilize the vertebrae, screened through the "*slinky*" maneuver. The "*slinky*" is a segmental mobilization of the spine that begins with sacral counternutation and reversal of lumbar lordosis but is ultimately dictated by motor patterning. When lower thoracic flexion is reached, the sacrum begins to counternutate, starting a "wave-like" chain reaction motion that continues up the entire spine, with distal segments flexing until the movement is resolved through reflexive extension that ends with cervical extension and completion of the movement.

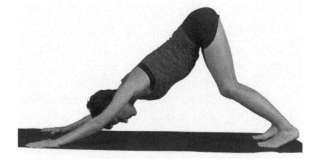

Figure 5.67
Downward-facing dog knee flexion

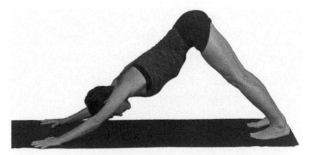

Figure 5.68
Downward-facing dog knee extension

TESMI (tissue extensibility and sensorimotor integration)

- Posterior RTC extensibility or pectoralis domination/"*peccing it*" causes the scapula to excessively protract and the humeral head to translate anteriorly and superiorly, losing form and force closure.

- Global myofascial and neurovascular health — Ask the patient to bear weight through an "*unbroken wrist*" (neutral position of the wrist, which is approximately 5–10 degrees of extension), and across the base of the wrist rather than fingers. Maintenance of forefoot and rearfoot neutral with dorsiflexion (locking) and plantarflexion (unlocking) of the subtalar joint, indicative of adequate mechanoreceptor activity and proprioceptive capability. Toe and plantar fascia and sciatic nerve mobility should allow for toe extension in dorsiflexion. Presence of any sciatic nerve tension, pain, or myofascial restriction, especially in the superficial back and deep front lines, giving regard to functional, arm, and spiral lines if asymmetries are observed.

Plank (Fig. 5.69)

Plank is a transitional pose that can determine placement of the hands and feet in downward-facing dog. It is also a part of four-limbed staff pose and includes variations such as side plank.

Assess and document:

OK (optimal kinematics)

- Hands that are shoulder width apart or wider, and, like the feet, do not require a change in position when transferring from downward-facing dog

- Spinal neutral and full plumb line alignment

- Ankle position in relative neutral, neither dorsiflexed nor plantarflexed.

MP (motor pattern)

- Ability to maintain spinal neutral with prolonged hold of plank

- Scapulothoracic joint control without scapular winging, protraction, or tipping

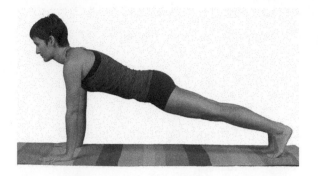

Figure 5.69
Plank

- Ability to inhale from downward-facing dog into plank and exhale back into downward-facing dog while maintaining spinal curves.

TESMI (tissue extensibility and sensorimotor integration) Global myofascial and neurovascular response.

Modified dolphin dive (caterpillar)
(Figs 5.70–5.72)

Modified dolphin dive is a critical maneuver that screens shoulder complex control, postural awareness, periscapular strength and scapulohumeral rhythm, and global proprioceptive awareness.

Assess and document:

OK (optimal kinematics)

- Segmental articulation of the spine in a controlled "dive" to prone lying. Modification is necessary for the majority of patient populations including: spinal articulation contraindication, lack of trunk control, acute stenosis, or weak shoulder complex as follows: perform from forearms (rather than from the hands) and with no spinal articulation as needed (for those with spinal extension contraindications) to safely transfer to the floor, maintain shoulder complex integrity, and improve shoulder complex strength and postural control

- The wrists experience full extension if performed from the hands. Maintain finger abduction. If

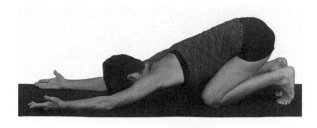

Figure 5.70
Modified dolphin dive (caterpillar) step 1

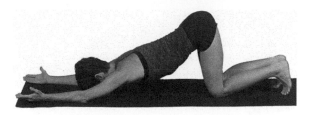

Figure 5.71
Modified dolphin dive (caterpillar) step 2

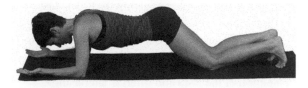

Figure 5.72
Modified dolphin dive (caterpillar) step 3. Prone lying is the terminal step in modified dolphin (not shown)

weight-bearing through the wrists is not possible, perform from the forearms

- Ability to keep the feet and tibia on the ground

- Freedom of the SIJ to move into nutation with symmetry at the PSIS and inferior lateral angles.

MP (motor pattern)

- Maintenance of TATD breath with control outside of spinal neutral (in spinal extension). If TATD breath cannot be maintained in previous postures, modify by lowering to the ground through a plank from the forearms and knees

- Maintenance of scapular depression and retraction without sole reliance on the upper trapezius and while avoiding elbow winging (glenohumeral joint internal rotation, also called "chicken winging"). The elbows remain close to the ribcage.

TESMI (tissue extensibility and sensorimotor integration) Global myofascial resilience and neurovascular response.

Cobra and Sphinx (using TATD breath) with/without GMAX recruitment and with/without knee flexion (Fig. 5.73)

Note previous sections concerning optimal kinematics and TESMI (tissue extensibility and sensorimotor integration).

Assess and document:

MP (motor pattern)

- Diaphragmatic isolation (noted by a smooth symmetrical lifting of the torso during inhale and descent during exhale) and symmetry

- Scapulothoracic proprioception and stabilization for adequate scapulohumeral rhythm via closed kinetic chain strength training

- Use of TATD breath during transition and hold phase, which includes proper use of all three diaphragms, as well as trunk stability synergist movement patterns (an inherent arm spiral and hip lock use with no dominant superficial movement strategy (gluteal or paraspinals)). If no arm spiral is used then teaching an active arm spiral may be necessary to safely complete assessment of this pose, which is the next pose assessed

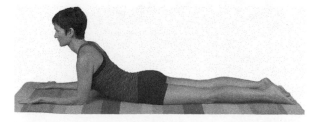

Figure 5.73
Sphinx (see Figs 5.27 and 5.28 for cobra)

- Co-contraction of quadriceps and hamstrings and anterior tibialis and gastrocnemius–soleus unit

- Spinal extension with voluntary control over the GMAX for neural patterning and dissociation of muscle groups for high level motor control

- Freedom of the sacroiliac joint to move freely into nutation with symmetry at the PSIS and inferior lateral angles with/without use of the GMAX

- Maintenance of form and force closure of gleno-humeral joint during glenohumeral joint extension with scapulothoracic depression, medial rotation, and mild retraction. The elbows are flexed and the arms are approximating with the ribcage and thorax

- Ability to perform cobra with and without bent knees to screen for presence of iliopsoas or rectus femoris restriction. The pelvis should not lift from the floor during cobra if iliopsoas length is adequate.

Sphinx: once options 1 and 2 have been mastered progress to propping on the forearms, in the absence of myofascial restriction, involuntary gripping of the gluteals, and initiation and maintenance of TATD breath.

Child's pose and reach, roll, and rise
(Figs 5.74–5.76)

Assess and document:

OK (optimal kinematics)

- Ability to perform child's pose (modify as necessary) without a dominant flexion moment at the spine

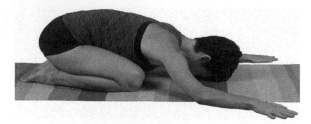

Figure 5.74
Child's pose *"reach, roll, and rise"* step 1, the *"reach"* portion (see also Figs 5.25 and 9.2)

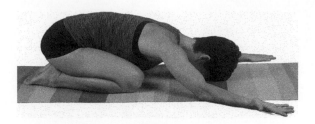

Figure 5.75
Child's pose *"reach, roll, and rise"* step 2, the *"roll"* portion

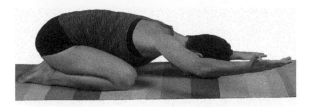

Figure 5.76
Child's pose *"reach, roll, and rise"* step 3, the *"rise"* portion

(i.e. inclusion of functional hip FABER). Lack of postural awareness, control, or mobility may create excess spinal flexion, cervical shear, or lateral shifting

- Flexion-based SIJ dysfunction via bony landmark palpation of the PSIS and inferior lateral angle

- The therapist will assess and document osteokinematic hip range of motion in flexion abduction and external as able (as tolerated by patient) for signs of femoroacetabular impingement

- Glenohumeral joint flexion ROM or scaption up to 180 degrees. Lack of arthrokinematic motion or soft tissue or myofascial restriction can impede overall osteokinematic ROM. If subacromial impingement is a concern, flex the elbows and eliminate shoulder flexion, substituting shoulder horizontal abduction instead

- Tibiofemoral flexion ROM

- The scapulae rest on the thoracic chest wall without excessive protraction, which could stem from loss of arthrokinematic or osteokinematic shoulder complex ROM

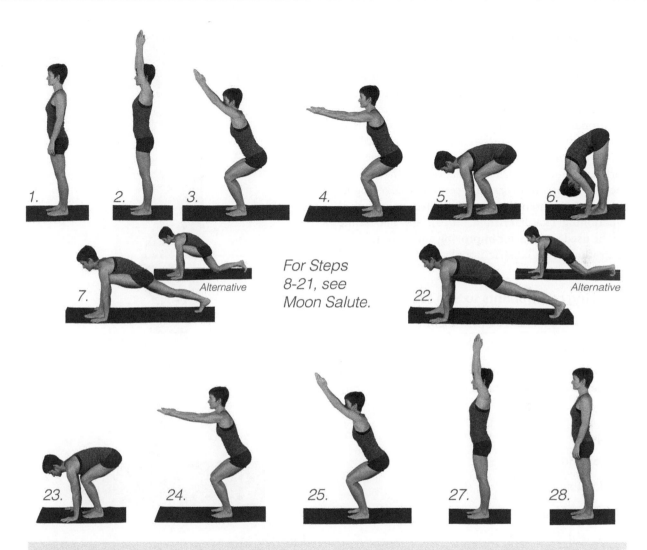

Figure 5.77
Sun salutation composition

- Ankle complex plantarflexion and arthrokinematic gliding. The ankles rest comfortably without excessive inversion and forefoot supination if lateral ankle instability is an issue.

MP (motor pattern)

- Ability to clear the arm from the floor 1–6 inches and minimize upper trapezius dominance without elbow flexion or raising the head from the floor

- Lower trapezius and serratus anterior function (action of glenohumeral flexion or scaption, elbow extension, and glenohumeral joint external rotation)

- The posterior ribcage expands via long, deep breathing (not TATD breath in regular child's pose).

TESMI (tissue extensibility and sensorimotor integration)

- Subscapularis or teres minor extensibility and response

- The front arm, spiral, functional, and superficial and deep front myofasical lines may be primarily implicated.

Sun salutation composition (Fig. 5.77)

The standing Sun salutation composition implicates visual, auditory, proprioceptive, and vestibular afferents, which provide vital information about tone, eye, and neck muscles, postural and equilibrium response, emotional development, behavior and cognitive status, in addition to the orthopaedic and systemic benefits listed under each posture. Use of yoga sequences, particularly in pediatric populations on the austism spectrum, can improve social-communicative, cognitive, spatial awareness, emotional affect, and physical functioning (Radhakrishna, 2010). The Sun salute can be used as a tool for improving attention and concentration in a pediatric population (Javadekar and Manjunath, 2012).

Standing components to Sun salutation

See Chapter 6 for instructions to postures 1–4.

1. Mountain

2. Upstretched mountain (arm floats/shoulder opener in standing spinal neutral with arm spiral)

3. Chair

4. Squat

5. Transitional lunge

6. Moon salutation.

Mountain (Fig. 5.78)

Assess and document:

OK (optimal kinematics)   Postural awareness and trunk control including bony landmarks:

- Bipedal balance (tandem stance) stability with eyes open and eyes closed

- Anterior — Symmetry of humeral and femoral head alignment, iliac crests and ASIS, patellar symmetry and resting position, forefoot and rearfoot symmetry

- Posterior — Symmetry of head alignment and shoulder positioning, scapulae and their resting position, iliac crests, carrying angle (cubitus valgus) of elbow is 5–10 degrees in males and 10–15 degrees in females. PSIS and inferior lateral angle of sacrum, knee crease, forefoot and rearfoot symmetry

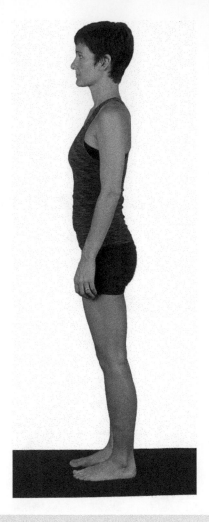

Figure 5.78
Mountain (see also Fig. 6.4)

bilaterally, navicular drop, position of lateral and medial malleoli; evaluate the resting position of the scapula to identify any idiosyncrasies in scapular positioning and provide feedback of any noted problems such as sloping shoulders, winging scapula, tipping scapula. Note the following: inability to self-correct forefoot and rearfoot malalignment (loss of arch height, rearfoot inversion/eversion, and forefoot supination/pronation)

- Lateral — Plumb line alignment (cervical and lumbar lordosis, thoracic kyphosis), scapulae position, and knee resting angle.

MP (motor pattern)

- Ability to recruit or relax postural stability muscles

- Ability to recruit or relax upper quarter muscles

- Use of TATD at an appropriate percentage of maximum voluntary isometric contraction to maintain lumbopelvic stability and safety.

TESMI (tissue extensibility and sensorimotor integration)

- All myofascial lines are relevant. Lack of mobility, resilience, or appropriate response from any part of the fascial meridians is visible in mountain

- Neurovascular issues such as numbness, tingling, hot/cold/change in sensations, or loss of motor function.

Upstretched mountain (Fig. 5.79)

See standing arm floats, shoulder opener, and arm spiral.

Chair (Fig. 5.80)

Assess and document:

OK (optimal kinematics)

- Form closure of hip joint in mountain, transition to, and chair pose. Palpate the greater trochanters bilaterally through the pose to assess form closure

- Hip and knee adduction moment as an indicator functional neuromuscular control (postural control and safety during transition from sit to stand or into/out of chair pose) of hip abductors, external rotators, and extensors (Stickler et al., 2015)

- Bipedal balance (tandem stance) stability with eyes open and eyes closed

- Ankle joint mobility.

MP (motor pattern)

- Shoulder complex proprioception and scapulohumeral rhythm (with arms at 90 degrees or more of elevation) and kinesis

- Force closure of hip joint in mountain, transition to, and chair pose offered via gluteals, hip lock, and TATD breath

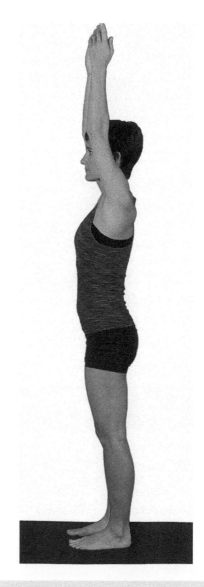

Figure 5.79
Upstretched mountain

- Endurance of lower and upper quarter.

TESMI (tissue extensibility and sensorimotor integration)

- Soleus response and/or superficial back line fascial mobility during hold phase and its effect on foot stability and fascia

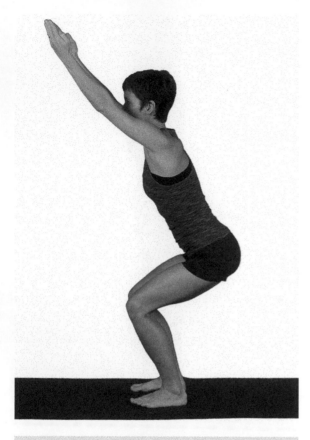

Figure 5.80
Chair

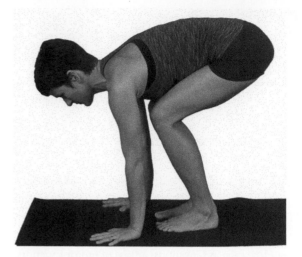

Figure 5.81
Partial squat for transitioning to lunge

- Global neural patterning — Hip lock, lower quarter co-contraction, TATD breath

- Shoulder external rotator strength via manual muscle testing (MMT)

- Vastus medialis and vastus lateralis (VMO/VL) recruitment

- Knee and foot proprioceptive input and balance with knee flexion (unique offering of chair).

Squat

Please note that this pose does not have to include full hip and knee flexion unless full ROM is functionally necessary. It can be partially performed and remain similar to chair pose as in Fig. 5.81. Refer to garland pose in Chapter 6 for full squat.

Assess and document:

OK (optimal kinematics)

- Perform femoral version/Craig test prior to squat. Hip osteokinematic FABER ROM limits are determined by femoral version angles and are known to be limited with presence of excessive femoral anteversion (Botser et al., 2012; Ejnisman et al., 2013)

- Spinal segmental mobility as in child's pose. Watch for loss of mobility, lateral shifting

- SIJ joint response (should be bilateral counternutation)

- Ankle joint mobility.

MP (motor pattern)

- Dynamic postural control during entry and exit into posture

- Lumbopelvic stabilization outside of spinal neutral

- Use or release of yogic locks throughout posture performance

- Ability to use either A-D (restorative version) or TATD breath (dynamic version).

TESMI (tissue extensibility and sensorimotor integration)

- Length/tension relationship of the pelvic floor. Mechanical loading may positively or negatively stress perineal scars

- Visceral fascia and internal organ positional response. Pelvic organ prolapse may need to avoid this posture

- Superficial back myofascial line resilience and response, including the soleus, may be primarily implicated.

Transitional lunge (Fig. 5.82)

Assess and document:

OK (optimal kinematics)

- Postural awareness and ability to self-correct

- Lower quarter joint mobility

- Hip impingement sign (modified Thomas test in a loaded position)

- Lower quarter balance with lower center of gravity.

MP (motor pattern)

- TATD recruitment outside of spinal neutral

- Quadratus lumborum response

- Smooth, controlled transition to other postures

- Tibiofemoral stability in flexion (anterior cruciate ligament protection benefit).

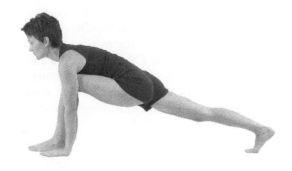

Figure 5.82
Transitional lunge (full) (see also Figs 6.14–6.17)

TESMI (tissue extensibility and sensorimotor integration)

- Groin and adductor resilience and response, as well as vascular structures at adductor foramen

- Myofascial tension may be of primary concern in the hip extension leg (superficial, deep front line), hip flexion leg (superficial back line, deep front line), and globally (spiral, functional, and/or arm lines)

- Hip extension leg — Iliopsoas, rectus femoris, tensor fascia lata (TFL), or quadratus lumborum extensibility

- Hip flexion leg — Hamstring, gastrocnemius/soleus extensibility

- Quadratus lumborum extensibility

- Vestibular health.

Moon salutation composition

The Moon salute is a quantitative and qualitative assessment of overall BPS health and well-being for ADL, independent ADL (IADL), and recreational or work-related task completion. It is a combination of the following postures and movements:

1. Arm spiral in a closed kinetic chain

2. Four-point position

3. Cat/cow (exhale/inhale)

4. Downward-facing dog preparation (exhale to entry and hold for 3–5 breaths)

5. Downward-facing dog (exhale to entry and hold for 3–5 breaths)

6. *Astang pranam* (inhale to entry and exhale to dive)

7. Cobra (exhale to complete movement; beginners should inhale into posture)

8. Child's pose reach, roll, and rise (exhale into child's pose; breathe normally with TATD breath while completing movement)

9. Child's pose (3–5 breaths before returning to four-point position on an inhale).

Chapter 5

FMA Geriatric Form (FMA-GF)

Assessment of the FMA-GF (see Fig. 5.5) can be done using the same assessment tools as the FMA-AF, but with greater attention to balance, vestibular, and stability impairment affecting functional mobility. Additionally, this form may place less emphasis on proximal stability, especially if there is a neurological component contributing to or driving patient disability. All supine postures can take place on a plinth or treatment table, and do not have to be evaluated through a standing to floor transfer. Seated postures can take place in a chair. Four-point Moon salutation can take place from a wall or chair. Plank to caterpillar begins the assessment for seated to floor or seated to supine transfer in order to evaluate prone lying via cobra. Child's pose and *"reach, roll, and rise"* can be performed either from prone if the patient is mobile enough to press from all fours back to a "high" child's pose, or one that does not require full knee flexion. Alternately, child's pose can be performed from the chair on a stable therapy ball or in standing through forward flexion at a chair. Standing Sun salutation composition takes place in standing with use of a chair to perform chair pose, and then adding the Moon salutation described from the previous column.

Standing posture rationale

Standing postures are introduced first if a person ambulates with/without an assistive device into the clinic. If they are being seen in in-patient or home health situations, seated postures are introduced first. Neurodevelopmental training suggests following developmental posture progression (Howle, 2007), which requires attending to sensorimotor needs in seated, kneeling, and half kneeling postures first based on observation of functional deficits. However, high intensity training in an upright position via standing posture progression can be undertaken by anyone who ambulates with or without an assistive device in

a safe way. Additionally, for each standing posture, the following sequence should be followed for populations needing adaptive yoga: (1) chair, (2) kneeling, (3) low lunge, and finally (4) high lunge. Chair postures are used for populations with demonstrated lack of postural control and awareness, debility, or fall risk. Kneeling and low lunge postures are used for those with trunk control but without the ability to control for a higher center of gravity and full degrees of freedom throughout the spine and extremities. Finally, the high lunge is the equivalent of the full posture.

With respect to use of yoga per the geriatric FMA, the combination of cognitive tasks and physical activity completion exacts a greater neuroprotective result than either task completed alone, something that the FMA can provide. There is value in rehabilitative therapies, such as occupational therapy, to have a patient recall movement sequences and integrate feedback, as well as in the therapist's observation of the person's ability to psychobiologically link purposeful movement. Future research should focus on continuing to investigate the acute effects of yoga on executive function and improved physiological and psychological parameters, as evidence by early support via the occupational therapy-based work of Gothe et al. (2013) and Rocha et al. (2012).

Review

This chapter offers a theoretical algorithmic framework for FMA using yoga postures that are recalibrated to embrace the evidence base in rehabilitation. The FMA is not deterministic, linear, or reductionist in focus; rather, it provides a method for streamlining clinical decision-making when assessing optimal kinematics, motor patterns, ability to adapt to imposed stresses, and TESMI. The FMA can be used alone or in conjunction with the prescription of postures that follow in Chapters 6–10, which include standing, seated, supine, prone, and semi-inversion postures.

Postures in this chapter, some of which are included in the functional movement assessment (FMA) algorithm, are foundational for yoga practice in rehabilitation, wellness, injury prevention, and sports conditioning. Their upright antigravity utility makes them adaptable and accessible for any patient population. Geriatric patient populations can benefit from using standing postures for balance training; however, those with limited ambulatory status can also reap benefit from standing postures via chair-based yoga or the use of props for modification, such as a wall, chair, plinth, or hydrotherapy for provision of external support.

Outline

- Neurophysiological rationale for using "step back" and "toe-out"
- Level I standing yoga postures
  - Mountain (FMA)
    - upstretched
    - extended
- Chair (FMA)
- Lunge (FMA)
- Warrior I
- Tree
- Swan dive
- Forward standing bend
- Eagle
- Triangle
- Garland (FMA)

Therapeutic benefits and general precautions and contraindications are listed in Table 3.9. Additional benefits and precautions are listed under each pose.

Neurophysiological rationale

The "step back"

Teaching standing postures should utilize myotatic stretch reflex (MSR) and Golgi tendon organ (GTO) reflex neurophysiology for strength and conditioning benefit(s). For this reason, those in rehabilitation for knee injury management or prevention, or who demonstrate lower quarter knee impairment(s), can particularly benefit from stepping back into the standing postures. Using warrior I as an example, the following rationale is used for anyone who needs to recover from, or prevent, lower quarter injury:

1. Begin at the front of the yoga mat.

2. Enter into standing postures from mountain through chair pose.

3. Step back (not forward) into warrior I. Stepping forward can transmit excessive shear force through the knee joint through propelling body mass forward in an open kinetic chain position and through addition of internal torque of the tibia in transit or during landing without co-contraction. This action can place the anterior cruciate ligament at high risk for injury (Fujiya et al., 2011).

4. Stepping backward into warrior I theoretically uses the MSR to engage the deep tendon patellar reflex and provide balance training for fall prevention.

5. Stepping backward into warrior I allows for slow stretch mechanoreceptors to adapt to movement and enhance the balance training and fascial response. When appropriate, speed can be introduced to stimulate fast twitch mechanoreceptors for higher-level athletic training and sports-specific conditioning. Stepping forward is reserved for sports-specific training in yoga.

6. The GTO, through slow entry into the pose rather than quick entry, mimics contract and relax

proprioceptive neuromuscular facilitation (PNF) patterning. If the transition to warrior I takes 6–10 seconds, and the pose is held for a 30-second minimum (Bandy, 1997), multiple physiological benefits are reaped, including joint stability (Flaxman et al., 2012), anterior cruciate ligament protection (Fujiya et al., 2011), and potential increase in flexibility and stability (Ryan et al., 2010) in the lower quarter.

7. Stepping back with the left leg, use isometric activation of the anterior tibialis (reciprocal inhibition) or isotonic activation of the gastrocnemius–soleus complex (autogenic inhibition) to facilitate muscle extensibility, balance response, and proprioceptive intelligence via mechanoreceptor training in the ankle.

8. Stepping back slowly allows for differential diagnosis of movement impairments that implicate force closure, form closure, neuromuscular patterning, and emotional motor considerations in the hip, pelvis, trunk, and lower quarter.

9. The vastus lateralis (VL) and vastus medialis oblique (VMO) work as general joint stabilizers through increasing joint compression and stability, and resisting hip adduction and hip adduction moments which create genu valgus and posterior femoral translation (Flaxman et al., 2012).

The "toe-out" (Fig. 6.1)

Toe-out is defined as "the angle formed by the long axis of the foot – that is, mid-heel to second toe, and the straight forward line of progression of the body" (Chang et al., 2007, p. 1271). Toe-out in standing balance poses should be monitored and encouraged for balance training and knee joint preservation. Less toe-out during gait has been correlated with knee adduction moment and subsequent progression of medial tibiofemoral osteoarthritis (Reeves and Bowling, 2011). Greater toe-out has been shown to mediate and possibly prevent tibiofemoral osteoarthritis by shifting ground reaction force vectors close to the knee joint center to reduce knee adduction moment (Chang et al., 2007).

Normal toe-out is typically accepted to be 7 degrees and bipedal stance of the feet approximately 6–10 cm apart. Increasing toe-out to 10–21 degrees, however, is posited to help reduce knee adduction moment and reduce medial knee osteoarthritis progression

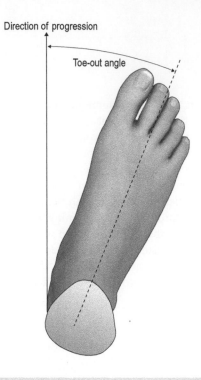

Figure 6.1

Toe-out angle. Grossly normal toe-out angle in absence of the presence of excessive femoral anteversion or femoral retroversion

(Reeves and Bowling, 2011). Assistance with this toe-out can be provided by focusing on lateral hamstring recruitment (Lynn and Costigan, 2008), including hip abductor and quadriceps strength training (Thorp et al., 2010). The correlation of knee pain and proximal hip musculature weakness includes patellofemoral pain syndrome (Fukuda et al., 2010; Bolgla et al., 2011; Dolak et al., 2011; Peters and Tyson, 2013) and the possibility for reducing knee valgus moment (Cashman, 2012) and exertional medial knee pain (Verrelst et al., 2014) underscores the importance of addressing the hip abductors, deep rotators, and gluteus maximus (GMAX) in standing balance postures.

A final consideration in using toe-out is for standing postures. If excessive femoral anteversion, femoral retroversion, acetabular version, and/or femoroacetabular impingement (FAI) or other type of impingement (i.e. ischiofemoral or subspinal) is present, standing postures must be adapted to accommodate these acetabular and femoral idiopathic morphologies. For example, excessive femoral anteversion results in hip external rotation loss and excessive internal rotation, in general. Therefore, toe-out and the accompanying hip external rotation may be less than in morphologically normal populations with 15 degrees of femoral anteversion. By contrast, femoral retroversion morphology may find more hip external rotation. Acetabular retroversion makes full hip flexion difficult because the anterior wall of the acetabulum protrudes (Patel et al., 2010; Incavo et al., 2011). In those with any of the aforementioned bony morphological conditions, modified standing postures are not just necessary but required. For example, in those with FAI, a modified squat is necessary, wherein the knees and hips do not fully flex and allow the posterior thigh to rest on the tibias.

This toe-out stance, provided respect for femoral and acetabular morphology is considered on an individual basis, is taught in all standing balance postures unless otherwise noted.

Level I standing postures

Level I standing postures serve as prerequisites to level II standing postures, which are outside the scope of this text. See Table 6.1 for an overview of standing postures.

Mountain pose with variations (*Tadasana [tah-dah-suhn]*) (Figs 6.2–6.6)

> **Code 6.1** (subscription code)
>
> Mountain and variations
>
>

1. Mountain
2. Upstretched mountain
3. Extended mountain.

Prerequisites

- Orofacial and respiratory assessment
- Abdominodiaphragmatic (A-D) breath
- Transversus abdominis (TA)-assisted thoracodiaphragmatic (TATD) breath
- Other yogic breath types in Chapter 4 are helpful but not required.

Table 6.1
Standing yoga poses

Pose	Figure	QR code
Mountain	Figures 6.2–6.3	Code 6.1
Mountain upstretched	Figure 6.4	
Mountain extended	Figure 6.5	
Chair	Figures 6.8–6.13	Code 6.2
Lunge	Figures 6.14–6.17	
Warrior I	Figures 6.18–6.20	Code 6.3
Tree	Figures 6.21–6.24	Code 6.4
Swan dive	Figures 6.25–6.28	
Forward standing bend	Figures 6.29–6.31	
Eagle	Figures 6.32–6.33	
Triangle	Figures 6.34–6.37	Code 6.5
Garland	Figures 6.39–6.42	

TI (therapeutic intention)

- FMA posture acts as a gateway posture for all postures (especially spinal extension) and for postural analysis and assessment. Mountain introduces a stable foundation that all postures evolve from and return to during practice

- Improve response of all three diaphragms via uptraining yogic locks for postural awareness and control in completion of activities of daily living (ADL)

- Awareness of three diaphragms for downtraining of yogic locks if orofacial obstruction (thoracic diaphragm dysfunction may manifest in sleep apnea or airway obstruction), respiratory diaphragm dysfunction (which may present with a range of issues outlined in Chapter 4), or pelvic floor (PF) diaphragm tension (non-relaxing pelvic floor) are present. Refer to Chapter 4 for assessment

- Daily mini-breaks at work

- All myofascial lines relevant. Lack of mobility, resilience, or appropriate response from any part of the fascial meridians would be visible in mountain

- Extended mountain (spinal extension in mountain) — Increase water diffusion of L5–S1 intervertebral disc via spine extension and/or posterior/anterior vertebral glides for posterolateral disc protrusion or herniation (Beattie, 2010)

- Extended mountain — Screening arthrokinematics of the shoulder and hip. Moving into the pose — Roll and

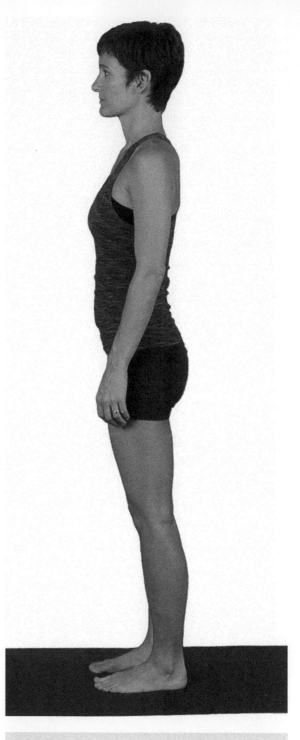

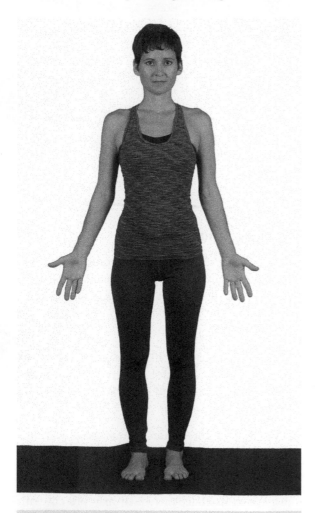

Figure 6.2
Mountain sagittal

Figure 6.3
Mountain lateral frontal

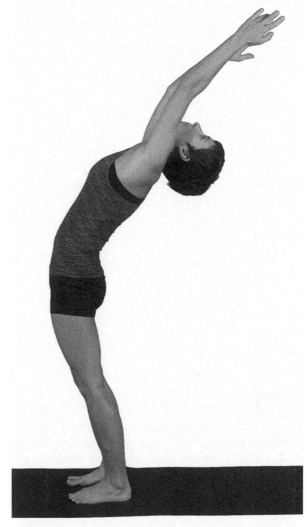

Figure 6.5
Mountain extended

glide should occur in all planes of motion in opposite directions when the concave surface (glenoid fossa and acetabulum) is fixed and the convex surface (humeral and femoral head) is moving. Once in the pose — Arthrokinematic roll and glide in all planes of motion should occur in the same direction when the convex surface is fixed and the concave surface is moving.

Mountain (see Figs 6.2 and 6.3)

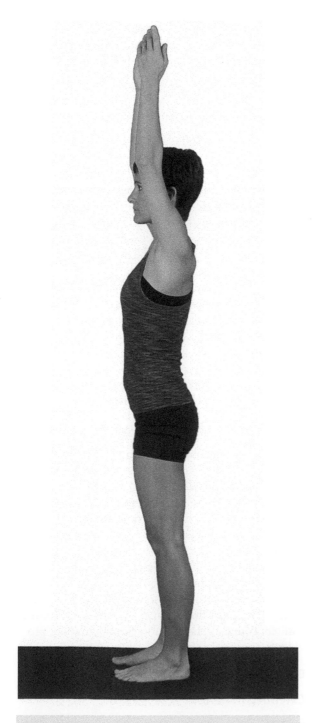

Figure 6.4
Mountain upstretched

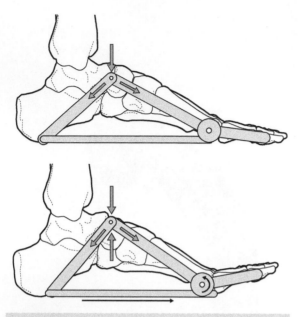

Figure 6.6
Windlass mechanism/truss crank

nonexistent diaphragmatic descent. Excessive supra-diaphragmatic pressure can create altered length/tension of orofacial structures and obstruct the airway.

UEs (upper extremities) — Reach earthward to initiate scapular depression through the shoulder complex as scapulothoracic stability is needed.

LEs (lower extremities) — Co-activate the muscles of the legs as needed to either (1) uptrain (facilitate) postural stability and response or (2) downtrain (relax) yogic locks for improved diaphragmatic translation, and vagal afferent activity, which would improve respiratory, fascial, visceral, cardiac, and psychoemotional responsiveness. Correct any malalignment of the forefoot and rearfoot, which typically presents as forefoot gripping, such as hammer toes or hallux valgus, or rearfoot eversion, such as navicular drop or a shift of the talus over the calcaneus, all of which would increase the windlass mechanism crank or stress over the plantar fascia (see Fig 6.6).

Alternate option

For a relaxation response, release co-activation and return to A-D breath as stated above.

Upstretched mountain (see Fig. 6.4)

Entry Inhale and abduct the arms without excessive recruitment of the upper trapezius or compensatory patterns such as scapular sloping, winging, or tipping. Externally rotate the glenohumeral joints when reaching 90 degrees abduction and supinate the forearms. Continue shoulder elevation until maximal functional range of motion (ROM) is reached. Employ oppositional force of the upper and lower quarters, as in reaching the limbs away from one another with active isometric co-contraction. Active glenohumeral external rotation during arm elevation, combined with concomitant scapulothoracic stabilization, provides the basis for arm spiral in this pose.

Exit Exhale and return to mountain.

Extended mountain (see Fig. 6.5)

Entry Inhale (for beginners) or exhale (for advanced) through upstretched mountain into spinal extension. Look for movement patterns that prevent form or force closure such as vertebral shearing, facet

SP (starting position) Stand with feet separated at pelvic width (6–10 cm approximately), which is a comfortable distance that maintains physical balance with a toe-out angle of 7 degrees. An angle of 10–21 degrees could reduce knee adduction moment in those at risk for medial knee osteoarthritis progression (Reeves and Bowling, 2011). If excessive femoral anteversion is present there may be 0 degrees toe-out. The arms rest naturally at the sides or in the anatomical position if periscapular awareness is desired.

Entry

TS (thoracic spine) — Maintain plumb line alignment and co-activation of the trunk and extremities if postural training is desired. Lengthen the posterior neck. Engage TATD breath at a maximum voluntary isometric contraction (MVIC) appropriate for safe task completion. The ribcage should be under involuntary oblique control. Watch for excessive external oblique employment, which can create excessive sub-diaphragmatic pressure through the pelvic floor and create a lower abdominal "pooching" with a splinting of the external obliques and asymmetrical or jamming, GMAX or paraspinal domination, lack of TATD breath, sacroiliac joint (SIJ) dysfunction, or diastasis rectus abdominis.

Exit   Exhale staying lifted through the chest and posterior ribcage. Inhale and reach the arms skyward. Return to mountain on exhale.

SRAs (static restorative approximations)   Note that the mountain pose may not always require "upright" against-gravity instruction. In those populations who cannot attain upright seated or standing, supine mountain instruction can be substituted, as follows, with the same instruction for finding spinal neutral:

- Supine mountain with ankles at neutral and feet pressed into the wall for co-activation of the lower quarter and proprioceptive feedback for carriage alignment

- Supine supported mountain with props, typically an appropriate angle of yoga couch

- Seated with feet on floor or, if the feet do not reach the floor, rest them on blocks. The feet find the floor actively if uptraining (strengthening) is needed or passively if downtraining (relaxation) is preferred. The feet are hip distance apart with the hands resting in the lap.

DMs (dynamic modifications)

- Stand:
  - with feet apart for genu valgus or varus or if there is a fall risk, balance impairment, or vestibular concern
  - at a wall or with a chair.
- Progression — Stand with feet together.
- Progression — Quadratus lumborum length *"tin soldier"* variation: ground the left heel and sidebend to the right, isolating the left quadratus lumborum by creating distance between the 12th rib and the iliac crest. Repeat on the opposite side.

TTCP (teaching and tactical cuing primer)

See Chapter 5 for mountain, upstretched mountain, and extended mountain. Manual cuing can include the following:

- Posterior and lateral rib expansion to temper anterior rib flaring, spinal extension compensatory

action, or faulty TATD breath mechanics, respectively

- Adopt plumb line alignment and neutral spine with TATD breath with upper and/or lower quarter stability and balance

- Watch for compensatory strategies such as loss of scapulohumeral rhythm or excessive recruitment of the deltoids or upper trapezius in order to elevate the shoulder above 45–60 degrees of scaption.

Contraindications   Fall risk, vestibular impairment; extended mountain – stenosis, spondylosis, spondylolisthesis; acute or unmanaged low back pain; lateral spinal shift; cervical kyphosis; fall risk; lumbar spine shearing, anterior cervical shear (forward head) precludes cervical extension.

Chair pose (Utkatasana [oot-kah-tah-suhn])
(Figs 6.7, 6.8–6.13)

Code 6.2 (subscription code)
Chair

Prerequisites   Same as mountain plus mountain pose.

TI (therapeutic intention)

- FMA gateway posture for entry into standing postures

- Facilitate and assess transition from standing to sitting and sit and stand safely in a variety of settings, ADL, and independent ADL (IADL) (work chair, school, shower, car, bed, etc.) plus ability to retrieve objects from the floor, get objects out of a lower cabinet, etc. Endurance in this pose is also necessary for athletes and individuals with active occupations requiring repetitive movement

- Weight-bearing method to measure hip abductor/external rotator strength (Lee and Powers, 2013)

- Assess arthrokinematics of the shoulder and hip. Moving into the pose — Roll and glide should occur in all planes of motion in opposite directions when the concave surface (glenoid fossa and acetabulum) is fixed and the convex surface (humeral and femoral head) is moving. Once in the

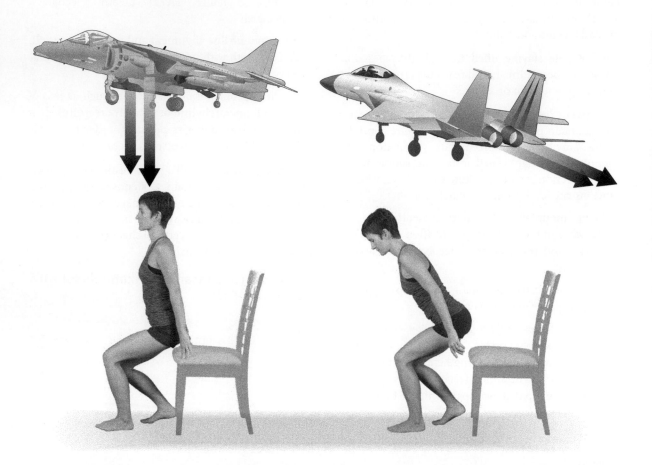

Figure 6.7

Static description of dynamic movement. While it is difficult to quantify the moment arms of a dynamic movement through static means, a loose analogy would to be compare a biomechanically efficient sit-to-stand with the action of an AV-8B Harrier jet versus an F/A 18 Hornet jet. It is impossible to correlate the aerodynamics of a jet with human movement, which is highly variable depending on the structural degrees of freedom, osteokinematic and arthrokinematic ranges of motion, and other myofascial, neuromuscular, and psychobiological features of the individual; however, some loose, grossly simplified similarities can be appreciated, as below.

"Aerodynamics" of biomechanically efficient and safe sit-to-stand transfer: "taking off." An AV-8B Harrier takes off vertically, utilizing the brute force of its engine in exchange for inefficient use of fuel and a high toll on its engine parts. By contrast, the pilot of a conventional jet aircraft smoothly advances the engine to full power as the plane accelerates down the runway, increasing airflow over the wings to the point that sufficient lift is produced to gently take the craft safely skyward with minimal wear and tear on the engine and the aircraft structure.

A similar effect could be loosely applied for sit-to-stand transfers. Vertical propulsion via momentum and upper body brute force is far less efficient and joint-preserving than a horizontal "take-off" that is "fueled" by local and global force closure via optimal neuromuscular patterning

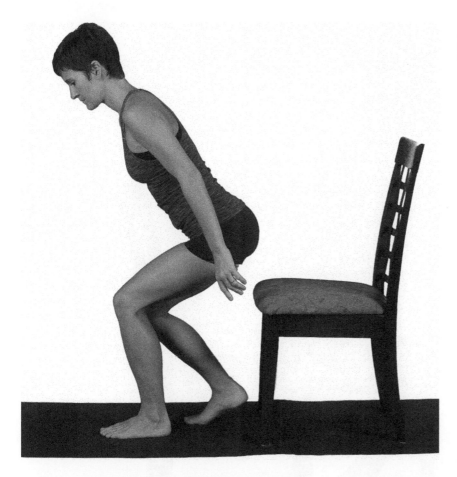

Figure 6.8
Chair, sit-to-stand 1

pose — Arthrokinematic roll and glide in all planes of motion should occur in the same direction when the convex surface is fixed and the concave surface is moving

- Unilateral chair (single leg squat) could be used for gluteus medius and maximus activation for proximal stability (Reiman et al., 2012)

- Reliable functional test for identifying hip abductor or trunk weakness. Testing biomechanical variables including hip flexion and adduction moment, knee flexion and adduction moment, as well as joint angles and vertical ground reaction force variables observed during single leg squat (unilateral chair) show good to excellent consistency with a low standard of error measurement (Alenezi et al., 2014). The unilateral chair also demonstrates reliability for use as a screen for hip abductor and trunk strength function when

the squat is performed five times in a chair at about 2 seconds per squat (Crossley et al., 2011). In women, nonoptimal frontal plane kinematics in single leg squat, specifically hip adduction and knee adduction moments, are correlated with lower extremity injury, hip abductor, hip external rotation, hip extensor, and lumbopelvic strength (Stickler et al., 2015), and nonspecific low back pain is associated with gluteus medius weakness (Cooper et al., 2016). Unilateral chair shows promise for potential use as a reliable functional measure to collect biomechanical variables

- Neuromuscular re-education for rotator cuff (RTC) and surrounding musculature (120 degrees without RTC impairment and 45 degrees or hands on ilia with RTC impairment)

- Identify altered movement patterns and muscle activity in populations with anterior cruciate ligament

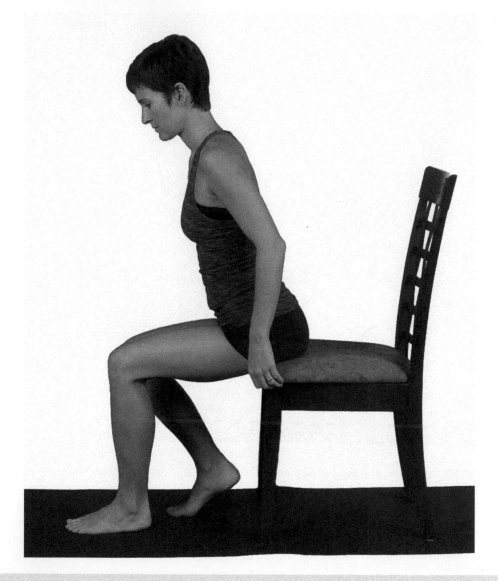

Figure 6.9
Chair, sit-to-stand 2

injury. In single and double leg squat, sensorimotor impairment and muscle weakness is evidenced
by imbalanced recruitment of agonist/antagonist
(quadriceps/hamstring and tibialis/gastrocnemius)
on the injured side, increased lateral displacement of
the hip–pelvis region, and increased knee adduction
(knee medial to supporting foot) moment (Trulsson
et al., 2015) (attributed to gluteus medius weakness)

- Lumbopelvic stability in pelvic neutral with knee
  and hip flexion
- Ankle joint mobility
- Soleus extensibility
- Neural patterning for: (1) hip synergistic isometric isolation and isotonic recruitment for gluteals,
  external rotators for hip impingement; (2) shoulder

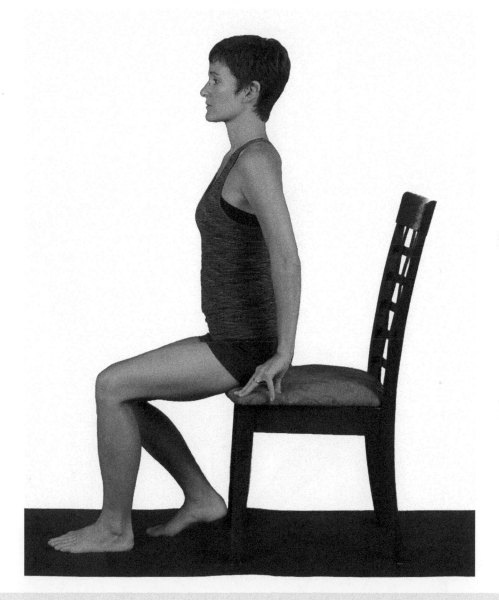

Figure 6.10
Chair, sit-to-stand 3

synergists isometric isolation and isotonic recruitment for shoulder impingement; (3) vastus medialis oblique and vastus lateralis balance

- All myofascial lines are relevant. Lack of mobility, resilience, or appropriate response from any

part of the fascial meridians would be visible in chair

- Proprioceptive and balance training and quadriceps to hamstring ratio strength training
- Functional transfer training (see Fig. 6.7 and Code 6.2).

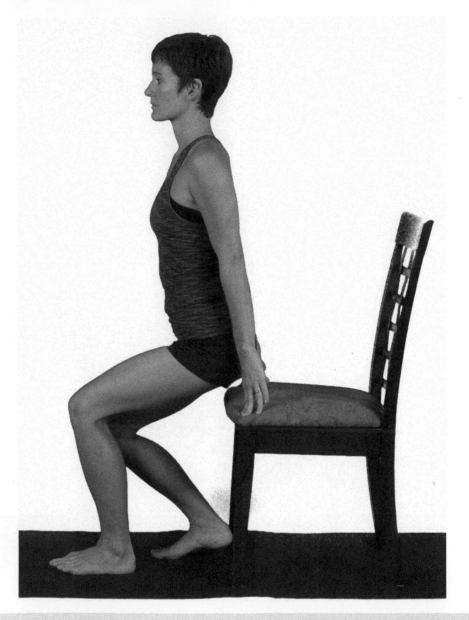

Figure 6.11
Chair, sit-to-stand 4

SP (starting position) Mountain with appropriate toe-out to optimize femoroacetabular positioning.

Entry

TS (thoracic spine) — Angle the trunk toward the thighs by using a hip flexion strategy. Keep the spinal column erect but honor spinal curves. Maintain TATD breath.

UEs (upper extremities) — Limit shoulder flexion to 120 degrees or less if active shoulder impingement or a rotator cuff lesion is present. Use arm spiral (minus forearm pronation) to assist with lower trapezius,

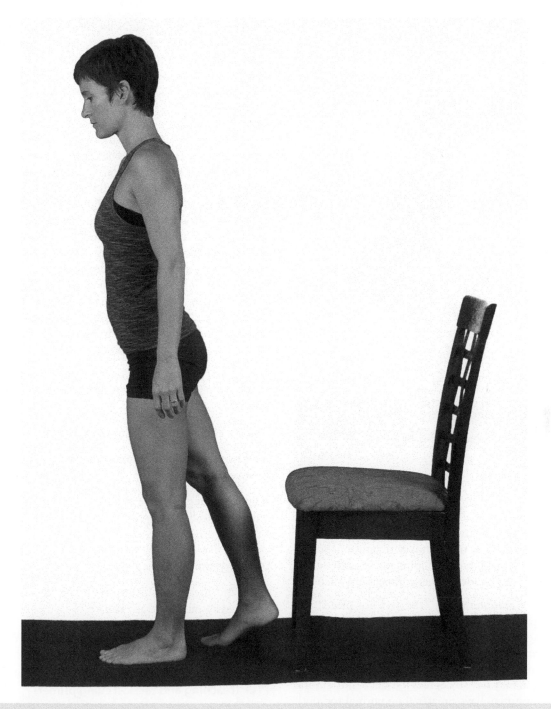

Figure 6.12
Chair, sit-to-stand 5

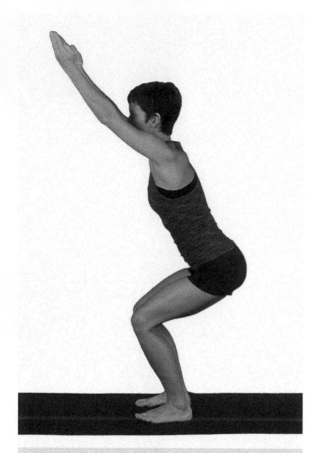

Figure 6.13
Chair pose

serratus anterior, and latissimus dorsi recruitment while dampening over-recruitment of the upper trapezius or muscles of secondary respiration. Screen for functional glenohumeral joint and shoulder complex kinematics by identifying compensatory actions.

LEs (lower extremities) — The feet are placed hip width apart in the toe-out recommended at the beginning of the chapter unless bony abnormalities are present in the pelvis, in which case toe-out will vary according to diagnosis (i.e. excessive femoral anteversion may have 0 degrees toe-out while femoral retroversion may have greater than normal toe-out). Note that modifications should be individualized based on the shape of the pelvis, which must be individually evaluated by a licensed healthcare provider.

Bend the knees only as far as the toes can still be seen while keeping the heels in contact with the floor and maintaining lower quarter alignment. Be cautious of overstretching the soleus. There should be no anterior or groin impingement symptoms during use of hip flexor strategy. Femoral and/or acetabular idiopathic morphology should have been screened for via the Craig test (Chapter 4) and or ROM testing (FMA, Chapter 5), respectively, in order to determine the amount of toe-out/foot placement for healthy hip flexion, abduction, and external rotation (FABER). If there is a lower quarter or lumbopelvic deficit, such as femoral instability in the acetabulum, knee pain, or back pain, keep the hands on the femoral heads and improve femoral head form closure abdominal, anterior, and posterior pelvic floor yogic locks (TATD breath) (Figs 4.12, 4.23) and hip lock (Fig. 4.22) force closure during entry, maintenance, and exit from chair. Pre-firing of TATD and the hip lock may be necessary to center the femoral head in the acetabulum and diminish pain and impairment.

Exit   Return to mountain or transition into another posture. Chair is the entry point for all level I standing postures.

SRAs (static restorative approximations)

- Perform in seated using imagery and minimal movement

- Legs-up-the-wall pose with knees flexed and feet flat into wall (90 degrees of hip and knee flexion and a neutral foot).

DMs (dynamic modifications)

- Aquatic therapy — Perform in the pool and/or against a wall on therapy ball.

- Stay higher in the pose and use less hip flexion.

- Keep arms lower than 90 degrees.

TTCP (teaching and tactical cuing primer)

- Avoid using the upper trapezii as primary movers, protracting the scapulae, or shortening the pectoralis group.

- Pre-firing muscle groups are critical in this foundational posture, not only for safe transitions into postures but for differential diagnosis of neuromuscular patterning deficits.

- If force closure is a problem in the trunk, shoulder, hip, or pelvis, use of guided imagery can assist in improving neuromuscular recruitment of primary and synergistic stabilizers.

Contraindications   Fall risk; can be modified for all populations using SRAs or DMs.

Lunge (transitional posture) (Figs 6.14–6.17)

Prerequisites   Same as chair pose plus:

- Chair pose

- Standing-to-floor transfer.

TI (therapeutic intention)

- Gateway posture for transfers and a prerequisite for Sun salutes

- Hip adductor, iliopsoas, hamstring, and gastrocnemius/soleus length

- Hip joint flexion, extension and arthrokinematic mobility requiring posterior glide, roll, and spin (flexion) and anterior glide, roll, and spin (extension)

- Reduction of fall risk in the elderly (Kerrigan et al., 2001)

- Assess arthrokinematics — Same as chair but including hip extension, abduction, and adduction (occurs during normal step forward during gait cycle) so roll and glide need to be adequate in all planes of motion (anterior, posterior, medial, lateral)

- Activation of vestibulocollic reflex for stabilization of the head in space and the cervicocollic reflex for stabilization of the head on the body

- Quadratus lumborum isolation and mobility

- Myofascial tensile force — Superficial and deep front line, compression of the bent lower quarter superficial back line, and tension on the straight leg superficial front and deep front line. The spiral band (crossed line) could also be commonly implicated

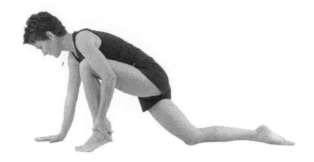

Figure 6.14
Lunge, modified with hand-assist 1

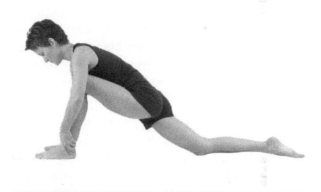

Figure 6.15
Lunge, modified with hand-assist 2

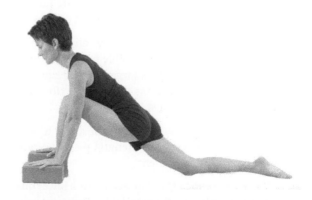

Figure 6.16
Lunge, modified from blocks

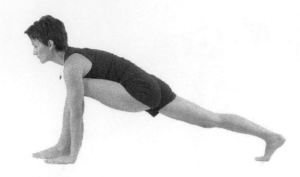

Figure 6.17
Lunge, full

- Anterior cruciate ligament preservation through activation of hip abductors, extensors, and external rotators to minimize excessive hip and knee adduction moment that increase risk of lower quarter injury and back pain (Stickler et al., 2015), particularly in women (Trulsson et al., 2015)

- Functional practice for floor-to-standing transfer.

SP (starting position) Forward standing bend, downward-facing dog, downward-facing dog preparation, or hands and knees with toe-out as necessary. This pose is used as a transition to other postures, or to target tissue length and response, endurance, and mobility for the lower quarter and spine.

Entry Inhale, lunge the left foot back. Remain here for 1–5 breaths. The hands can support the lunge on the floor, from blocks placed on the floor, or in a chair.

TS (thoracic spine) — Plumb line alignment and spinal neutral may not be possible but TATD breath should still be used in this larger neutral zone. For those with contraindications to spinal flexion, kneel to transition to maintain spinal neutral.

UEs (upper extremities) — Use arm spiral to foster joint stability, periscapular strength, proprioception, and to prevent impingement.

LEs (lower extremities) — Co-activate the lower quarter intermittently (6–10 seconds) for lower extremity flexibility or stability. Glide through complete ankle ROM to test joint function. Utilize hip lock to seat the femoral head and prevent hip anterior impingement.

Exit Exhale, and bring the left foot forward, returning to forward standing bend.

SRAs (static restorative approximations)

- Knee-to-chest with/without knee extension

- Hip telescoping

- Reclined supported tree.

DMs (dynamic modifications)

- Kneel to transition.

- Help the foot through with the hand.

- Use blocks under hands.

TTCP (teaching and tactical cuing primer)

- Plantarflex the back ankle on initial lift-off.

- Dorsiflex the foot prior to placement of the foot on the ground between the hands.

- Balance each side by alternating which foot lunges back/forward.

- Use visual imagery for motor function enhancement.

- Facilitate muscular and fascial pelvic flexibility by using visual imagery to separate the left and right, anterior and posterior pelvic floor and adductors.

- The ankle is in subtalar neutral, neither dorsiflexed nor plantarflexed during the final static manifestation of the lunge.

Contraindications Restriction in mobility that impairs alignment; acute low back pain; spinal flexion contraindications, or degenerative joint disease of the spine, hip, or knees; hip labral injury, avoid full hip extension; femoroacetabular impingement, caution with hip flexion, adduction, and internal rotation (FADDIR) motions.

Warrior I pose (Virabhadrasana I [veeruh-buh-drah-suhn]) (Figs 6.18–6.20)

Code 6.3 (subscription code)
Warrior I

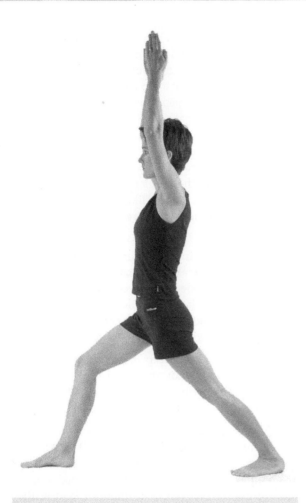

Figure 6.18
Warrior I, full

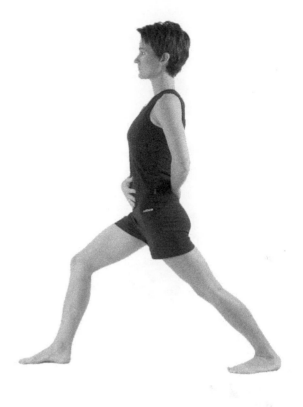

Figure 6.19
Warrior I, biofeedback for spinal neutral and TATD breath

Prerequisites Same as chair pose.

TI (therapeutic intention)

- Isolate psoas and gastrocnemius while maintaining spinal neutral

- Gateway posture for spinal extension when performed crescent-style

- Entry-point for standing postures, especially triangle and revolved triangle (not included in level I postures)

- Assess arthrokinematics — Same as lunge

- Agonist/antagonist development to prevent lower quarter injury and medial knee pain (Verrelst et al., 2014) and back pain during unilateral squat portion (Trulsson et al., 2015) — Quadriceps balance (vastus lateralis to vastus medialis oblique) and quadriceps-to-hamstring ratio development, hip external rotator and gluteus medius isolation, strength + endurance (power); address patellar tracking via proximal strengthening to minimize patellofemoral pain syndrome (Peters and Tyson, 2013)

- Coordination of TATD to diminish back pain risk

- Neural patterning (i.e. dissociation) between hip external rotators and GMAX

- Optional: vestibulo-ocular reflex (VOR) training — Address functional motor patterning of lumbopelvic region to treat pelvic or hip pain or VOR

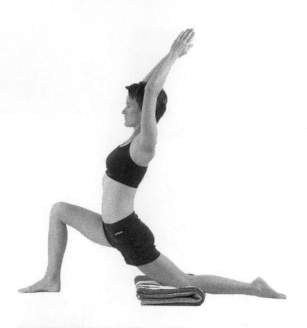

Figure 6.20
Warrior I, modified in kneeling with blankets

through the addition of trunk rotation or sidebending during warrior I

- Myofascial tensile force — The most commonly implicated lines are the *back leg* – superficial back line; *front leg* – superficial front, lateral, spiral (depending on back leg stance), functional line (anterior and posterior), and deep front lines or bands; and arm lines (if arms are used)

- Confidence, stamina, determination

- Metaphor for the facing the past, present, and future.

SP (starting position)   Chair.

Entry   From chair pose, using TATD breath at a maximum voluntary isometric contraction (MVIC) appropriate for safe and stable task completion, step back 3–4 feet (depending on height) with the left foot, with the feet placed a normal standing distance apart (almost a "heel bisecting heel" alignment but with heels about 2 inches apart in the sagittal plane). Turn the left foot 0–10 degrees or normal toe-out as therapeutically determined. Back foot toe-out should be determined by pre-screening the hip joint (see

chair) and according to the presence of any pain. Back foot toe-out should be normal (approximately 7 degrees) in those who should avoid knee torque, those who have excessive hip anteversion, hip labral injury, SIJ torsion or pain, low back pain, or pelvic floor dysfunction or pain, or in populations who need to address psoas length and pliability. This toe-out, depending on the length-tension of soft tissues and femoroacetabular morphology, could require minor external rotation in the back leg. Those with excessive femoral anteversion are less likely to experience hip external rotation due to femoral neck torsion morphology.

Inhale, bend the front knee and flex the front hip only as much as can allow for maintenance of spinal neutral and a grounded back heel. If the heel cannot contact the floor, shorten the lunge and/or fill the space with a blanket under the midfoot/arch. Arm position can vary with therapeutic need.

TS (thoracic spine) — Keep the pelvis in a neutral position to avoid torsion in the SIJ and back knee. Draw the anterior ribs into a V-shape and broaden the posteroinferior ribs via TATD breath.

UEs (upper extremities) — The arms have many options for positioning. They can be used to assist in external stabilization of the pose, by holding a chair, for example; or, they can be in an upstretched mountain position, prayer hands position, or kept at the waist. Arm positioning is optional and is a matter of therapeutic intent.

LEs (lower extremities) — Isolation of the psoas — Bend the rear knee and lift the heel to return the pelvis to neutral. Return the knee and heel to their original position maintaining spinal neutral. The psoas and potentially the iliacus are on greater stretch as a result of this maneuver. Press the heels into the ground and separate the groin to isometrically co-contract hip synergists and lumbopelvic stabilizers.

Exit   Return to standing on exhale.

SRAs (static restorative approximations)

- Supine hip telescoping with knee-to-chest

- Supported modified pigeon.

DMs (dynamic modifications)

- Perform in kneeling or supported kneeling through chair-, wall-, or ball-assist.

- Crescent pose — The back heel is suspended and balance occurs on the back toes and front foot only.

TTCP (teaching and tactical cuing primer)

- Warrior I is not a backbend; rather, crescent pose utilizes spinal extension. Warrior I is separate from crescent pose.

- Power comes from the feet pressing away from one another to co-contract the lower quarter.

- If patellofemoral or SIJ dysfunction is an issue, maintain a vastus medialis oblique, hip lock, hip abductor (including GMAX) focus through repeated entry and exit (Fukuda et al., 2010; Bolgla et al., 2011; Dolak et al., 2011; Peters and Tyson, 2013).

- Offer manual resistance to isolate hip external rotators in both chair and warrior I.

- Provide gentle manual resistance on the proximal portion of the femur/thigh in a posterior direction while standing behind the student to provide inhibition to the hamstrings, quadriceps, or to facilitate contraction of the gluteals as needed to center the femoral head in the acetabulum.

Contraindications   Hip osteoporosis; anterior hip instability or impingement; Achilles tendon degeneration or inflammation.

Tree pose (Vrksasana [vrk-shah-suhn])
(Figs 6.21–6.24)

Prerequisites   Same as chair pose.

TI (therapeutic intention)

- FMA for gluteus medius dysfunction

- Unilateral stance for balance testing/training

- Arthrokinematic screen for hip joint mobility and lateral glide of stance hip joint (when opposite foot is placed close to the hip). Stance leg — Roll and glide in all planes of motion will occur in the same

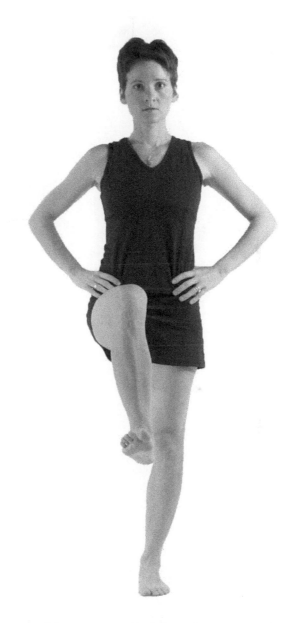

Figure 6.21
Tree, step 1

direction when the convex surface is fixed and the concave surface is moving. Airborne leg — Roll and glide will occur in all planes of motion in opposite directions when the concave surface is fixed and the convex surface is moving

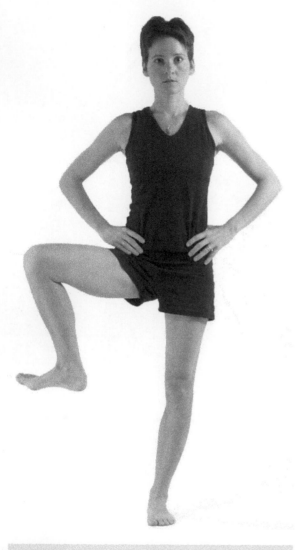

Figure 6.22
Tree, step 2

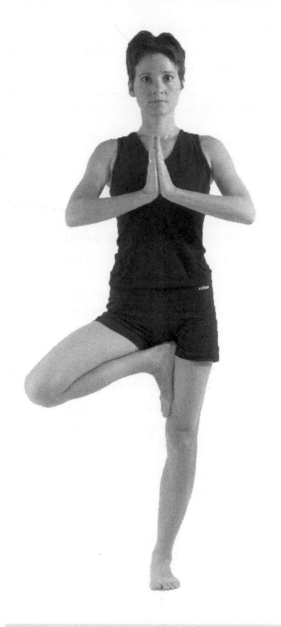

Figure 6.23
Tree, step 3

- *Differential diagnosis*: the isometric press of the foot into the stance thigh will potentially increase pain if labral tear (due to loss of hip pressurization or seal) or capsular deficiency (due to intra-articular instability) is present

- Screen for form closure (femoral head centering in acetabulum of stance leg) via trunk stabilizers and hip rotator cuff/synergists, as well as GMAX. Training these muscles can reduce risk of knee osteoarthritis,

patellofemoral pain syndrome (PFPS) through unloading the knee and reducing tibiofemoral valgus moment in the frontal plane (Pollard et al., 2010)

- Vestibular functioning and central stability, which can give the clinician vital information about tone, eye and

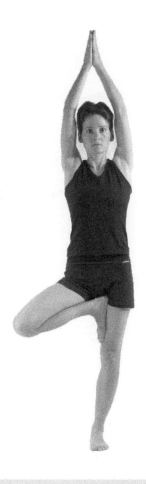

Figure 6.24
Tree, step 4

neck muscles, postural and equilibrium responses, emotional development, behavior and cognition

- *Trendelenburg test*: contralateral (from stance leg) gluteus medius tear or pain provocation without pelvic drop (moderate sensitivity and specificity); ipsilateral pain provocation for greater trochanter (high sensitivity and specificity) with pain but no pelvic drop, osteoarthritis (low sensitivity), or labral tear screen (low sensitivity) (Cook and Hegedus, 2013)

Code 6.4 (free code)
Modified Gillet test in tree pose

- Modified Gillet test (Code 6.4): the conventional test only assesses whether the ipsilateral posterior superior iliac spine (PSIS) drops during hip flexion (a normal response); this has poor reliability and very poor sensitivity (Cook and Hegedus, 2013). However, a modified version provides more useful and detailed information about innominate and thoracolumbar mobility (Lee, 2011, p. 190) and can be completed during tree

- All myofascial lines are relevant. Lack of mobility, resilience, or appropriate response from any part of the fascial meridians would be visible in chair. The spiral band (crossed line) may be most affected, however

- Screen for ilium arthrokinematics with sacrum (nutation and counternutation)

- Mental adaptability and perception.

SP (starting position) Mountain.

Entry With normal or increased toe-out as determined in the toe-out screen section, lift the right knee until the hip and knee are parallel. Take hip external rotation without trunk rotation. Gaze at a fixed point. Press the hands and legs toward the midline.

TS (thoracic spine) — Plumb line alignment and level iliac crests should be maintained, avoiding quadratus lumborum over-recruitment.

UEs (upper extremities) — Take any position using arm spiral.

LEs (lower extremities) — Place right ankle onto the left leg above or below the knee. The toes spread wide but remain pliable while the lower quarter co-activates to create joint stability and balance.

Exit Bring the arms by the sides. Lift the foot from the leg, remaining in hip external rotation and flexion for a breath. Return to hip and knee flexion at 90 degrees for another breath. Return the leg to the floor. Remain in mountain for several breaths.

SRAs (static restorative approximations)

- Supine supported tree

- Seated head-to-knee.

DMs (dynamic modifications)

- Leave foot lower on the leg or with toes touching floor

- Chair-, wall-, or partner-assist

- Use the airborne foot (placed at the groin for advanced practitioners) to press the hip joint laterally and provide a gentle lateral glide moment

- Reverse kinetic chain screen: hip hike "*tin soldier*" and swim the pelvis over the acetabulum bilaterally to screen for presence of arthrokinematic hip joint deficits. Any deficits that affect joint capsule integrity or intra-articular joint pressurization may create pain, impingement, or visible loss of ability to hip hike and swim through a full ROM.

TTCP (teaching and tactical cuing primer)

- Strengthen the upper extremity by palms meeting overhead.

- If impingement is a concern, leave the arms below 60 degrees of shoulder elevation and/or perform low shoulder lock or arm spiral.

- The trunk and lower quarter is anchored to the earth. The upper body and spine may be blown by the winds of life, allowing for adaptation, resilience, and growth.

- Toe-out is encouraged, as stated at the beginning of the chapter.

Contraindications Recent ankle sprain or chronic instability; loss of proprioceptive or motor control at hip, knee, or ankle; internal or external snapping hip, hip joint pathology such as instability or hip labral tear.

Swan dive and forward standing bend pose (Uttanasana [ooh-tah-nah-suhn])
(Figs 6.25–6.28 and Figs 6.29–6.31)

Prerequisites Same as chair pose plus chair pose.

TI (therapeutic intention) – Swan dive

- Transition through Sun salutes or floor-to-standing transfer

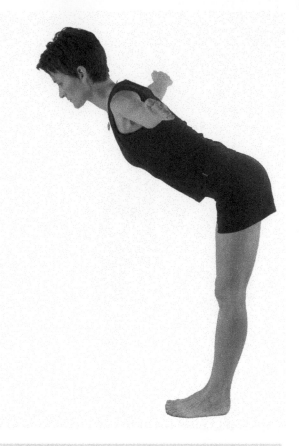

Figure 6.25
Swan dive, full step 1

- Teach proper ergonomics and functional load transfer for ADL completion

- Assess arthrokinematics of the shoulder and hip — Moving into the pose for the shoulder — Roll and glide should occur in all planes of motion in opposite directions when the concave surface (glenoid fossa) is fixed and the convex surface (humeral head) is moving. For the hip (and for the shoulder once in the pose and the hands are supported in a closed kinetic chain) — Arthrokinematic roll and glide in all planes of motion should occur in the same direction when the convex surface (humeral and femoral head) is fixed and the concave surface (glenoid fossa and acetabulum) is moving

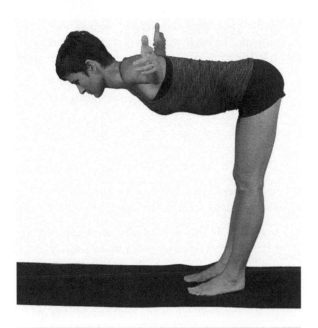

Figure 6.26
Swan dive, full step 2

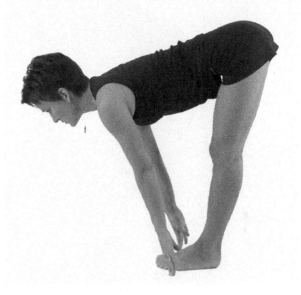

Figure 6.28
Swan dive, full step 4

- Isolated and coordinated co-activation of quadriceps, hamstrings, hip external rotators, and gluteals through the transfer, coupled with TATD breath for stability and safety

- Myofascial tensile force — Superficial back line may be likely most affected

- Swan dive has been historically used as a standing flexion test for SIJ dysfunction via palpating and noting symmetry of PSIS movement (a normal response). However, this test provides poor sensitivity and specificity and is of very poor diagnostic value (Cook and Hegedus, 2013), especially when used as a single screen.

TI (therapeutic intention) – Forward standing bend

- Functional mobility assessment of scoliosis, postural movement strategy, and SIJ mobility

- Cervical spine traction (in full flexion if head is in gravity-dependent position)

- Hamstring length

- Myofascial mobility of superficial back line

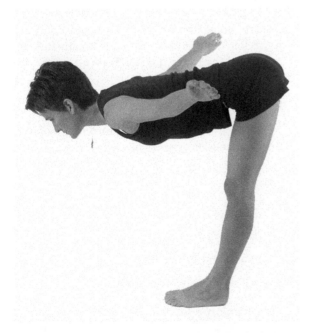

Figure 6.27
Swan dive, full step 3

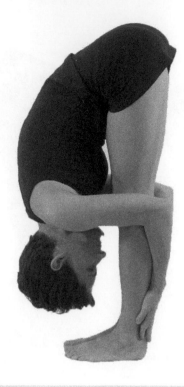

Figure 6.29
Forward standing bend, full step 5

- Dura mater mobility

- Power (strength + endurance) for inversions (if hands can reach the floor and mimic a "pick up" or "lift off."

SP (starting position) Mountain, transitioning from forward standing bend, or chair.

Entry Inhale to upstretched mountain. Exhale and bend knees or keep knees extended at zero degrees and "dive" without trunk flexion and with hip flexion. The arms should be at 90 degrees abduction or less through the transition.

TS (thoracic spine) — Maintain spinal neutral and plumb line alignment through swan dive until the full manifestation, wherein lumbar flexion, or a reversal of lumbar lordosis, must occur to have hands contact the floor. If contraindicated, maintain spinal neutral throughout and use a wall, chair, or blocks. Maintain TATD breath to facilitate spinal unloading and full

use of the respiratory diaphragm, both of which are instrumental in back pain prevention and management. Palpate the following areas and watch for postural anomalies:

- SIJ — Palpate posterior superior iliac crests and inferior lateral angle. Ilia glide over the inferior lateral angle should be symmetrical and smooth in both directions of swan dive (see Table 3.8 and Fig. 3.23 for arthrokinematic SIJ mechanics)

- Lumbar and thoracic transverse processes — Identify primary and/or secondary curves

- Ribcage — Obvious signs of rib humps indicative of rotational idiosyncrasy or scoliosis.

UEs (upper extremities) — Hands rest to the ground or prop.

LEs (lower extremities) — The trunk and lower quarter co-activates to facilitate force and form closure, especially trunk and pelvic synergists (hip external rotators). Do not hyperextend the knees.

Exit Inhale and draw the head away from the sacrum. If hamstrings allow, find spinal neutral, without bending the knees. Inhale and continue to upstretched mountain via TATD breath and co-activation of the lower quarter, return to standing mountain.

SRAs (static restorative approximations)

Swan dive — Can be taught using furniture walking/transfer methods or props as needed.

Forward standing bend — Facilitate safe floor-to-standing transfers.

- Knees-to-chest

- Windshield wipers

- Supported hand-to-big toe

- Forward seated bend from chair.

DMs (dynamic modifications)

Swan dive

- Supine-to-sit and sit-to-stand transfers should be mastered before attempting swan dive

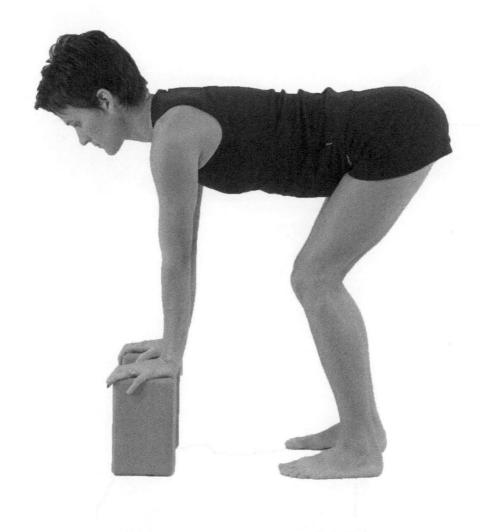

Figure 6.30
Forward standing bend, modified with bent knees and hands on blocks

- Lateral articulation (in those without compromised spinal integrity or osteoporosis).

Forward standing bend

To limit ROM in the pose use:

- Hands on blocks

- Bent knees

- Forward seated bend from chair.

Other modifications:

- Restorative option 1 — Framed arms in a "V" shape, using the ulnar side of the forearm with hands clasped behind head to create a traction moment for the cervical spine, superficial fascial back line, and dura mater

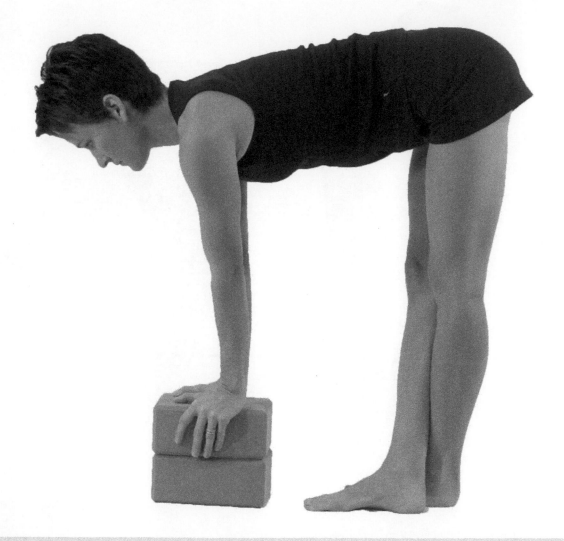

Figure 6.31
Forward standing bend, modified with crossed legs to isolate unilateral posterior tissue(s)

- Restorative option 2 — Framed arms that inter-twine to hang earthward to create a general traction and spinal release moment
- Cross one leg over the other to isolate unilateral hamstrings and posterior tissue(s). The hamstring in front receives the more intense tensile force.

TTCP (teaching and tactical cuing primer)

- The greater trochanter aligned approximately over the ankles
- The full expression has hands beside the feet, which requires more than normal wrist extension

- Work floor-to-standing transfers for older population
- Employ the hip external rotators, TATD breath, gluteals, and hamstrings for synergistic support
- Prevent orthostatic hypotension with muscle pumping action of lower extremities.

Contraindications Posterior hip joint instability, subspinal or ischiofemoral impingement (hip) hip dysplasia such as shallow acetabulum and/or excessive femoral anteversion or acetabular version; pregnancy (full forward flexion); uncontrolled hypertension in forward bend; unmanaged glaucoma; fall risk, osteoporosis, osteopenia, or poor postural control resulting in chronic low back pain requires supported substitution of these poses with standing-to-floor transfer education. In most cases, chair-supported (furniture walking) standing-to-floor transfer education is safely indicated.

Eagle pose (Garudasana [gah-roo-dah-suhn])
(Figs 6.32–6.33)

Prerequisites

- Same as chair pose plus chair pose.

TI (therapeutic intention)

- Extensibility of posterior shoulder RTC bilaterally, hip RTC of non-weight-bearing leg, and soleus of weight-bearing leg
- ROM — Hip FADDIR; shoulder – flexion, horizontal adduction, and internal rotation with isometric external rotation and scapulothoracic stabilization
- Assess arthrokinematics of the shoulder and hip — The convex humeral and femoral head(s) roll anteriorly and glide posteriorly in the glenoid fossa and acetabulum, respectively. Moving into the pose (except stance leg) – Roll and glide will occur in all planes of motion in opposite directions when the concave surface (glenoid fossa and acetabulum) is fixed and the convex surface (humeral and femoral head) is moving. Once in the pose (and stance leg moving into the pose) – Roll and glide in all planes of motion will occur in the same direction when the convex surface is fixed and the concave surface is moving
- Modified Hawkins–Kennedy test — The original test is a passive test by which the examiner places

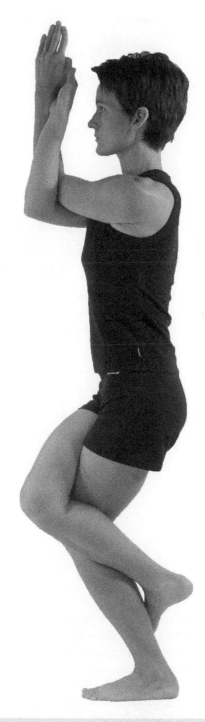

Figure 6.32
Eagle, full erect

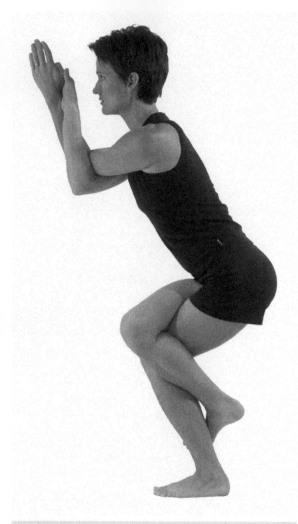

Figure 6.33
Eagle, full angled. See Figs 5.55–5.59 for scaffolded eagle arm entry

- Myofascial tensile force — Superficial back, posterior spiral and functional lines, and arm lines most readily affected

- Hip and knee stability and balance.

SP (starting position) Mountain. If only using arms, perform in seated.

Entry Flex shoulders and elbows to 90 degrees, engaging periscapular stabilizers. Place left elbow into the bend of the right without protracting scapulae. Intertwine the arms until palms touch. The shoulders remain in plumb line alignment. The scapulae actively depress, medially rotate, without excessive retraction. The elbows are roughly parallel with the ground. Bend the right knee and cross the left leg over the right. In most cases, the left toe tip touches the floor and does not intertwine around the right leg.

Balance on the right leg.

For advanced practitioners who can perform the pose with knee joint gapping or torsion, hip impingement, or knee abduction (valgus) moment, wrap the left lower leg around the right until the left shin rests against the right calf or the left foot hooks on the right medial ankle. In the full manifestation the legs intertwine.

TS (thoracic spine) — Plumb line alignment and TATD breath.

Vestibular note — Allow each eye to gaze ipsilaterally on either side of the arms.

Exit Release legs and arms.

SRAs (static restorative approximations)

- Shoulder opener over blanket

- Threading-the-needle

- Supine position.

DMs (dynamic modifications)

UEs (upper extremities)

- Bring shoulder across the chest to target length of the posterior RTC.

- The pectoral group is only eccentrically lengthening during the final arm posture. The pectorals are not to be used as a primary concentric movement strategy other than to initially cross one elbow over the other.

the patient's arm in 90 degrees of shoulder flexion with stabilization of the scapula, and forced humeral internal rotation in an attempt to reproduce pain. It has "mediocre" diagnostic value at best (Cook and Hegedus, 2013, p. 178). However, for a person with shoulder impingement, this pose will likely be positive for pain provocation. If done incorrectly (without the dynamic stabilization instructed), it could also cause shoulder impingement due to faulty mechanics

LEs (lower extremities)

- Keep non-weight-bearing toe or foot on the floor and do not entirely intertwine lower extremities unless lumbopelvic integrity and stability has been established. The knee and hip can be flexed to advance the posture.

- Use props to maintain balance (external support).

TTCP (teaching and tactical cuing primer) Do not force the palms together.

Contraindications RTC impingement or active lesion/syndrome; osteoarthritis, shoulder reconstruction; knee hip osteoarthritis, hip labral insufficiency, suspected tear, FAI, subspinal (hip) impingement, external or internal snapping hip, hip or shoulder joint instability, or hypermobility.

Triangle pose (**Utthita trkonasana [ooh-tee-tuh tree-koh-nah-suhn]**) (Figs 6.34–6.37)

> **Code 6.5** (subscription code)
> Triangle
>

Figure 6.34
Triangle, full

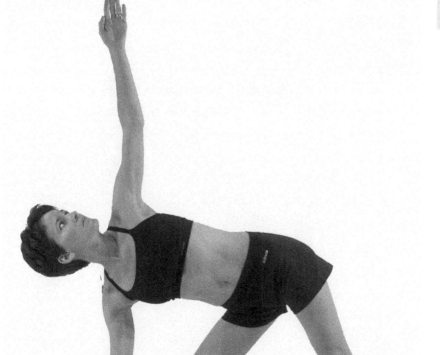

Figure 6.35
Triangle, modified (higher height) with block

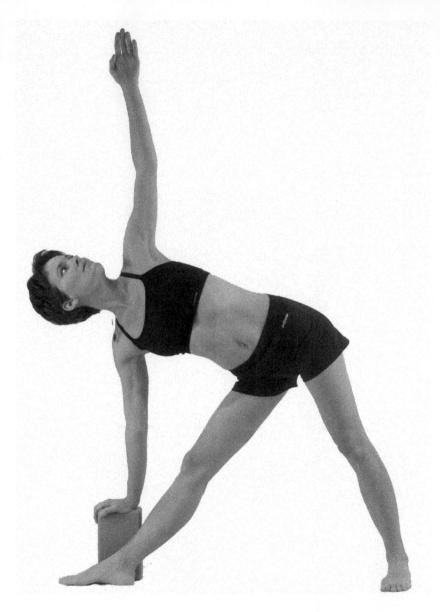

Prerequisites   Same as chair pose plus:

- Chair pose
- Warrior I.

TI (therapeutic intention)

- Developing hip (FABER) strategy in those who experience back pain

- Development of hip joint mobility and hamstring extensibility, proprioceptive awareness with active insufficiency of hip abductors in return to standing

- Teaches proper lifting techniques

- Thoracolumbar segmental mobility (only for full manifestation of pose which would require some lateral vertebral gliding and minor sidebending and

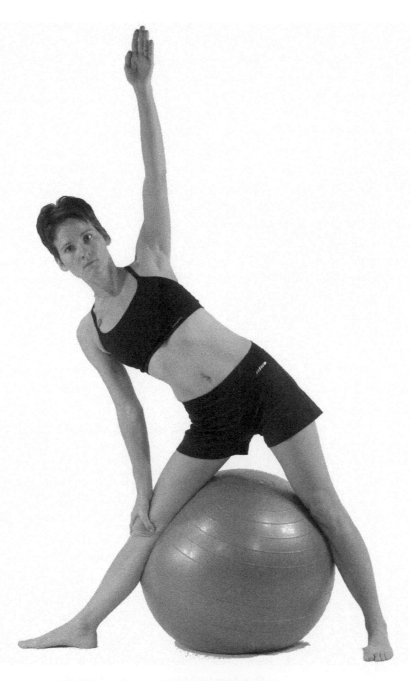

Figure 6.36
Triangle, modified (higher height) with ball

rotation), T1–T8 rotation and sidebending (75%) and L1–S2 for sidebending (27%) and rotation (13%) (Neumann, 2010) plus associated required ribcage elasticity

- Assess arthrokinematics of the shoulder and hip — Moving into the pose (shoulder only) — Roll and glide should occur in all planes of motion in opposite directions when the concave surface (glenoid

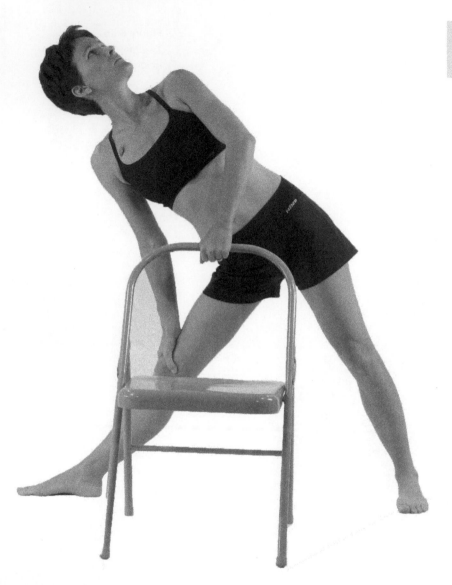

Figure 6.37
Triangle, modified (higher height) with chair

fossa and acetabulum) is fixed and the convex surface (humeral and femoral head) is moving. Moving into the pose (hip) and once in the pose (lower shoulder only) — Arthrokinematic roll and glide in all planes of motion should occur in the same direction when the convex surface is fixed and the concave surface is moving. The upper shoulder will continue to function in an open chain, which means it will follow the roll and glide in opposite directions

- Modified pose would follow Fryette's first, third, and fourth laws
- Full pose would follow Fryette's second, third, and fourth laws
- Shoulder ROM in arm spiral bilaterally
- Cervical retraction
- Ilia and hip dissociation education
- Quadratus lumborum, psoas as lumbar stabilizer

- Triangle is a triplanar pose (frontal, sagittal, and transverse) in its full form, therefore, all myofascial lines share primary affect potential.

SP (starting position)   Warrior I.

Entry   From a warrior I (right foot forward), turn the "steering wheel" of the pelvis right to deepen the right hip crease.

TS (thoracic spine) — The pelvis is neutral while moving outside the frontal plane and into the sagittal and transverse planes. The pelvis is, therefore, in neutral but outside of a frontal plane. (The cue of the pelvis being aligned *"between two panes of glass"* is not biomechanically possible or safe and should not be used.) The final posture does require minimal side-bending and contralateral rotation and little to no spinal flexion moment. The cervical spine retracts before attempting to rotate to the left. Stabilize the lumbar spine and pelvis to minimize iliolumbar ligament injury risk. The ilia of the superior innominate should be allowed to glide anteriorly to maintain *"triplanar pelvic neutral."*

UEs (upper extremities) — Place the right hand on the thigh or shin in arm spiral. Open up the chest to the left. The left palm is facing the anterior trunk with the arm in spiral. Create a blade (fingers together and straight) with the left hand. The arms are co-contracting at the bicep/tricep in arm spiral. Practice scapular depression and medial rotation rather than retraction.

LEs (lower extremities) — Utilize hip external rotation through the front leg that allows the foot to face straight ahead on the mat; use isometric hip external rotation through the back leg to center the femoral head and prevent terminal tension and subsequent laxity of the iliofemoral ligament. The GMAX can be used to assist with femoral head positioning as needed but should not dominate as the only isometric strategy. The back hip is not rotated but is adducted. See exceptions in DMs (dynamic modifications). The knees are in zero degrees extension. The ankle of the front leg is in sagittal plane (rearfoot) neutral with frontal plane plantarflexion. The back ankle may be in 15 degrees toe-in with rearfoot neutral or up to 15 degrees toe-out if knee adduction moment or FAI

is an issue. Weight is equally distributed throughout the edges of the feet.

Exit   Engage the back leg. Employ TATD breath, hip lock, hip abductors, and the GMAX as needed to provide trunk and lumbopelvic support. The front leg adductors and hamstrings are eccentrically working. Lift the arch of the foot to increase action of the TA and pelvic floor. Inhale, return to standing through TATD and lower extremity co-contraction and left arm assist.

SRAs (static restorative approximations)

- Supine hip telescoping with knee-to-chest
- Supine supported tree
- Supine supported hand-to-big toe.

DMs (dynamic modifications)   Rest hand further up thigh or shin to avoid the "trifecta of injury" (Fig. 6.38) — Loaded spinal flexion, rotation, and sidebending over a long lever arm without adequate spinal stability.

- FAI — Bend one or both knees or toe-out to minimize front hip FABER and back hip adduction, which can cause mechanical FAI
- Excessive femoral anteversion — FABER ROM may be limited owing to femoral neck torsion and require hand support high on the front femur, chair, or wall, bending both knees, and/or toe-out
- Femoral retroversion — FADDIR ROM may be limited owing to femoral neck torsion and require flexion of the back knee with toe-out and/or increased dynamic stability of the hip rotator cuff in the front leg
- SIJ dysfunction — The back hip may internally rotate owing to the inability of the hip to dissociate from ilium movement, which could cause SIJ torsion moment(s)
- Posterior joint compression — The back hip may internally rotate or the knee may flex to minimize posterior labral compression force due to hip joint immobility or ROM loss
- Chair-assist — Seated or with right hand on chair when right leg is in front

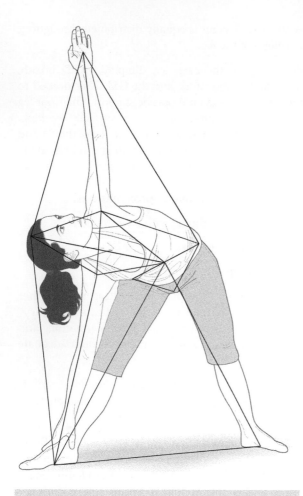

Figure 6.38

"Trifecta of injury" versus "triplanar pelvic neutral"

- Wall-assist — But do not lean the pelvis against it as this interferes with spinal neutral and creates a torsion moment in the SIJ

- Ball between the thighs at or away from a wall.

Advanced modifications

- Place little to no weight through the bottom hand to challenge lumbopelvic and hip stabilizers.

- Arm variations: using arm spiral:

  - internally rotate and horizontally adduct the arm behind the body to rest on the hip crease, or

  - fully elevate/flex/abduct the shoulder.

TTCP (teaching and tactical cuing primer)

- Triangle is not a sidebend, although a minimal amount of sidebending occurs in the final manifestation. The spine receives priority and ultimately informs the pose.

- The superior ribs should not flare and rise.

- The ilia should be free to move anteriorly and toward the opposite ilia, while the front hip is free to externally rotate.

- Hip release — The therapist uses light pressure to deepen the bottom hip crease with the foot or hand while taking two fingers of the other and lightly applying distraction to the lower arm by holding the fingertips to encourage a gentle FABER strategy in the hip instead of a dangerous flexion moment in the spine.

- The top upper extremity should not horizontally abduct in 90 degrees abduction.

- Use synergistic support for lumbopelvic stabilization via TATD breath during transition.

- Compensatory patterns include:

  - trunk flexion, sidebending, or rotation; torsion of the sacrum

  - excessive recruitment of deltoid and upper trapezius

  - use of secondary muscles of respiration.

Contraindications Acute low back pain; osteoporosis with poor body awareness, hamstring or hip instability injury; FAI; external or internal snapping hip; subspinal impingement (hip); immediate postpartum; loss of thoracolumbar kinematics (Fryette's law 1).

Garland pose (Malasana, variation [mah-lah-suhn]) (Figs 6.39–6.42)

Prerequisites Same as triangle.

TI (therapeutic intention)

- An FMA gateway posture for overall health and wellbeing. This pose is often avoided in Western cultures due to lack of trunk and lower quarter mobility

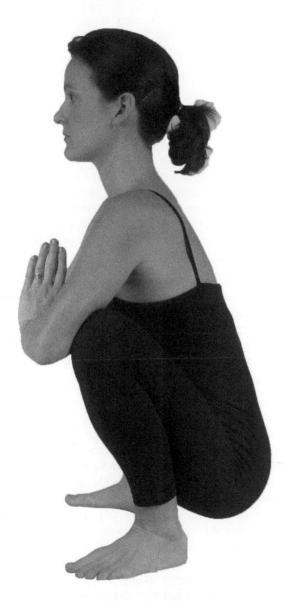

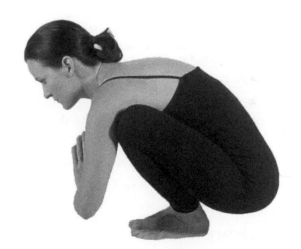

Figure 6.40
Garland, modified with heels on scaffolded blankets

Figure 6.39
Garland, full erect

Figure 6.41
Garland, full with spinal flexion moment

- ADL posture required to improve dressing ADL (such as putting on socks and pants), home care IADL, such as housekeeping, playing and caring for children, etc.

- Assess arthrokinematics of the shoulder and hip — Moving into the pose — Roll and glide should occur in all planes of motion in opposite directions when the concave surface (glenoid fossa and acetabulum) is fixed and the convex surface (humeral and femoral head) is moving. Once in the pose (and at end range of entering the pose for the hip) — Arthrokinematic roll and glide in all planes of motion should occur in the same direction when the convex surface is fixed and the concave surface is moving

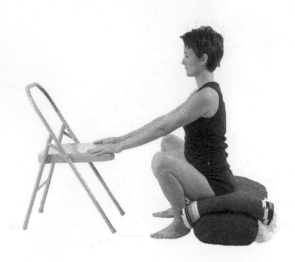

Figure 6.42
Garland, modified with blankets, chair, bolster, and/or wall as needed

- Gastrointestinal motility and gas relief via abdominal/visceral mobilization and massage; release of puborectalis for diminishing levator ani tension to allow for defecation

- Concentric diaphragmatic strengthening via increased resistance to diaphragmatic descent due to abdominal content compression

- Dynamic postural control outside of spinal neutral

- Advanced awareness of yogic locks

- Hip ROM in FABER

- Spine ROM in flexion

- SIJ counternutation

- Fascial superficial back line mobility

- Pelvic floor loading via increased intra-abdominal pressure and length-tension for perineal scar mobilization or downtraining of the pelvic floor

- Myofascial tension — Superficial back, functional and spiral lines (if asymmetry is present), and perineum and pelvic fascia will likely be affected first

- Fryette's second, third, and fourth laws would be applied to this posture

- Used as restorative or dynamic pose

- Childbirth preparedness.

SP (starting position)   Mountain.

Entry   With feet hip distance apart and between zero and 45 degrees toe-out, flex the knees and hips to enter into chair pose. The knees can separate for a larger excursion in the squat. Maintain spinal neutral and TATD breath. It is critical to screen the hip as stated during the "toe-out" section prior to using this posture.

Arm placement — Maintain scapular depression and medial rotation rather than scapular retraction or protraction. *Options*: (1) bring elbows on the inside of the knees and press the knees gently into FABER position for shoulder lock. The spine elongates isotonically. (2) Place no pressure on the inside knee joint via a gentler shoulder lock.

TS (thoracic spine) — Play with cat/cow position to determine ideal spinal neutral based on which position the pelvic floor (through TATD breathing) fires optimally. The length/tension relationship of the pelvic floor determines its ability to generate tension, in combination with the surrounding fascia. Ideal squat alignment depends on the pelvic floor length/tension relationship, pelvic anatomy, and femoral neck length, orientation, and version. These factors, including neurovascular and fascial, impact foot, knee, hip, and pelvic positioning in squat. Test the ability to engage and release TATD breath freely in a squat, to determine optimal joint placement.

UEs (upper extremities) — Keep the chest from collapsing via positional pressure from the arms. For visceral massage, the knees and thighs compress the abdomen in a full squat and the arms "hug" the knees to increase abdominal compression.

LEs (lower extremities) — The hip joint is in some degree of FABER depending on the individual's hip alignment (see Craig test, Chapter 4).

Exit   Using TATD breath, return to mountain or other posture.

SRAs (static restorative approximations)

- Seated in chair in "*squatty potty*" with feet on blocks to simulate lower quarter flexion and release puborectalis

- Wall-supported squat, seated on blankets

- Supine supported knee-to-chest or happy baby.

DMs (dynamic modifications)

- Heels on blankets to protect Achilles tendons/fascia

- Folded blankets under the sitting surface for spine support

- Partial squat/chair

- Chair- or wall-assist.

TTCP (teaching and tactical cuing primer)

- Lengthen the neck and elongate the trunk to maintain posture

- Modified pose — Heels grounded

- Advanced pose — Heels suspended.

Contraindications   Osteoporosis; acute low back pain, first trimester pregnancy; high risk pregnancy; third trimester pregnancy before baby has turned head down; hip intra-articular pathology; FAI, subspinal impingement (hip), hip instability; osteoarthritis or excessive femoral anteversion limiting hip FABER; pudendal nerve impingement or neuralgia.

Review

The standing postures presented in this chapter are considered level I, or foundational postures; they provide the opportunity for systems-based improvement and maintenance of health and well-being through incorporation of mindful movement of the postures, breath, and evidence-based rehabilitation concepts. Because of their upright nature, they are perhaps more accessible than any other category of postures as a first line of integrative management in rehabilitation.

Postures in this chapter are foundational seated and kneeling positions, included for their adaptability for a broad range of patient populations and also required for progression to more difficult postures. They are categorized into two levels, I and II, progressing in mechanical difficulty and neuromotor complexity. Patient populations will present with a wide range of disabilities, and for this reason it is important to meet individuals where they are, rather than having them conform to any preconceived notions of yoga posture practice. Meditation and equanimity during difficulties are a tenet of yoga posture practice, and although meditation is typically thought of as a seated pursuit, note that any posture in yoga carries equal meditative potential. The postures in this chapter also offer multiple static restorative approximations (SRAs) for the clinician to adapt to patient needs as they deem necessary, making seated and kneeling yoga postures accessible to any patient population.

Outline

- Level I seated yoga postures
  - Easy seated pose
  - Perfect pose
  - Thunderbolt
  - Staff
  - Head-to-knee
  - Cobbler's
  - Wide-angle forward seated bend
  - Gate
  - Cow pose (arms only)
  - Seated twist — Lord of the fishes
- Level II seated yoga postures
  - Forward seated bend
  - Hero

- Boat
- Seated twist — Sage
- Camel
- Review

Note: Half-lotus and lotus poses are excluded from this text because of their high-risk nature. Although "quintessential" in historical yoga practice, the postures are not requisite. Those with hip, knee, or ankle intra-articular injury, or degenerative conditions such as osteoarthritis, joint or ligamentous instability, or joint hypermobility conditions, such as Ehlers–Danlos syndrome, should avoid these postures. They offer limited therapeutic benefit for populations who suffer from comorbidities such as back or pelvic pain or dysfunction. The end range of motion (ROM) required in hip flexion, abduction, and external rotation (FABER) further increases risk for those with excessive hip anteversion. Fortunately, modifications and SRAs can be substituted that create success in these postures, such as supported strap-assisted supine half-lotus or supported easy-seated pose.

Therapeutic benefits and general precautions and contraindications are listed in Table 3.9. Additional benefits and precautions are listed under each pose. See Table 7.1 for an overview of seated postures.

Level I seated yoga postures

Easy seated pose (Suhkasana [sue-kah-suhn]) *and perfect pose* (Siddhasana [see-dah-suhn]) (Figs 7.1–7.3)

Prerequisites

- Orofacial and respiratory assessment

- Supine abdominodiaphragmatic (A-D) breath functional movement assessment (FMA) column (1)

Table 7.1
Seated yoga postures

Pose	Figure	QR code
Level I		
Easy seated pose	Figures 7.1–7.3	
Perfect pose	Figures 7.4–7.6	
Thunderbolt	Figures 7.7–7.8	
Staff	Figures 7.9–7.11	Code 7.1
Head-to-knee	Figures 7.12–7.18	
Cobbler's	Figures 7.19–7.23	Code 7.2
Wide-angle forward seated bend	Figures 7.24–7.27	
Gate	Figures 7.28–7.32	Code 7.3
Cow pose (arms)	Figures 5.51–5.54	Code 7.4
Level II		
Seated twist – Lord of the fishes	Figures 7.33–7.40	
Forward seated bend	Figures 7.41–7.45	
Hero	Figures 7.46–7.47	
Boat	Figures 7.48–7.51	Code 7.5
Seated twist – Sage	Figures 7.52–7.55	
Camel	Figures 7.56–7.59	

- Transversus abdominis-assisted thoracodiaphragmatic (TATD) breath (yogic locks 3–6) with neutral spine maintenance
- Craig test/femoral version screen
- Standing to floor transfer if performing from floor
- Other yogic breath types in Chapter 4 are helpful but not required.

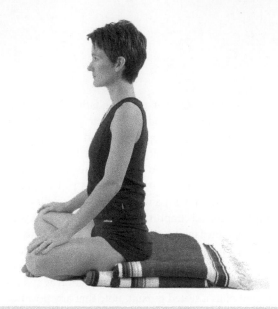

Figure 7.1
Easy seated pose, modified on scaffolded quarter-fold blankets

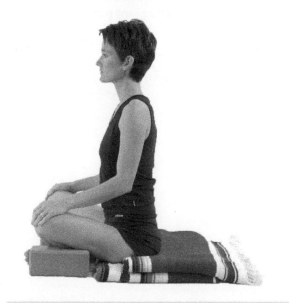

Figure 7.2
Easy seated pose, modified on scaffolded quarter-fold blankets with block support under knees

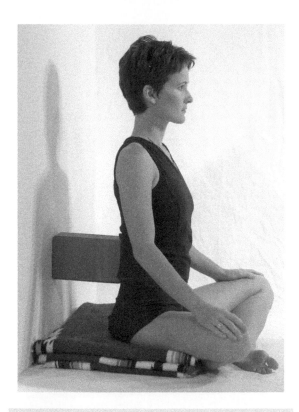

Figure 7.3
Easy seated pose, modified on quarter-fold blankets with block-assist at wall

TI (therapeutic intention)

- Hip osteokinematic FABER range of motion (ROM)

- Knee osteokinematic ROM in flexion, minimal tibial external rotation without excessive lateral joint gapping, tensile force on the lateral collateral ligament of the knee, or medial meniscus compression

- Ankle osteokinematic ROM in plantarflexion and inversion

- Assess arthrokinematics of the shoulder and hip — Moving into the pose — Roll and glide should occur in all planes of motion in opposite directions when the concave surface (glenoid fossa and acetabulum) is fixed and the convex surface (humeral

and femoral head) is moving. Once in the pose — Arthrokinematic roll and glide in all planes of motion should occur in the same direction when the convex surface is fixed and the concave surface is moving

- Myofascial tensile force — Superficial back, superficial and deep front (sartorius, psoas, diaphragm), functional, and spiral lines/bands may be most affected.

SP (starting position)   Seated and, for most populations, a minimum of two quarter-folded blankets and/or two blocks or a chair.

Entry   With a cradling motion, reach under the left leg, grasp the calf and dorsum of the left foot and bring the foot to rest near the right groin in hip FABER. Place the rearfoot near or at the lateral border of the right perineum and the forefoot against the right thigh. The spine should maintain plumb line alignment. Screen for sacroiliac joint (SIJ) dysfunction (unlocking of the sacrum bilaterally or unilaterally), or presence of torsion at the posterior superior iliac spines (PSIS) and the inferior lateral angle of the sacrum.

Easy seated pose option — Cradling the right foot, bring the plantar surface of the foot and place it atop the left thigh near the left groin and lateral edge of the left perineum.

Perfect pose option — Cradling the right foot, bring the plantar surface of the right foot and sit it on top of the left thigh, placing the right foot between the left distal calf and proximal thigh (Figs 7.4–7.6).

LEs (lower extremities) — In the absence of a functional hip FABER range, improper load transfer could be dispersed through the hip joint creating adverse shear, tensile, or compressive force at the anterior labrum owing to its vulnerable morphological make-up and connection with the ligamentum teres. Adverse load transfer would continue into the tibiofemoral (knee) joint, leading to excessive tibial external rotation, lateral gapping, and excessive tensile force on the lateral collateral ligament. This adverse load could lead to excessive medial meniscal compression or a

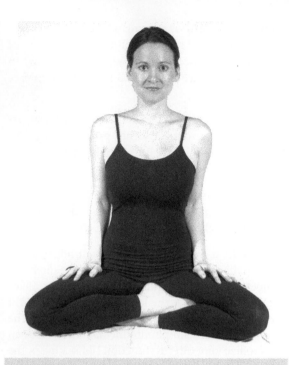

Figure 7.4
Perfect pose, full

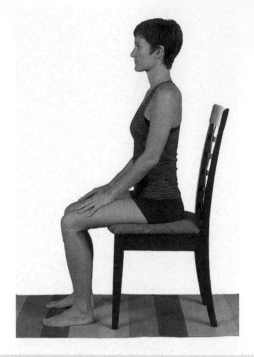

Figure 7.6
Perfect pose, modified seated in chair

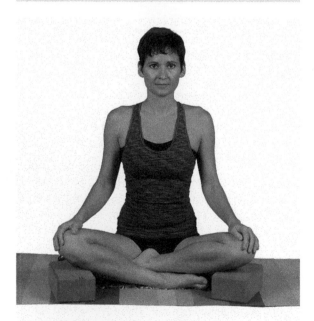

Figure 7.5
Perfect pose, modified with quarter-fold blankets and block support under knees

torsion moment. The ankle, as a result, could also experience altered load transfer via excessive tensile lateral force on the anterior talofibular ligament, thus increasing risk for lateral ankle sprains via ligamentous plastic deformation. As a first limiter of anterior displacement and plantarflexion of the talus (Golanó et al., 2010), the anterior talofibular ligament is the most frequently injured ligament and should be protected during this pose.

Exit   Guide the top leg out of the position first, not utilizing hip flexors. Repeat on the opposite side.

SRAs (static restorative approximations) (Chapter 8)

- Supported supine tree

- Supported supine cobbler's.

DMs (dynamic modifications)

- Substitute knee-to-chest, hip telescoping, and/or windshield wipers (Chapter 8).

- Lower quarter restriction — Use blankets (two-tier is recommended), wedges, blocks, or a combination to elevate the sitting surface and support the lower quarter under the knees to minimize FABER. Alternatively, add the additional support of sitting against a wall.

- Chair assist — Sit in a chair if hip or lumbopelvic, including SIJ, ROM limitations preclude floor sitting.

TTCP (teaching and tactical cuing primer)

- This posture should be comfortable and not challenging to the low back, sacrum, hip, knee, or ankle.

- To avoid hip flexor activation, lean into the ipsilateral leg to downtrain psoas activity and increase safety.

Contraindications Knee meniscus injury; previous medical history including knee injuries or surgeries; excessive hip anteversion, hip intra-articular injury that limits ROM or functional mobility; hypermobility of the knee joint creating excessive tibial external rotation; lateral collateral ligament laxity; hormonally induced ligamentous laxity.

Thunderbolt pose (Vajrasana [wajh-jer-ah-suhn]) (Figs 7.7, 7.8)

Prerequisites Same as easy seated pose.

TI (therapeutic intention)

- Osteokinematic ROM in hip and knee flexion and some hip and tibial internal rotation; ankle plantarflexion and inversion

- Lower extremity anterior compartment pliability

- Lower quarter muscle compression (responsiveness for cardiovascular health)

- Assess arthrokinematics of shoulder and hip — Same as easy seated pose

- Myofascial tensile force — Superficial and deep front, functional (gluteals particularly), and spiral lines (if arms are used)

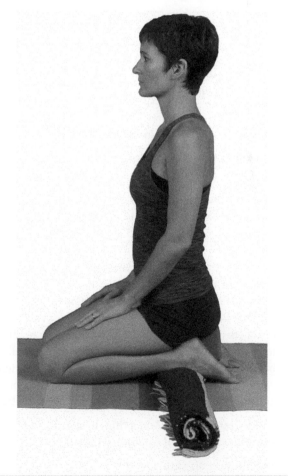

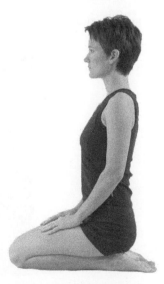

Figure 7.7
Thunderbolt, full

Figure 7.8
Thunderbolt, modified block-supported with ankle roll

- Gastrocnemius/soleus compression for gastrointestinal motility via corresponding Marma point(s) (*indrabasti*)

- Entry point for hero and reclined hero.

SP (starting position)   Four-point with knees hip width apart.

Entry   Use soft tissue mobilization to address tension, tender points, trigger points, or edema from the calves before entering the pose. Place the hands on the floor to guide the pelvis back toward heel sitting. The palms rest down on the thighs or in a hand posture. Maintain trunk plumb line alignment. The hips flex to 90 degrees or slightly more with the knees in full flexion and the ankles in full plantarflexion. All lower quarter joints may experience some internal rotation, especially for those with excessive femoral anteversion.

Exit   Place the hands in front of the body on the floor and transition into four-point position, a lunge, or tall kneeling.

SRAs (static restorative approximations) (Chapter 8)

- Knee-to-chest

- "*Sleepy knees or kissing knees*" — From hook lying, separate the feet wider than hip width (mat width if able) and allow the knees to rest together.

DMs (dynamic modifications)

- Knee restriction — Sit on one or more blocks positioned on the floor between the heels to provide a solid, safe support that lessens the need for knee flexion. Blankets can be draped over blocks at the distal legs or more blocks can be stacked to further lessen required knee flexion. Avoid placing a blanket between the distal thigh and proximal calf, which would create athrokinematic gapping of the knee joint and could contribute to cruciate ligament instability.

- Ankle restriction — Add a thin, tightly rolled blanket under the axis of rotation at the ankles.

- Substitute chair sitting.

TTCP (teaching and tactical cuing primer)   Use myofascial release over the superficial or deep front line if restriction is present.

Contraindications   Ankle sprains, knee pain, osteoarthritis, meniscus lesion or surgeries or loss of ROM (ostekinematic or arthrokinematic); ankle joint restriction or instability; history of foot drop or diabetic neuropathy.

Staff pose (*Dandasana [dahn-duh-suhn]*)
(Figs 7.9–7.11)

Code 7.1 (subscription code)
Staff

Prerequisites   Same as easy seated pose plus:

- Seated shoulder lock

- Seated arm spiral

- Hook lying knee lifts helpful to screen for lumbopelvic stabilization.

TI (therapeutic intention)

- Gateway pose for arm balances (lift-off option) and development of clinical normal (90 degrees hip flexion with spinal neutral maintenance) hamstring length

- Pelvic/perineum awareness and mobility

- Hip osteokinematic flexion ROM

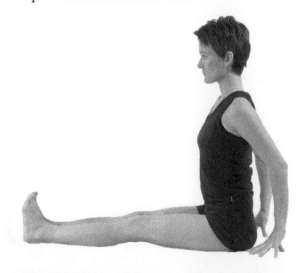

Figure 7.9
Staff, full with "*spider legs*" fingers

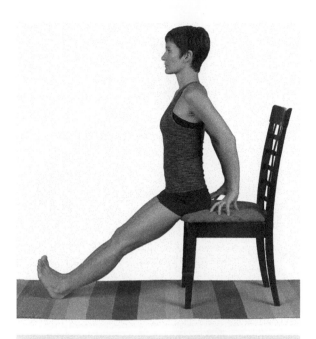

Figure 7.10
Staff, modified seated in chair with *"spider legs"* fingers

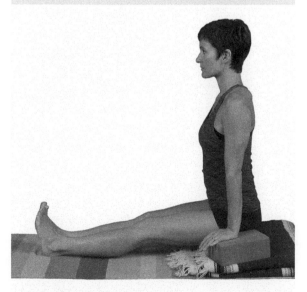

Figure 7.11
Staff lift off with block support

- Assess arthrokinematics of shoulder and hip — Same as easy seated pose

- SIJ proprioception and biofeedback for postural control

- Lower limb tension test (sciatic nerve)

- Myofascial tensile force — Superficial back line and possibly the superficial and deep front line if the psoas or rectus femoris tries to "drive" the posture or if diaphragmatic function is nonoptimal

- Gateway pose ego soother (*ahamkara* control)

- Teach prevention of iliolumbar ligament "stretch" by emphasizing fascial and muscular response and maintaining spinal curve alignment.

SP (starting position)   Seated.

Entry   Bring legs hip width apart or, for pregnancy, excessive abdominal girth, or femoral retroversion, the legs will need to be separated and possibly slightly externally rotated. Co-activate the quadriceps and hamstrings to extend them without hyperextension using proprioceptive neuromuscular facilitation (PNF) patterns outlined in Chapter 3. Maintain plumb line alignment. Engage TATD breath. The knees should not extend past zero degrees. The ankles should be kept in neutral, neither dorsiflexed nor plantarflexed. The wrists can either support the pose in full extension with palms pressing into the floor in an arm spiral fashion (preferably on blocks to maintain coracoacromial arch space for rotator cuff (RTC) clearance, especially if the torso is short or the arms are long), or support the pose with domed "*spider legs*" finger position 5 inches behind the pelvis. "*Spider legs*" fingers is a finger-tip touch to provide biofeedback without weight-bearing and stressing the vulnerable joints in the hands.

Exit   Gateway pose to other seated poses. Typically used as a transition.

SRAs (static restorative approximations)

- Legs-up-the-wall

- Modified supported reclined hand-to-big toe.

DMs (dynamic modifications)

- Use a two-tier approach or yoga couch to elevate the sitting surface

- Substitute chair sitting with strap on balls of the feet

- Legs separated to allow for larger trunk or waist girth

- *Progression*: Lift-off — With the hands resting on blocks beside the pelvis, lift the body (the heels will remain on the ground) from the earth through shoulder depression. Work up to holding for five breaths at a time. Repeat three times.

TTCP (teaching and tactical cuing primer)

- There must be enough freedom in the pose for performance of an anterior pelvic tilt (cat pose) and return to spinal neutral. Modify the pose to allow for a neutral pelvis, rather than allowing perpetual practice in posterior tilt, which could compromise the iliolumbar ligaments, ligamentous support, and form closure of the SIJ, ability of the pelvic floor to sustain an even contraction throughout the diaphragm, respiratory diaphragm descent, spinal disc integrity, and overall spinal posture and proprioceptive awareness.

- Manual pulling of the tissues (i.e. separating the ischial tuberosities and associated fascia and soft issue) is not recommended. The aggressive action may cause the practitioner to miss vital tissue extensibility or sensorimotor feedback.

Contraindications   Recent hamstring strain; inability to find pelvic/spinal neutral in supine hook lying or standing; non-mastery of mountain; loss of lumbar lordosis.

Head-to-knee pose (Janu sirsasana [jah-noo sheer-sha-suhn]) (Figs 7.12–7.18)

Prerequisites   Same as staff.

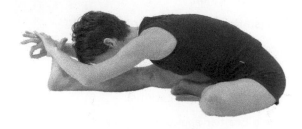

Figure 7.12
Head-to-knee, full at zero degrees pelvic obliquity (symmetrical pelvis)

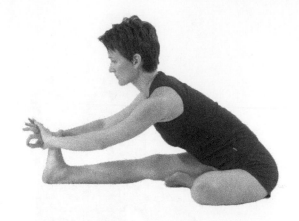

Figure 7.13
Head-to-knee, modified (preferred) at zero degrees pelvic obliquity

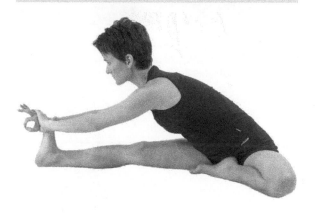

Figure 7.14
Head-to-knee, full 120 degrees pelvic obliquity (asymmetrical pelvis)

TI (therapeutic intention)

- Gateway pose for hip FABER ROM and neural patterning for trunk control in inversions and semi-inversions requiring FABER

- Unilateral osteokinematic ROM in hip FABER and gross spinal flexion (in full expression, which is rarely taught)

- Unilateral hamstring flexibility (straight leg)

- Lower quarter co-contraction for joint stability and PNF to increase tissue extensibility (straight leg)

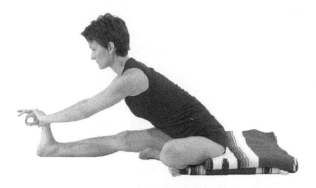

Figure 7.15
Head-to-knee, modified with scaffolded quarter-fold blankets

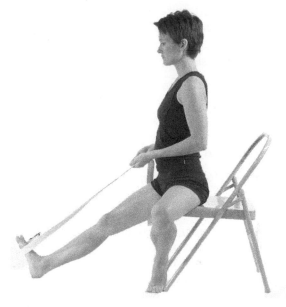

Figure 7.17
Head-to-knee, modified seated in chair with belt-assist

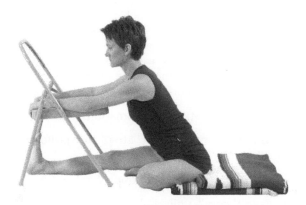

Figure 7.16
Head-to-knee, modified with scaffolded quarter-fold blankets and chair support to minimize flexion moment at spine

- Unilateral adductor extensibility (bent leg)

- Unilateral neural mobilization and test of the sciatic nerve and spinal meninges (straight leg)

- Myofascial tensile force — Superficial back, posterior spiral and arm, and inferior functional lines or bands; possibly tensile force through the superficial and deep front line if the psoas tries to "drive" the posture or if diaphragmatic function is nonoptimal. Perineal tensile force is possible

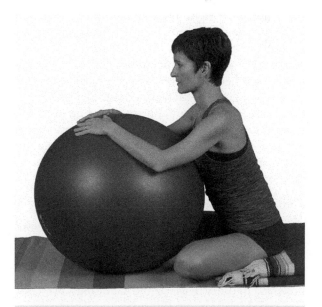

Figure 7.18
Head-to-knee, modified with scaffolded quarter-fold blankets and therapy ball to minimize flexion moment at spine

- Symmetrical SIJ movement (neutral in modified position and counternutation in full pose) in zero degree version *OR* asymmetrical SIJ mobilization if 120 degree version is performed

- Contact of perineum into blankets and spread of ischial tuberosities has potential for uptraining (Kegel or anterior and posterior root lock) or downtraining (reverse Kegel) of the pelvic floor for neuromuscular re-education

- Preparation for full lotus (*padmasana*).

SP (starting position)   Staff.

Entry   From staff, if needed, bring the right leg into slight abduction and/or external rotation in the presence of femoral retroversion. Otherwise, the right leg can remain in a hip width position as in staff pose. With spinal plumb line alignment, draw the left knee into the chest and sit the heel on the floor. Place the left knee in hip FABER, keeping the anterior superior iliac spines (ASIS) in the frontal plane. If the left lateral knee and femur do not rest entirely to the floor, support with a block or a blanket over a block. Co-activate the right lower extremity and draw the foot into neutral position as if standing upright. Prevent chest collapse and increased pelvic floor pressure. Full expression allows for spinal flexion but the initial modified position does not. The use of spinal flexion as a primary strategy is considered a substitution and compensation for poor hamstring or fascial extensibility in the presence of poor postural awareness and control. The upper extremities maintain an active arm spiral in a closed kinetic chain (hands on floor or holding the strap or the ball of the foot).

TS (thoracic spine)

Zero degree version — In the primary action of this pose the ASISs are roughly in the frontal plane. In a modified form (the preferred alignment) of the pose, preservation of the lumbar lordosis and sacral nutation is preferred in order to isolate the hamstrings, posterior fascia, and sciatic nerve. If the spine is not given priority, then an iliolumbar ligament "overstretch" strategy could occur via reversal of the lumbar lordosis and unlocking or counternutation of the SIJ will occur, which prevents form and force closure. In the full posture manifestation (less used except in populations

where lumbar lordosis reversal and increased thoracic kyphosis is preferred), the lumbar lordosis is reversed and the SIJ is unlocked/counternutated.

One hundred and twenty degree version — If a 120 degree angle is adopted in this pose, the SIJ is asymmetrically mobilized and again, the iliolumbar ligaments on the contralateral (tensile) side could experience excessive tensile force. The 120 degree angle approach is not preferred for beginners because of its asymmetrical properties, which can increase injury due to the long moment arm at the spine when combined with a flexion, rotation, and sidebending moment, or "*trifecta of injury.*" Increased risk for disc injury can occur in an asymmetrical position. The ischial tuberosities and soft tissue of the gluteus maximus and surrounding musculature should flare posterolaterally through subtle effort and awareness, rather than by manual manipulation.

Exit   Inhale and return to spinal neutral, eliminating spinal flexion. Exhale and re-engage TATD breath to make a safe transition to staff. Maintain co-contraction through the lower extremities for joint stabilization and support. Repeat on the opposite side.

SRAs (static restorative approximations) (Chapter 8)

- Supine tree with/without strap for piriformis mobilization

- Unilateral happy baby with strap

- Legs-up-the-wall, unilateral (tree)

- One hundred and twenty degree version — Other asymmetrical yoga postures such as threading-the-needle can be substituted to unload the spine and decrease the risk of injury that would result from impaired load transfer and loss of form and force closure.

DMs (dynamic modifications)

- Two-tier blanket-assist

- Block-assist (under bent knee)

- Strap-assist (on ball of straight leg foot)

- Chair- and strap-assist (seated from chair plus strap)

- Ball-assist

- Ninety degree angle position

- Alternate position — 120 degree angle position is used for entry into higher-level application asymmetrical seated postures which use Fryette's laws of spinal motion and combined spinal flexion, rotation, and sidebending, such as revolved forward seated bend, revolved head-to-knee, and/or revolved wide-angle forward seated bend.

TTCP (teaching and tactical cuing primer)

- Establish and maintain postural control and prevent involuntary posterior pelvic tilting, or what Lee (2014) calls gluteal gripping or back clenching.

- Think of this pose as a tree, folded in half.

- The psoas should not be "holding" the pose or posture. Use autogenic or reciprocal inhibition to downtrain the psoas (can be applied to all seated postures). See a full explanation in forward seated bend pose.

- Breath challenge during forward flexion increases lung capacity and alveolar ventilation.

- Maintain scapulothoracic stabilization via arm spiral.

Contraindications Same as forward seated bend, plus hip intra-articular injury due to hip anteversion or dysplasia should avoid full hip FABER without modification(s).

Cobbler's pose (*Baddha konasana [bah-duh coh-nah-suhn]*) (Figs 7.19–7.23)

Code 7.2 (subscription code)
Cobbler's

Prerequisites Same as staff plus supine cobbler's pose.

TI (therapeutic intention)

- Gateway pose for hip motor control/neural patterning in arm/hand balances and squats

- Osteokinematic ROM in hip FABER

- Hip adductor/groin extensibility

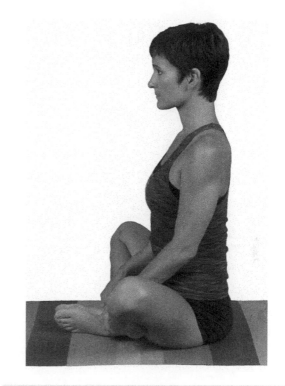

Figure 7.19
Cobbler's, full frontal plane

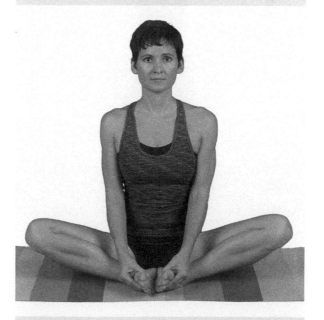

Figure 7.20
Cobbler's, full sagittal plane

Chapter 7

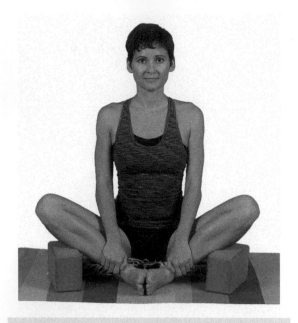

Figure 7.21
Cobbler's, modified with quarter-fold blankets and block support under knees in sagittal plane

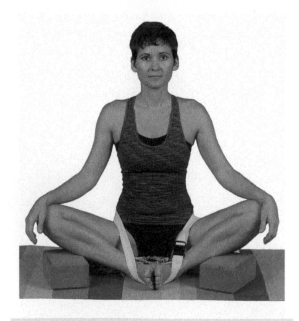

Figure 7.22
Cobbler's, modified and bound with strap on quarter-fold blankets and block support under knees in sagittal plane

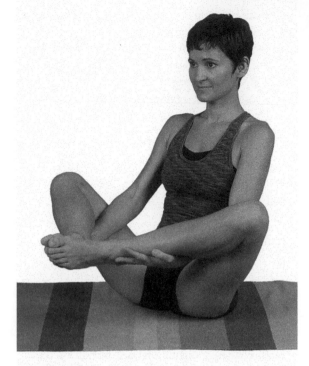

Figure 7.23
Suspended cobbler's

- Assess arthrokinematics of shoulder and hip — Same as easy seated pose

- Myofascial tensile force — Deep front, spiral, arm, and functional line or band and the perineal and inferior pelvic fascia may be most implicated

- Heightened awareness of inferior locks (abdominal, root, and hip) and neuromuscular training via overflow mechanism, especially in "floating cobbler's"

- Preparation for lotus.

SP (starting position)   Seated.

Entry   Bring the soles of the feet together and move the hips into a FABER position. Avoid actively forcing the legs closer to the floor. If lengthening of the adductor tissue is desired, use of proprioceptive neuromuscular facilitation (PNF) is preferred to reciprocal inhibition from the hip external rotators. However, this PNF method should be avoided if FABER is limited in the patient due to injury or congenital or acquired

200

malformation such as excessive femoral anteversion. Maintain plumb line alignment as able, given that some loss of lumbar lordosis occurs with this pose due to sacral unlocking (counternutation). This pose should facilitate hip FABER and not compromise the integrity of TATD breath, although outside of spinal neutral. Avoid spinal flexion as a primary strategy for pose completion. The upper extremities maintain arm spiral with the hands clasping the feet or with hand support of the posture on the floor or via blocks.

Cautions

- High-risk posture for fibrocartilaginous tears of the upper and lower quarter (i.e. shoulder and hip joints) — Use the Craig test to screen for femoral version angles.

- Rule out joint hypermobility before prescribing the posture.

- There should be no external force (manual force by practitioner) placed caudally or inferiorly through the hip joints or knees in this position. The hips are in a close-packed position where little to no joint mobilization can occur, which increases hip labral injury risk (especially in populations with hip dysplasia, acetabular undercoverage, hypermobility syndrome, or excessive femoral anteversion, for example).

Exit Inhale and return to spinal neutral. Exhale and re-engage TATD breath to make a safe transition to seated.

SRAs (static restorative approximations)

- Supine supported cobbler's

- Supine supported bound (strap) cobbler's (not for those with excessive hip femoral anteversion)

- Seated supported bound (strap) cobbler's.

DMs (dynamic modifications)

- Use blankets and blocks under the knees and/or femurs or sit against the wall for postural support

- Unilateral cobbler's/head-to-knee in chair

- *"Suspended cobbler's"* (combination of boat plus cobbler's) for root lock or pelvic floor strength.

TTCP (teaching and tactical cuing primer)

- The pelvis is vulnerable in this position due to end ROM in FABER. Practice this posture with caution and non-violence (*ahimsa*) to prevent injury.

- Manual cuing for hip and hip flexor release or down-training — Use the web space of the hand in the hip crease for soft tissue (iliopsoas, sartorious, tensor fasciae latae (TFL)) feedback without hip joint mobilization. PNF can also be used (autogenic is preferred since reciprocal would increase FABER force).

Contraindications Same as forward seated bend and head-to-knee pose plus hip intra-articular injury due to excessive femoral anteversion, femoral retroversion, or hip dysplasia should avoid full hip FABER without modification.

Wide-angle forward seated bend pose (Upavista konasana [oopha-veesh-tuh coh-nah-suhn]) (Figs 7.24–7.27)

Prerequisites Same as easy seated pose and cobbler's pose.

TI (therapeutic intention)

- Gateway pose for hip adductor extensibility

- Hamstring extensibility

- Osteokinematic ROM in spinal flexion, hip flexion, some hip external rotation, SIJ counternutation

- Assess arthrokinematics of shoulder and hip — Same as easy seated pose

- Myofascial tensile force — Superficial back, posterior arm, perineal and pelvic fascia, spiral, and functional lines or bands

- Perineal and pelvic floor muscle proprioception

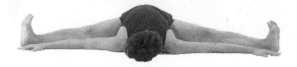

Figure 7.24
Wide angle forward seated bend, full with cervical rotation

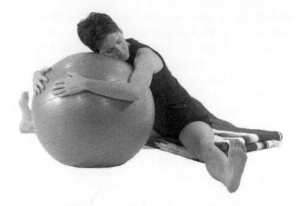

Figure 7.27
Wide angle forward seated bend, modified quarter-fold blankets and ball support to minimize flexion moment at spine

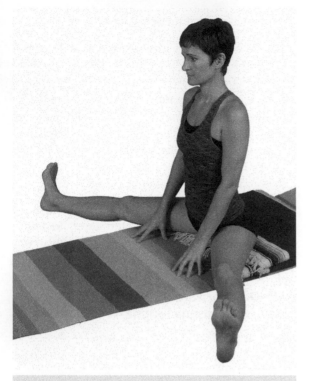

Figure 7.25
Wide angle forward seated bend, full modified with scaffolded quarter-fold blankets

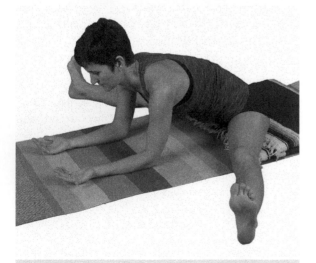

Figure 7.26
Wide angle forward seated bend, modified with scaffolded quarter-fold blankets and arm spiral assist from forearms

- Sciatic nerve neural mobilization
- Contact of perineum into blankets and spread of ischial tuberosities has potential for uptraining (anterior and posterior root locks) or downtraining (reverse Kegel/piston breath allowing for involuntary natural descent of three diaphragms on inhalation and return on exhalation) of the pelvic floor for neuromuscular re-education.

SP (starting position) Seated.

Entry Draw knees to the chest, keeping the hip flexors at rest. Reach under the medial distal femur and separate the legs 3 or more feet apart into a seated "V" shape. Rock the pubic symphysis forward while widening the ischial tuberosities posterolaterally without manual force. With the exhale, walk the hands out in front of the body for a supported forward bend and use props for safety. Full expression of the pose allows for spinal flexion; however, the pose can be modified for any population. Focus on lengthening of the posterior tissue rather than the compensatory action of spinal flexion. The cervical spine, in full postural expression, experiences full extension unless the head is turned to the side to rest on the floor. The trunk should always be supported by the contact of the hands on an external support (chair, blocks, wall, ball, or another person) due to increased injury risk from the long lever arm of the spine and the cantilevered head weight onto the lumbopelvic spine and hip adductors.

Exit Inhale to return, using TATD breath and spinal neutral.

SRAs (static restorative approximations) Supine supported happy baby with/without strap-assisted knee extension.

DMs (dynamic modifications)

- Prop-assist — Support the pose with blankets under the trunk and pelvis.

- Wall-, ball-, or chair-assist for trunk support.

TTCP (teaching and tactical cuing primer)

- Watch for hip external rotator or internal rotator restriction by looking at which direction the toes point and the hips rotate. The toes or hips may internally rotate with adductor, internal rotator, fascia restriction, or excessive femoral anteversion, or they may externally rotate with abductor, extensor, external rotator, fascia restriction, or femoral retroversion.

- Neural mobilization of the sciatic nerve may occur through ankle dorsiflexion.

- Watch for pelvic and hip movement dissociation. Inadequate dissociation can compromise load transfer through the lumbopelvic region, as well as length/tension relationship of the pelvic floor muscles.

Contraindications Same as all forward flexion seated postures plus adductor strain or groin injury, hernia.

Gate pose (Parighasana [pah-ree-gah-suhn]) (Figs 7.28–7.32)

Code 7.3 (subscription code)
Gate

Prerequisites Same as easy seated pose plus:

- FMA column (3); (4) 1, 2; (6) 1-2, 4

- Floor-to-kneeling transfer.

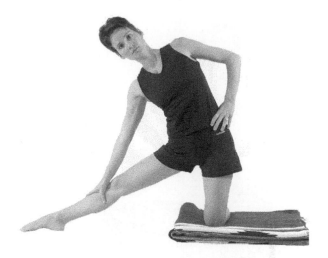

Figure 7.28
Gate, full with modified arm at waist on quarter-fold blanket

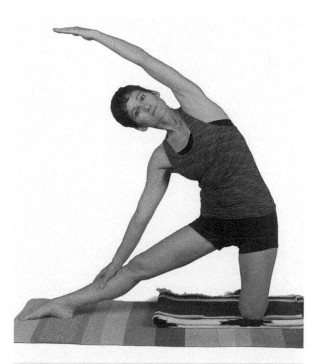

Figure 7.29
Gate, full on quarter-fold blanket

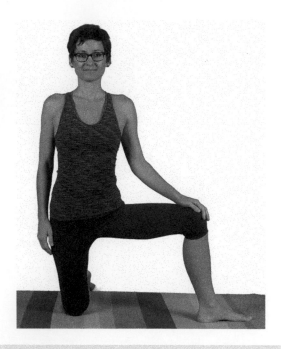

Figure 7.30
Gate, modified with bent knee without blanket

TI (therapeutic intention)

- Dynamic postural control (during entry and exit) outside of spinal neutral (sidebending)

- Intercostal, quadratus lumborum, paraspinals extensibility (bent knee side) and anterior tibialis extensibility (extended leg)

- Osteokinematic hip FABER (extended leg) and hip adduction (kneeling leg) and arthrokinematic mobility

- Assess arthrokinematics of the shoulder and hip — Moving into the pose — Roll and glide should occur in all planes of motion in opposite directions when the concave surface (glenoid fossa and acetabulum) is fixed and the convex surface (humeral and femoral head) is moving. Once in the pose — Arthrokinematic roll and glide in all planes of motion should occur in the same direction when the convex surface is fixed and the concave surface is moving. The upper shoulder should continue to

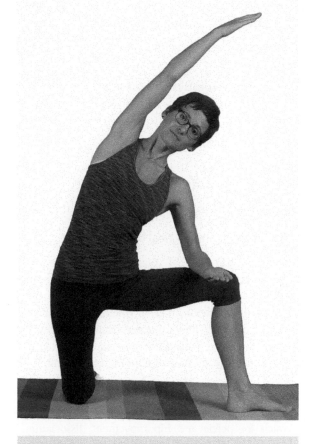

Figure 7.31
Gate, modified full with bent knee without blanket

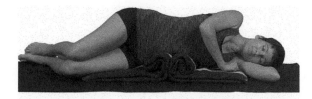

Figure 7.32
SRA (static restorative approximation) for gate, sidelying over Ganesha-fold blanket

function in an open-chain, which means it will follow the roll and glide in opposite directions

- Visceral mobilization

- Asymmetrical posture for ribcage mobility

- Shoulder complex osteokinematic ROM and proprioception in arm spiral

- Lumbopelvic stabilization outside of neutral in osteokinematic sidebending

- All myofascial lines are relevant. *Most likely affected fascia*: Extended leg — Posterior tensile force in the lower quarter, except for the contralateral trunk deep front line, which would experience tensile force. Arm line — Tensile force bilaterally. Functional line — Lower quarter tensile force and ipsilateral trunk compressive force. Spiral line — Concomitant tensile and compressive force, depending on location of the restriction(s)

- Segmental mobility via facet opening of contralateral side of spine to sidebend and activation of multifidus bilaterally

- Round ligament mobilization and premenstrual syndrome meditation via fascial attachment of round ligament to perineum.

SP (starting position)   Kneeling.

Entry   Bring the right lower extremity into hip FABER with an extended knee and ankle plantarflexion. With limited hip FABER, the knee can remain flexed at 90 degrees. The toes work to touch the floor actively. The left weight-bearing or kneeling knee remains under the hip, creating a small hip adduction moment. The left upper extremity is in arm spiral with a supinated forearm. The right upper extremity is in arm spiral with the palm supported by the upper or lower leg (not on the knee). Reach through the left arm with minimal upper trapezius recruitment. Right sidebend the torso without flexion or rotation. Support the torso with the left arm. The right arm supports the pose by reaching oppositionally into flexion (skyward).

TS (thoracic spine) — Thoracic sidebending and rotation follows no consistent arthrokinematic coupling patterns, according to a 2007 systematic review (Sizer et al., 2007). Nonetheless, osteokinematic sidebending is thought to generally total 25 total degrees at the thoracic spine, with the majority occurring at T11–T12 and the remaining coming from L1–L5 (Neumann, 2010). Osteokinematic rotation occurs

mostly from T1 to T8 (Neumann, 2010). Note that any thoracic rotation demands similar rotational mobility from the ribcage (Sahrmann, 2011). Thus, any scoliosis or structural impairment in the thoracic and lumbar spine will be apparent in gate pose and present as asymmetry in movement or diaphragmatic descent. The pelvis enters the sagittal plane as in triangle pose and extended side angle pose.

UEs (upper extremities) — Screen for scapular dyskinesis including premature or delayed scapular mobility and also scapular tipping, winging excessive upper trapezius recruitment, which would indicate arthrokinematic joint restriction.

LEs (lower extremities) — Patella of the non-weight-bearing knee remains superior-facing to allow the foot to rest flat on the floor and facilitate anterior tibialis lengthening.

Exit   Inhale and let the left arm and TATD breath facilitate safe pose transition. Repeat on the opposite side.

SRAs (static restorative approximations)

- Chair supported spinal sidebend

- Supine mountain *"toy soldier"* hip hike (isolation of the quadratus lumborum)

- Sidelying over *"Ganesha-fold"* (see Fig. 7.32).

DMs (dynamic modifications)

- Limit trunk sidebend

- Limit left arm abduction

- Flex the non-weight-bearing knee to 90 degrees

- Place a blanket under the left knee for those with osteoarthritis or bony landmark discomfort.

TTCP (teaching and tactical cuing primer)

- Do not support the weight of the body only through the external support of the hand or knee. The pose is supported internally through TATD breath and no lower extremity hyperextension moment should be created through use of the knee as a fulcrum.

- Keep the flexed knee leg aligned so that the hip is not flexed and the femur remains perpendicular to the earth. Those with hip femoroacetabular impingement (FAI) must adapt the posture to avoid impingement by flexing both knees to 90 degrees and taking less trunk sidebending.

Contraindications   Hip FAI or labral tear; hip or knee osteoarthritis; lumbar spinal fusion; excessive femoral anteversion.

Open faced cow arms pose (arms only) (Gomuhkanasana arms [gaa-moo-kha-nah-suhn]) (see Figs 5.51–5.54)

Code 7.4 (subscription code)
Open faced cow arms

Prerequisites   Same as easy seated pose plus FMA column (3), (4) 1-3.

TI **(therapeutic intention)**

- Gateway pose for upper quarter proprioception

- Shoulder ROM — Upper arm FABER via scaption, lower arm extension, horizontal adduction, internal rotation

- Assess arthrokinematics of the shoulder — Roll and glide should occur in all planes of motion in opposite directions when the concave surface is fixed and the convex surface is moving

- Pectoralis major and minor extensibility

- Trunk and shoulder regional dissociation

- Myofascial tensile force — Superficial and deep front, spiral, arm (anterior for front arm and posterior for back arm), and functional lines or bands

- *Optional*: addition of contralateral cervical rotation away from upper arm can add myofascial tension over the face and scalene area.

SP **(starting position)**   Seated or standing. Seated eliminates degrees of freedom in the pelvis and lower extremities that would cause substitution or compensatory strategies. Traditionally the legs are aligned to fold over one another in a "V" shape with the heels on contralateral sides of the body with hip FABER. However, the risk of FAI and intra-articular hip injury may preclude this positioning for many populations. As a result, the traditional leg posture is not required, and any leg position, including staff, easy seated pose, standing mountain, or kneeling may be used.

Entry   From arm spiral, use a "*two-finger approach*" — Take the first two fingers of the right arm and palpate the left anterior humeral head as the left arm maximally internally rotates and pronates. Only move the left arm as far into rotation and pronation as can be completed without anterior translation of the humeral head (loss of form closure which will be palpable by the two finger placement). Next, supinate and externally rotate the right arm in scaption. The right arm moves into FABER with elbow flexion to reach between the scapulae while the left arm moves to the sacrum and then up the back between the scapulae via scaption.

TS (thoracic spine)

Maintain spinal plumb alignment throughout the pose.

UEs (upper extremities) — Scaption is the preferred action of the glenohumeral joint. The "bottom" shoulder should not compensate for internal rotation by shortening the pectoralis, protracting the scapula, or allowing humeral head anterior translation, which would decrease subacromial space. Do not allow the upper trapezius of the right shoulder to dominate the movement strategy. The elbows move in opposition to one another.

Exit   Release after 2 minutes and repeat on the opposite side.

SRAs (static restorative approximations)

- Supine arm spiral or arm floats ("*snow angels*")

- Supine "*accordion-fold*" for shoulder and pectoralis mobilization and/or arm spiral.

DMs (dynamic modifications)

- Use a yoga belt or strap in the "top" arm by dropping the strap behind the back. Grasp it with the "bottom" arm.

- Perform in seated to limit pelvic and lower quarter degrees of freedom.

TTCP (teaching and tactical cuing primer)

- Manually cue the shoulders to remain broad and level bilaterally during the pose

- Tactile feedback — Spinal alignment and glenohumeral and scapulothoracic position ("*two-finger approach*"; use of scapular assistance test (SAT) or scapular repositioning test (SRT) to assist in scapular upward rotation or scapular repositioning, respectively).

Contraindications Anterior or inferior glenohumeral instability; active RTC lesion or impingement; recent shoulder surgery; shoulder replacement.

Spinal twist/Lord of the fishes pose (Ardha matsyendrasana [r-dha maht-seeyan-druh-suhn]) (Figs 7.33–7.40)

Prerequisites Same as easy seated pose plus FMA column (3), (4).

TI (therapeutic intention)

- Gateway pose for gastrointestinal motility, visceral mobilization, and downward flow of energy (*apanavayu*)

- Spinal rotation, some lumbar flexion (if not contraindicated), and sidebending

- Assess arthrokinematics of the shoulder and hip — Moving into the pose — Roll and glide should occur in all planes of motion in opposite directions when the concave surface (glenoid fossa and acetabulum) is fixed and the convex surface (humeral and femoral head) is moving. Once in the pose — Arthrokinematic roll and glide in all planes of motion should occur in the same direction when the convex surface is fixed and the concave surface is moving if the humerus is bound or in a fixed closed kinetic chain and the femur is not moving

- Shoulder complex ROM — *Anterior extremity*: external or internal rotation (dependent on

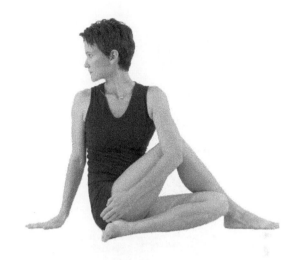

Figure 7.33
Lord of the fishes, full arm variation 1

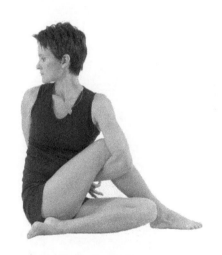

Figure 7.34
Lord of the fishes, full bound arms

position taken), scaption, and horizontal abduction; *posterior extremity*: internal rotation, extension, horizontal abduction and arthokinematic inferior glides (if bound position taken) or arm spiral (without binding arms)

- Hip joint flexion, adduction, and internal rotation (FADDIR) (top leg) and FABER (bottom leg)

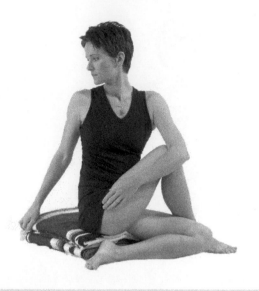

Figure 7.35
Lord of the fishes, modified on quarter-fold blankets with arm variation 1

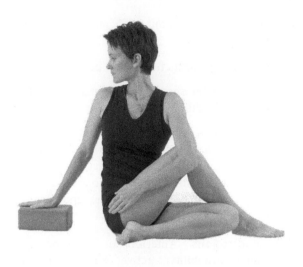

Figure 7.37
Lord of the fishes, full arm variation with block-assist

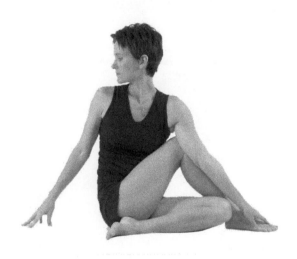

Figure 7.36
Lord of the fishes, full arm variation 2

- Spinal segmental mobilization and arthrokinematic motion theoretically in Fryette's mechanical laws 1 (if rotation occurs in spinal neutral) and 2 (if rotation occurs outside of spinal neutral). See gate pose arthrokinematics for a review of thoracic coupling

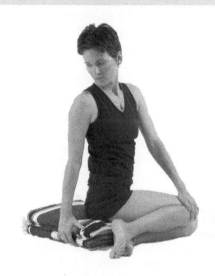

Figure 7.38
Lord of the fishes, modified in side-sitting with quarter-fold blankets

- SIJ counternutation (in full twist)

- Quadratus lumborum extensibility bilaterally depending which side of trunk sidebending or caudad pelvic grounding is emphasized

- All myofascial lines are relevant, especially the spiral and functional bands or lines

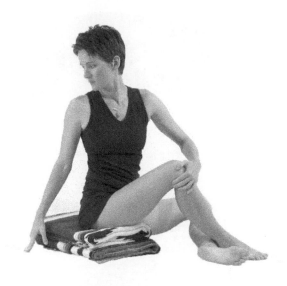

Figure 7.39
Lord of the fishes, modified with quarter-fold blankets and partial twist

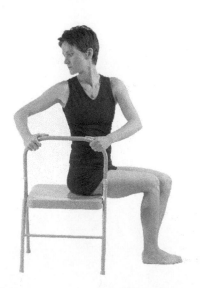

Figure 7.40
Lord of the fishes, modified seated in chair

- Increased resistance to diaphragmatic descent could strengthen diaphragm and improve breath awareness.

SP (starting position)   Seated.

Entry   Flex the right knee and rest the right foot on the inside or outside of the left knee. If able, lift the right ischial tuberosity and bring the left hip into FABER while placing the left heel under an elevated right ischial tuberosity. The right pelvis remains elevated until the pelvis turns to a "one o'clock" position, which maintains SIJ relatively neutral during the twist. The right leg rests, foot flat and knee flexed, on the outside of the left distal femur, as able. The twist occurs in the direction of the top leg. Arm options are listed below.

TS (thoracic spine) — Before initiating spinal rotation, lift and shift the ipsilateral hip and SIJ posteriorly (right twist – right hip and SIJ; left twist – left hip and SIJ). This "*takes the SIJ with you*" instead of creating torque moment through the L5–S1 and the SIJ.

UEs (upper extremities) — Shoulders remain level.

Exit   Initiate the exit from the pelvis up, on an inhale or an exhale. The cervical spine is the last to de-rotate and exit the pose. Repeat on the opposite side.

SRAs (static restorative approximations) (Chapters 8 and 9)

- Supine supported spinal twist such as resting windshield wipers

- Prone supported spinal twist such as threading-the-needle.

DMs (dynamic modifications)

- Windshield wipers (Chapter 8)

- Arm options (for right twist):

  - left arm on outside of thigh, palm facing in to thigh

  - left arm holding right foot

  - reach under right knee with left arm and behind the back with right arm to clasp hands

  - right arms resting to floor behind body

- Use blocks and blankets under the main weight-bearing hip (for right twist, place under left hip)

- Chair-assist

- Limiting ROM excursion:

  - do not cross right over left leg in a right twist

  - stack the legs and perform a partial version of half lord of the fishes/seated spinal twist. In a right twist the right leg would stack with knees bent on top of the left leg. Spinal rotation would occur to the right.

TTCP (teaching and tactical cuing primer)

- The sacrum and ilia (which comprise the SIJ) must move with the pose, rather than the pose moving against the SIJ or shearing or forcing excessive movement in the lumbar spine or SIJ.

- Intention is breath cultivation, not depth of twist.

Contraindications　Osteoporosis caution for flexion; knee surgery, injury, edema, or osteoarthritis follow DMs (dynamic modifications) for supporting the knee in 15–20 degrees of flexion; first trimester pregnancy; high risk pregnancy; cervical spinal shearing or malalignment; caution with gastroesophageal reflux disease; SIJ dysfunction; degenerative joint disease, degenerative disc disease; hip intra-articular (labral tear, FAI, etc.) or iliopsoas injury a caution. Those with excessive femoral anteversion or femoral retroversion may need to avoid end-range external rotation and internal rotation, respectively.

Level II seated yoga postures

Forward seated bend pose (Paschimottanasana [pahs-chee-moe-tuh-nuh-suhn]) (Figs 7.41–7.45)

Prerequisites　Same as easy seated pose plus:

- FMA column (3), (4) 1-2

- Screen for hip stability (ask about history of dysplasia or Ehlers–Danlos syndrome that would increase subluxation risk).

TI (therapeutic intention)

- Gateway pose for seated postural control

- Lumbopelvic control in larger neutral zone (outside of spinal neutral and in lumbar flexion)

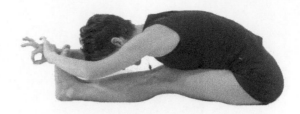
Figure 7.41
Forward seated bend, full flexion

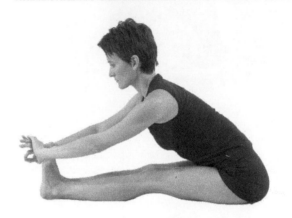
Figure 7.42
Forward seated bend: full (preferred) without end-range flexion

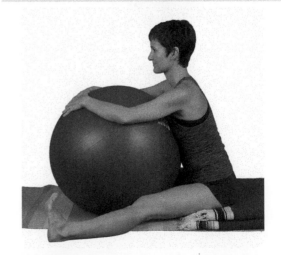
Figure 7.43
Forward seated bend, modified with scaffolded quarter-fold blankets and therapy ball to minimize flexion moment at spine

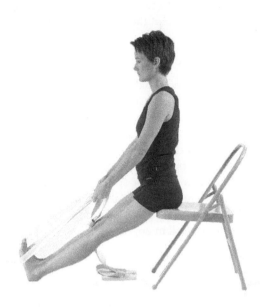

Figure 7.44
Forward seated bend, modified seated in chair

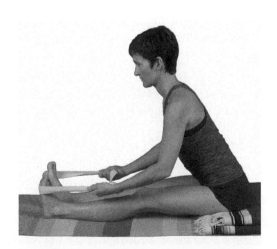

Figure 7.45
Forward seated bend, modified with scaffolded quarter-fold blankets and strap

- Assess arthrokinematics of shoulder and hip — Same as easy seated pose

- Neural mobility — Lower limb neural tension test for the sciatic nerve; slump test variation

- Myofascial tensile force — Superficial back line and possibly the superficial and deep front line if the psoas or rectus femoris tries to "drive" the posture or if diaphragmatic function is nonoptimal. The posterior spiral or functional lines could be implicated if spinal malalignment is present

- Hamstring length greater than 90 degrees clinical normal

- Ego soother (*ahamkara* control)

- Protection from psychoemotional vulnerability or past violent trauma

- Patient education:

  - using hip strategy over lumbar flexion strategy

  - ergonomic tasks such as sitting posture and lifting technique.

SP (starting position) Staff.

Entry Inhale, sit in plumb line alignment/spinal neutral.

Although the full pose allows for spinal flexion, avoid dependence on spinal flexion as the primary strategy, which ignores hamstring extensibility, overstretches iliolumbar ligaments and contributes to poor lifting technique.

TS (thoracic spine) — Paraspinals can develop endurance for spinal support, a standardized test that can assist in prediction of long-term outcomes in chronic low back pain (Delitto et al., 2012). Establishing motor memory for healthy ergonomics and lifting strategies is a logical application. Another intention could be for patients with lumbar stenosis; however, other postures (child's pose or legs-up-the-wall in lumbar flexion/posterior pelvic tilt) limit degrees of freedom in the spine and extremities and offer a safer method for forward flexion. The ischial tuberosities and gluteal soft tissue may flare posterolaterally but manual adjustment of the gluteals is discouraged in order to improve subtle body awareness of myofascial restriction(s). The SIJ remains in a neutral position until the final expression, where counternutation occurs. However, the final expression in full spinal flexion is rarely taught since most patient populations already abuse spinal flexion and have flexion-based postural disorders.

UEs (upper extremities) — Use arm spiral to engage periscapular stabilizers with hands on the floor, feet, or yoga strap/block in a closed kinetic chain.

LEs (lower extremities) — Co-activate the quadriceps and hamstrings, anterior tibialis and gastrocnemius/soleus, and peroneals and posterior tibialis to assist in autogenic or reciprocal lengthening of the hamstrings and gastrocnemius/soleus complex. Maintain neutral foot alignment as in mountain. Bring legs hip-width apart or, for pregnancy, excessive abdominal girth, or femoral retroversion, the legs will need to be separated and possibly slightly externally rotated.

Exit Inhale, look up and return to spinal neutral, eliminating spinal flexion. Exhale and re-engage TATD breath to safely transition from staff by returning to 90 degrees of hip flexion. Maintain co-contraction through the lower extremities for joint stabilization and support during exit.

SRAs (static restorative approximations)

- Legs-up-the-wall

- Supine forward seated bend modification.

DMs (dynamic modifications)

- Yoga couch to elevate seated surface

- Ball-assist — The legs may be separated to allow for trunk or abdominal bulk or girth, as, for example, in pregnancy or distension due to obesity, and supported with a ball

- Chair-assist

- Strap-assist — Place over the ball of the foot, not the arches

- If hands can reach the feet hold the outer corners of the feet to balance medial and lateral hamstring extensibility via maintenance of foot neutral. If the great toes are clasped the tendency is to allow the foot to supinate, which allows for asymmetrical semitendinosus, semimembranosus (medial hamstrings) and the biceps femoris (lateral hamstring) lengthening.

TTCP (teaching and tactical cuing primer)

- Establish and maintain proper lumbopelvic and spinal alignment to prevent posterior pelvic tilting,

guarding of the SIJ (counternutation), lateral spinal shift, or overuse of the gluteals, paraspinals, or external oblique.

- This posture is mountain pose folded in half.

- Iliopsoas should not hold or "drive" the pose. This strategy occurs when short hamstrings or pelvic asymmetry creates a spinal flexion or torsion moment that is given priority over spinal alignment. The iliopsoas responds reciprocally to hold the posture. Intra-articular hip injury can also cause over-recruitment or spasm of the hip flexor as a protective mechanism. Autogenic or reciprocal inhibition could downtrain the iliopsoas that provides physical work in opposition.

Contraindications Osteoporosis and osteopenia patients should only perform honoring plumb line alignment without spinal flexion; degenerative disc disease, degenerative joint disease; active low back pain or sciatica; active SIJ dysfunction; caution for positive slump test; caution for GERD (gastroesophageal reflux disease).

Hero/vitality pose (Virasana [vee-rah-suhn])
(Figs 7.46 and 7.47)

Prerequisites Same as easy seated pose plus FMA columns 2–5. If dynamic stability is not possible, TATD breath columns (3–5) can be eliminated and replaced with external support in reclined hero.

TI (therapeutic intention)

- Hip osteokinematic ROM in FADDIR and arthrokinematic motion for lateral and posterior joint capsule to improve hip FADDIR

- Knee and ankle osteokinematic ROM in knee flexion, some tibial internal rotation, ankle supination, inversion, and plantarflexion

- Assess arthrokinematics of shoulder and hip — Same as easy seated pose

- Postural awareness and lumbar and lumbosacral junction (L5–S1) segmental mobility

- Lower quarter self-massage for edema management and gastrointestinal motility

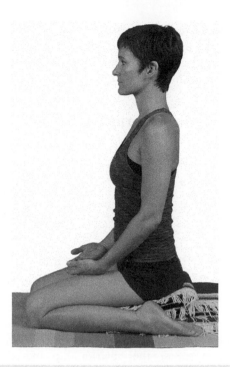

Figure 7.46
Hero, modified on reverse yoga couch

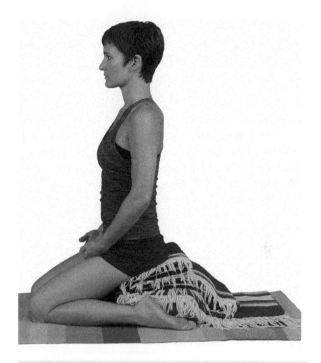

Figure 7.47
Hero, modified on reverse yoga couch with blocks

- Root lock awareness for uptraining (Kegel) or downtraining (reverse Kegel)

- All myofascial lines are relevant. Lack of mobility, resilience, or appropriate response from any of the fascial meridians would be visible in hero

- Progression towards full lotus.

SP (starting position)   Kneeling or four-point position, with a minimum of three tri-fold blankets, from two to four blocks, a chair, and a wall available as needed. This pose is modified from its original form to protect the knees.

Entry   Kneeling, keeping knees at hip width (can be together if excessive femoral anteversion is present), spread the feet slightly wider than the pelvis so can rest on the buttocks or one or more blocks that are placed between the feet. For those with femoral retroversion, this pose may need to avoid hip internal rotation. This pose is different from thunderbolt based on the distance between the feet. The feet are together in thunderbolt, while separated in hero.

Massage the gastrocnemius, treating any trigger or tender points with soft tissue mobilization techniques such as firm pressure and kneading, but do not roll the muscle belly of the calf laterally as it can place the tibia in excessive internal rotation, putting the meniscus at risk. Place the hands over the hip joints to feel the slight internal rotation of the hip and spreading of the ischial tuberosities. *Option*: myofascial release can be performed over the front line of the knees and the back line of the body without manipulation of the underlying muscle mass. Sit back on the blocks. Reclined hero is introduced in Chapter 8.

Exit   Return to kneeling. Never circumduct the knee to transfer to sitting. This creates shear plus torsion moments in the knees and increases ligamentous and meniscus injury risk.

Cautions

- High-risk posture — Hero posture is not often used or taught due to high probability of contraindication in patient populations. When it is taught it is modified from its traditional form (where the ischial tuberosities are firmly planted between the heels, also known as "W" sitting).

- This pose is absolutely contraindicated for any intra-articular fibrocartilaginous knee or hip injury or for any child whose epiphyseal plates have not closed due to the pose's potential to create excessive femoral anteversion or tibial torsion, which can contribute to abnormal load transfer in the lower kinetic chain and lumbopelvic spine and contribute to premature aging of the joints.

SRAs (static restorative approximations)

- Block- or blanket-assist to elevate sitting surface
- Chair-sitting substitution
- Wall-assist — Sit against wall
- "*Sleepy or kissing knees*" (hook lying hip internal rotation).

DMs (dynamic modifications) and TTCP (teaching and tactical cuing primer)

- Knee support — Props should be used to protect the knees. Hero is rarely performed in its full expression secondary to lack of therapeutic application and concomitant risk of fibrocartilaginous injury at the knee and hip joint(s). Use as many yoga couch blanket-folds as needed to place between the heels to elevate the sitting surface and support the posture.

- Ankle support — Use a thinly rolled blanket under the axis of rotation in the ankle to avoid neurovascular impediment, excessive anterolateral ligamentous instability, or to accommodate missing or uncomfortable end-ranges of plantarflexion.

Contraindications Degenerative joint disease or degenerative disc disease causing acute pain or neurovascular signs or symptoms; knee meniscus injuries and ligamentous injuries; severe osteoarthritis; not to be performed during pregnancy without props due to joint laxity; children in bone growth stage secondary to risk of femoral torsion; caution for "yoga foot drop" secondary to nerve compression of the common peroneal nerve as it traverses the fibular head; SIJ dysfunction; stenosis; intra-articular hip injuries, such as FAI or hip labral tear, and congenital or acquired hip joint malformation, such as dysplasia; femoral retroversion.

Boat pose (Navasana [nah-vah-suhn])
(Figs 7.48–7.51)

Code 7.5 (subscription code)
Boat

Prerequisites Same as easy seated pose plus:

- Entire FMA (1–6) including yogic locks (TATD in/outside of neutral spine, which constitutes locks 3 of 6)

- Absence of iliopsoas as a primary driver of movement that contributes to existing pathology of, or compresses, the anterior hip morphology. The Craig test/femoral version screen is recommended if intra-articular hip injury is suspected.

TI (therapeutic intention)

- Advanced gateway pose for inversions
- Advanced pelvic floor strengthening and neuromuscular education

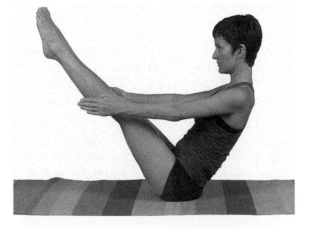

Figure 7.48
Boat, full

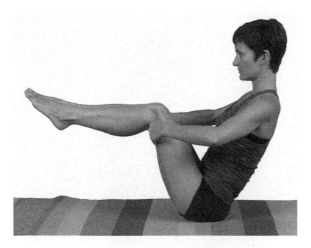

Figure 7.49
Boat, half and modified with arm spiral hold

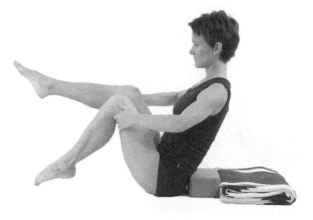

Figure 7.51
Boat, partial and modified with arm spiral hold and blanket/block support for safety and biofeedback

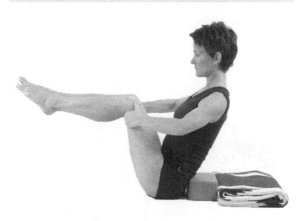

Figure 7.50
Boat, half and modified with arm spiral hold and blanket/block support for safety and biofeedback

- Assess arthrokinematics of shoulder and hip — Same as easy seated pose. If the humerus or femur becomes fixed (not moving), then roll and glide will occur in the same direction

- Myofascial tensile force — Superficial back, possible lateral and spiral, posterior arm, and functional lines/bands may be most likely implicated

- Lumbopelvic proprioception and spinal neutral neuromuscular education.

SP (starting position) Seated.

Entry Draw the knees toward the chest where the hip angle is 90 degrees or more of flexion, hip width apart. Maintain plumb line alignment to the hip as able, including glenohumeral joint neutral. Engage TATD breath and on exhale lift the heels from the ground, keeping the toes on the ground. Reach under the knees with the blades of the hands, palms facing the body. Stay on the front side of the ischial tuberosities and maintain spinal neutral as much as possible. Beginners can remain here. Maintain TATD breath and assure that increased intra-abdominal pressure is not adversely affecting pelvic organ positioning or pelvic floor integrity. Those with FAI may need to avoid full hip flexion while those with femoral retroversion may need to externally rotate at the hip joint.

Intermediate — Practice lifting one lower leg parallel to the floor. Then lift the other leg or practice lifting them alternately.

Intermediate progression — Lift both lower legs parallel to the floor, without holding knees with the hands.

Advanced — Knee extension for full boat. The shoulders flex and take arm spiral with a neutral wrist and forearm.

Exit Lower the legs to the floor and maintain TATD breath. The arms may lift to 90 degrees flexion with palms turned to face legs or in pronation. The glenohumeral joints remain in arm spiral. The lower extremities remain co-contracted at upper and lower legs without rigidity.

Alternate — Bring heels together and toe-out to 45 degrees for less hip flexor recruitment, as necessary.

SRAs (static restorative approximations)

- Supine hook lying
- Prone TATD initiation.

DMs (dynamic modifications)

- Prop-assist — Use a block behind the sacrum (top of the block should meet the base of the sacrum to provide balance, support, and proprioceptive feedback)

- Pose substitution:
  - long sitting with unilateral lower extremity lift (hip flexion and knee extension or straight leg raises (SLRs))
  - side plank from knee and hand (blanket support under the knee).

TTCP (teaching and tactical cuing primer)
Engaging the pelvic floor may assist in downtraining the sternocleidomastoid, platysma, and other secondary muscles of respiration or in resolution of diastasis rectus abdominis (DRA) impairment.

Contraindications   Inability to sustain TATD contraction in downward-facing dog preparation for 10 seconds or 5 breaths; caution with GERD; knee osteoarthritis; anterior intra-articular hip injury or FAI; pelvic organ prolapse, DRA, incontinence, or related pelvic pain due to pelvic floor loss of integrity.

Sage pose (Bharadvajasana [bahrahd-vah-jah-suhn]) (Figs 7.52–7.55)

Prerequisites   Same as easy seated pose plus entire FMA (1–6) including yogic locks (TATD breath constitutes or requires performance of locks 3 through 6).

TI (therapeutic intention)

- The only pose which couples thoracic rotation with contralateral cervical rotation and scalene,

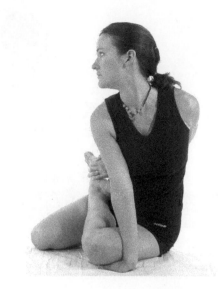

Figure 7.52
Sage, full

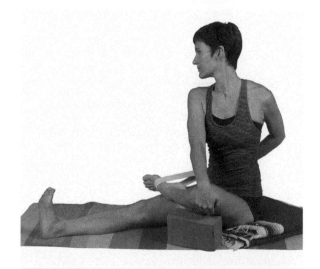

Figure 7.53
Sage, modified with scaffolded quarter-fold blankets and extended knee with strap to bind foot, and block support for leg

subclavius, and pectoralis minor isolation, including potential glenohumeral joint inferior glide

- Spinal osteokinematic ROM in mild thoracic flexion, and global rotation and sidebending

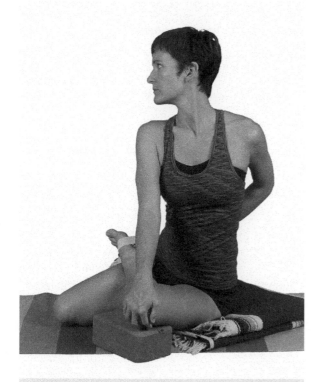

Figure 7.54
Sage, modified with scaffolded quarter-fold blankets and flexed knee, strap to bind foot, and block support for leg

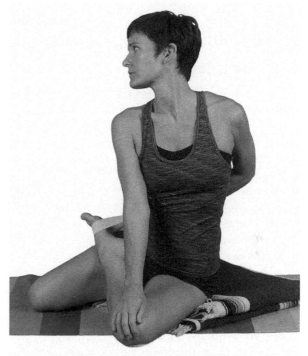

Figure 7.55
Sage, modified with scaffolded quarter-fold blankets and flexed knee with strap to bind foot

- Gastrointestinal motility, visceral massage and downward flow of energy/motility (*apanavayu*)

- Hip osteokinematic in FABER

- Assess arthrokinematics of shoulder and hip — Same as easy seated pose. Once in the pose — Arthrokinematic roll and glide in all planes of motion could occur in the same direction if the convex surface of the shoulder's humeral head or hip's femoral head remains fixed and the concave surface of the glenoid fossa or acetabulum is moving

- Knee osteokinematic ROM in knee flexion, self-limited tibial external rotation (half-lotus leg), and self-limited tibial internal rotation (grounded leg)

- Ankle osteokinematic ROM in plantarflexion and inversion/supination

- Intercostal, quadratus lumborum, and paraspinals extensibility on side of tensile force

- Resisted diaphragmatic strengthening

- Forearm and wrist ROM and tissue extensibility in all planes of motion

- Pectoralis major and minor extensibility

- All myofascial lines are relevant (especially the spiral arms, lateral band/raphe), and deep front lines or bands including the scalenes, hyoid area, platysma, subclavius, upper trapezius, sternocleidomastoid, and diaphragm. Depending on the position taken, the lower quarter counterpart lines may also be equally affected with tensile force

- Posterior upper extremity — Glenohumeral osteokinematic extension, external rotation, and horizontal adduction ROM

- Anterior upper extremity — Glenohumeral joint flexion, external rotation, and horizontal adduction

- High level lumbopelvic awareness and postural control

- High level scapulothoracic stabilization.

SP (starting position)   Staff.

Entry   Bring both knees bent and the feet to the right side, as in a left side sit. If desired, reach under and lift the left leg, sitting the foot into the right groin or to the edge of the right knee. Otherwise, stay in a side-sitting position with the right ischial tuberosity cleared from the floor. Bring left arm behind the trunk and grasp the forefoot or use a strap to facilitate binding by placing the strap over the left forefoot. Bring the right hand, palm facing the ground and fingers under the left distal thigh, to the ground through left thoracic trunk rotation. Rotate the cervical spine to look over the right shoulder. The spine should remain as neutral as possible during rotation. There may be some thoracic flexion or reversal of lordosis coupled with upper thoracic and cervical extension during the spinal rotation and sidebending; however, the posture should not be performed using spinal flexion as the dominant movement strategy. The SIJ should travel with spinal rotation, thereby minimizing or eliminating SIJ torque moment.

UEs (upper extremities) — The hand under the distal femur should resist scapular protraction, while working toward full wrist extension and combined glenohumeral external rotation, flexion, and horizontal adduction. The bound glenohumeral joint (posterior shoulder) adducts, internally rotates, and extends. Both upper extremities actively work toward scapulothoracic stabilization.

LEs (lower extremities) — This full pose requires full knee flexion and half-lotus but can be easily modified with a variety of modifications (see DMs). Loss of lower quarter mobility may necessitate screening for athrokinematic motion and/or use of manual therapy or joint mobilizations.

Exit   Inhale and find more spine length and height. Exhale and release the left arm and return to facing forward. Repeat on the opposite side.

SRAs (static restorative approximations)   Supine windshield wipers with contralateral cervical rotation (i.e. spinal twist to the left and cervical rotation to the right).

DMs (dynamic modifications)

- Blanket-assist — Elevate the sitting surface.

- Block-assist — Place a block under front hand instead of reaching to the floor.

- Partial pose — Eliminate arm-binding.

TTCP (teaching and tactical cuing primer)

- Lift the chest to avoid improper load transfer and form/force closure of the shoulder complex and/or spine.

- If joint mobility is not available, modify the pose rather than using upper quarter force to attain joint mobility (which could compromise fibrocartilaginous tissue in the hip and knee, and ligamentous stability in the spine, pelvis, knee, and/or ankle). Do not force the twist using the levers of the arms and legs; instead initiate the twist from the abdominal musculature and with a thoracic rotation moment.

Contraindications   Carpal tunnel syndrome; degenerative disc disease, degenerative joint disease, SIJ dysfunction or acute low back pain; intra-articular hip or knee dysfunction or injury; osteoporosis or osteopenia; pelvic organ prolapse; FAI or hip dysplasia.

Camel pose (Ustrasana [oos-trah-suhn]) (Figs 7.56–7.59)

Prerequisites   Same as sage pose.

TI (therapeutic intention)

- Lumbopelvic control and postural awareness outside of spinal neutral (spinal extension)

- Assess arthrokinematics of shoulder and hip — Same as easy seated pose. Once in the pose — Arthrokinematic roll and glide in all planes of motion could occur in the same direction if the convex surface (humeral and femoral heads) remain fixed and the concave surface (glenoid fossa and acetabulum) is moving

- Management of excessive anterior pelvic tilt or bilateral chronic SIJ nutation by encouraging bilateral sacral counternutation during the initial posture entry

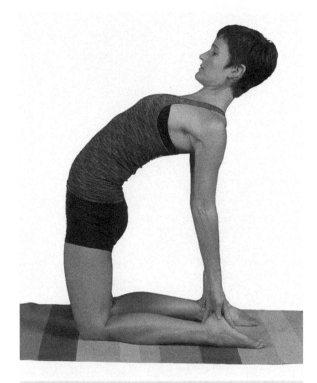

Figure 7.56
Camel, full with hands on plantarflexed heels or feet

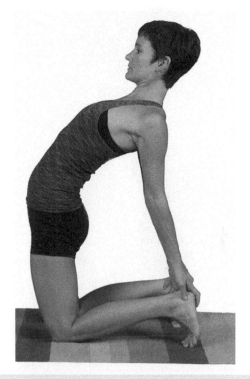

Figure 7.57
Camel, full with hands on dorsiflexed heels

- Abdominal, psoas major and minor, iliacus, and quadriceps length

- Management of degenerative disc disease (posterolateral or posterior) causing bulging or herniated discs in modified position(s)

- Segmental spinal mobilization in extension

- Osteoporosis or osteopenia extension-based exercise

- Indirect sciatic nerve decompression

- Osteokinematic ROM — Ankle plantarflexion, glenohumeral joint extension, internal rotation (starting position) and external rotation (finishing position)

- Concomitant anterior abdominal length and eccentric strength (on entry); concentric strength in active insufficiency (on exit)

- Myofascial tensile force — Superficial and deep front, spiral, functional, and arm lines or bands could be most affected.

SP (starting position)   Kneeling.

Entry   With knees hip width apart, bring the hands to the sacrum, palms resting against the sacrum with fingers facing up or down. Slightly posteriorly, tilt the pelvis then extend the spine and lift the chest superiorly by pressing into an imaginary resistance at the sternum. Keep the pelvis over the knees via hip and trunk extension. The sacrum nutates at end range, but nutation should not be an initial movement strategy (i.e. via gross anterior pelvic tilting). Rather, achieve thoracic extension in initial pose entry. Enter and exit the pose without spinal rotation or sidebending. If cervical extension is chosen retract the cervical spine prior to extension. For populations with vascular or postural comorbidities, avoid cervical extension and maintain cervical retraction (*mild jalandhara bandha*) and/or flexion (*full jalandhara bandha*) throughout the entire pose, which avoids vertebral artery compromise. Bring the palms, one at a time, to blocks beside the ankles, to the heels, or to the soles of the feet (advanced).

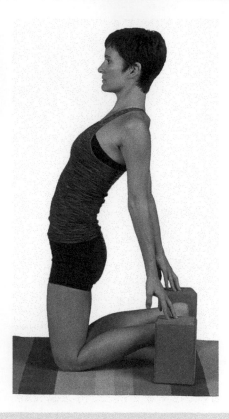

Figure 7.58
Camel, modified with hand support on blocks

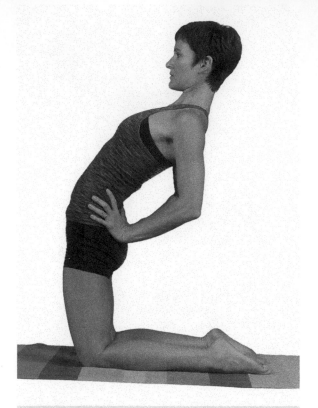

Figure 7.59
Camel, modified with hand support on lumbosacral junction

TS (thoracic spine) — Maintain gluteal relaxation if SIJ dysfunction is present or if gluteal gripping is dominating the movement. Employ gluteals if there is femoral head anterior translation, shallow acetabulum or hip instability, weak gluteals, hypermobile SIJ, and/or when bridge pose has been mastered with healthy dissociation of the gluteus maximus from the hamstrings as a hip extender.

UEs (upper extremities) — The upper extremities fully participate in posture support via glenohumeral joint extension and internal rotation in the starting position, and shoulder extension and external rotation in the dynamic position.

LEs (lower extremities) — Do not flex the knees past 90 degrees in order to reach the feet. Rather, use a support under the hands to minimize injury risk to spine.

Exit   Return the palms, one at a time, to the sacrum. Employ TATD breath and co-activation of the lower

extremities to lift the trunk to an upright position through the sternum, pressing into the imaginary resistance.

SRAs (static restorative approximations)

- Supine over thoracic spine tri-fold blankets
- Supine over ball
- Supported bridge
- Supported half bow pose.

DMs (dynamic modifications)

- Wall-assist — Facing the wall, with both ASISs against the wall, extend the spine without allowing the ASISs to lose contact with the wall.
- Manual assist for lumbar spine stability — Keep the hands on the sacrum.

- Manual assist for cervical spine stability — Keep the hands on the back of the head in a glenohumeral FABER position.

- Block-assist — Use blocks on the outside of each foot.

- Foot-assist for stability — Turn the toes under, thereby elevating the heels and making it easier to reach your feet.

TTCP (teaching and tactical cuing primer)

- Promote thoracic and lumbar segmental extension and avoid shearing or lateral shifting

- Manual cuing for stability of the pose, decompression of the sacrum, and reduced compression and shearing at the lumbar spine — Create tensile force through the lumbar spine via lifting at the inferior angle of the scapulae

- Manual cuing for neuromuscular education and decompression of the sacrum — Using your knees, approximate the ASISs bilaterally.

Contraindications   Stenosis, acute low back pain, spondylolisthesis, pregnancy; spondylosis; degenerative joint disease; lumbar posterior or lateral shear; anterior glenohumeral or hip joint instability; lumbar fusion, weak pelvic floor, cervical fusion, DRA.

Review

The seated and kneeling postures presented in this chapter are categorized into two different levels, moving from simpler positions with smaller degrees of freedom (level I) to more complex biomechanical positions requiring greater degrees of freedom and neuromotor skill (level II). Seated postures are a natural progression to transfer from standing into supine postures, hence their location in the text between standing and supine postures. Seated postures also offer the opportunity to teach safe progression and transfer to supine postures. For those who cannot perform standing postures, both standing and seated and/or kneeling postures can be performed from a chair or plinth.

Postures in this chapter are foundational supine pose and presented in two segments. The first group (level I) consists of postures included in the primary adult functional movement assessment (FMA) algorithm

used for assessment and management. They are also suggested prerequisites for the second group (level II) of supine postures, which also includes some restorative postures. Supine postures are some of the most accessible yoga movements for their ability to be performed in both supine and inclined positions as well as from the floor or a treatment table or plinth.

Therapeutic benefits and general precautions and contraindications are listed in Table 3.9. Additional benefits and precautions are listed under each pose. See Table 8.1 for an overview of supine yoga postures.

Prerequisite interventions

Three-tier approach (yoga couch) (Figs 8.1 and 8.2; Code 8.1)

Code 8.1 (free code)
Yoga couch

Prerequisites

- Orofacial and respiratory assessment

- Supine abdominodiaphragmatic (A-D) breath (other breath types in Chapter 4 may be helpful but are not required)

- Transversus abdominis-assisted thoracodiaphragmatic (TATD) breath for transfer from supine-to-sit and vice-versa

- Standing-to-floor transfer if performing from floor.

TI (therapeutic intention)

- An alternative to corpse pose that creates a safe therapeutic landscape and clinical environment for those who cannot lie supine

Table 8.1

Supine yoga postures

Pose	Figure	QR code
Prerequisite interventions		
Three-tier approach blanket fold - yoga couch	Figs 8.1–8.2	Code 8.1
Corpse and safe supine-to-sit transfers	Figs 8.3–8.4 and 5.7	Code 8.2
Functional movement assessment algorithm postures (level I)		
Knee-to-chest and hook lying knee lifts	Figs 5.8–5.9 and 5.34–5.35	Code 5.7
Hip telescoping	Figs 5.10–5.14	
Windshield wipers	Figs 5.19–5.24	Code 5.3
Supine arm spiral	Figs 5.29–5.30	Code 5.4
Supine arm floats	Figs 5.31–5.33	
Happy baby	Figs 8.5 and 5.16	
Bridge	Figs 8.6–8.7, 5.36	
Two-foot	Figs 5.37–5.42	
Additional supine postures (level II)		
Reclined supported tree	Figs 8.8–8.10	
Reclined cobbler's	Figs 8.11–8.12	
Strap-assisted half-lotus	Fig. 8.13	
Half upward-facing bow	Figs 8.14–8.15	
Tabletop or Eastern-facing	Figs 8.16–8.19	
Reclined hero	Figs 8.20–8.21	Code 8.3
Hand-to-big toe	Figs 8.22–8.24	
Upward-facing forward seated bend	Figs 8.25–8.27	
Upright extended foot	Figs 8.28–8.31	

- Positioning favorable for execution of manual therapy in supine that would include mobilization with movement such as deep breathing, upper quarter mobilizations, and myofascial release and manual therapy for the cervical spine

- All fascial lines are relevant. Lack of mobility, resilience, or appropriate response from any part of the fascial meridians would be visible in this pose.

SP (starting position) A Mexican-style blanket should be folded in half on the short edge and then

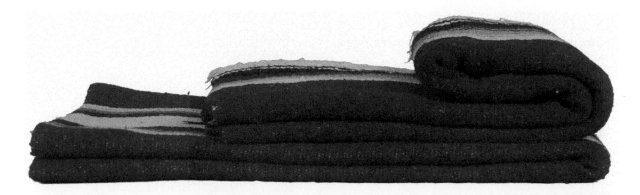

Figure 8.1
Yoga couch, low

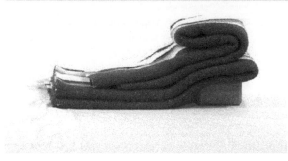

Figure 8.2
Yoga couch, high

folded into thirds. Once folded into thirds the blanket can be folded in half on the short edge again. Repeat with a second blanket. The top blanket should be folded by one-third to support cervical lordosis, unless excessive thoracic kyphosis is present and not reversible; in which case the blanket is used for both cervical lordosis support and head elevation to prevent undesired extension moment at the cervical spine.

Entry   Rest in supine on the blankets. Lie on the side first, then log-roll the torso and head onto the blankets. The pelvis rests on the floor, the lumbar lordosis is supported by the bottom tier of the "couch," and the bottom of the ribcage meets the bottom of the second tier. The top tier (third) adjusts to fill the cervical lordosis and support the head and subsequent spine in plumb line alignment. The torso rests at an approximately 30-degree incline from the horizontal.

The glenohumeral joint rests in an open-packed position with the arms in 45 degrees of abduction and the forearms in supination. The lower extremities have approximately 18 inches distance between the heels and the hips resting in natural external rotation of approximately 15 degrees.

Exit   On exhale, draw the heels into the body to feet flat position, one leg at a time and with minimal muscular effort. Sway the knees side to side slightly until momentum gently assists in rolling to the right or left side (left side for warmth, focus, and digestion, and right side for cooling and relaxation). Bring the left arm (or right arm if rolling to the left side) to rest in a fetal position on the right side. Turn the torso toward the ground in order to get the arms underneath the trunk. Use the strength of the arms to press up to a seated position, allowing the head to follow and right itself last from flexion only, rather than from side-bending, rotation and flexion. Keep the eyes closed throughout this transition as able, unless the vestibular system is compromised and requires visual input.

SRAs (static restorative approximations)/DMs (dynamic modifications)

- Increase the elevation. If a 30-degree incline is insufficient, move the pose against a wall for physical support of the blanket structure, elevating the trunk to a 45–60 degree incline

- *"Sleepy knees or kissing knees"* (Chapter 7)

- Legs resting in a chair
- Knee flexion 15–20 degrees (open-packed position) for edema or osteoarthritis
- If shoulder extension is desired to address myofascial restriction or pectoralis group length, the arms rest on the floor at approximately 20–30 degrees of shoulder extension
- If shoulder extension is not desired, blocks can be placed under the arms to maintain shoulder neutral.

TTCP (teaching and tactical cuing primer)

- This pose should not challenge the body to the point of discomfort. It should be a restful position.
- This pose should facilitate A-D breath and a meditative state.

Contraindications — Vestibular dysfunction, allergies, asthma or chronic obstructive pulmonary disease (COPD), vertigo, dizziness, pregnancy may need higher incline angle. Those with joint instability or inflammation may need additional support and/or positioning in open-packed joint positions to rest in yoga couch.

Corpse pose and safe supine-to-sit transfer (Savasana [sha-vah-suhn]) (Figs 8.3 and 8.4)

> **Code 8.2** (subscription code)
> Corpse

Prerequisites   Same as yoga couch.

TI (therapeutic intention)

- Heighten awareness of environment without being distracted by it
- Increase perception and awareness of the self, encourage self-evaluation and feelings of well-being (Anderzén-Carlsson et al., 2014)
- Assimilation of practice
- Traditional finishing posture for yoga practice
- Reduction of anxiety (Chugh-Gupta et al., 2013)

- All fascial lines are relevant. Lack of mobility, resilience, or appropriate response from any part of the fascial meridians would be visible in this pose
- Reduction of flexion synergy in hyper-recruitment pathologies such as cerebral palsy, post-stroke, or traumatic brain injury, or multiple sclerosis
- Reduction in menopausal symptoms for breast cancer survivors (Cramer et al., 2015)
- Safe transfers from supine to sit and sit to supine.

SP (starting position)   Supine lying.

Entry and exit   See yoga couch and eliminate blankets so there is no trunk elevation or shoulder extension.

SRAs (static restorative approximations)/DMs (dynamic modifications)

- Use yoga couch
- *"Sleepy knees/kissing knees"* (Chapter 7)
- Blanket coverage for warmth (physical) or protection (psychoemotional), especially for those who have suffered emotional trauma or physical violence trauma, feel ungrounded or vulnerable
- If this is uncomfortable for the spine, place a blanket roll under the knees or bend the knees, and/or place a small towel roll under the base of the skull and/or the suboccipital region
- Return to yoga couch.

TTCP (teaching and tactical cuing primer)

- Avoid using neck flexion as a primary movement strategy to exit the pose because it creates cervical spine shear force. Psychoemotionally, leading with the head and neck implicates the *"thinking mind,"* and the brain is resting during this pose.
- Avoid sitting straight up from corpse, which creates shear in the unstable, unsupported supine, particularly at distal ends of the kinetic chain (cervical and lumbar spine).

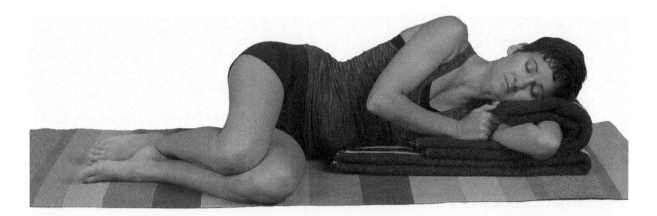

Figure 8.3
Corpse, sidelying on low yoga couch (see also Fig. 5.7 for safe supine-to-sit transfer)

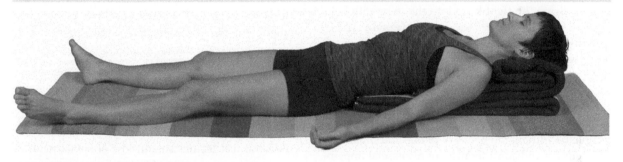

Figure 8.4
Corpse, supine lying on low yoga couch

Contraindications Asthma, COPD, anxiety, anxiety from trauma, nausea, pregnancy, and/or vestibular dysfunction. Those with joint instability or inflammation may need additional support and/or positioning in open-packed joint positions to rest in corpse.

Knee-to-chest pose (lumbopelvic and lower quarter mobility) and hook lying knee lift (lumbopelvic control) **(Apanasana [ah-pah-nuh-suhn])** (see Figs 5.8 and 5.9)

Prerequisites Same as yoga couch plus:

- Yogic locks (TATD constitutes 3 of 6) – TATD breath for transfer from supine to sit and vice-versa; only used when using pose for stability

- Arm spiral (for proper arm placement and stability)

- Craig test/femoral version screen.

TI (therapeutic intention)

- Gateway pose for spinal proprioception and neuromuscular education movement in and outside of spinal neutral

- Myofascial mobility — Superficial back, spiral, posterior arm, and posterior functional lines/bands

- Hip osteokinematic flexion

- Arthrokinematics of the shoulder and hip — Moving into the pose (through the entire pose) — Roll and glide will occur in all planes of motion in opposite directions when the concave surface (glenoid fossa and acetabulum) is fixed and the convex surface (humeral or femoral head) is moving. Once in the pose — Arthrokinematic roll and glide in the hip in all planes of motion will occur in the same

227

direction when the convex surface is fixed and the concave surface is moving

- Differential diagnosis of hip versus spine mobility and ilium gliding

- Lumbosacral proprioception and control

- Alternative to mountain and standing balance postures

- Screen for femoroacetabular impingement (FAI) via increased anterior pelvic tilt angle (Chapter 5).

SP (starting position)   Supine lying over quarter-fold blanket, supine without blanket support, or yoga couch (unable to lie in supine).

Entry   Bring the right knee into the chest with help from the hands behind the knee. Maintain TATD breath. Keep the extended knee and lower quarter co-activated for synergistic trunk support and input and to facilitate functional carryover into standing postures. The extended leg remains active, as if in standing. Preserve lumbar lordosis integrity. All hamstring length range of motion (ROM) measures are completed with maintenance of plumb line alignment for accuracy and consideration of myofascial impairment or neural tension.

Hook lying knee lift (**see Figs 5.34, 5.35 and Code 5.7**)

To test how the weight of the lower extremities is handled by the trunk (lumbopelvic stabilizers) and concomitantly, how the load of the lower extremities is transferred to the trunk in an open kinetic chain movement, a hook lying knee lift can be performed. While this movement does not provide information about how the load is transferred in a closed kinetic chain moment or action (i.e. walking), it can give an objective measure if the individual can lift the foot off the ground without contralateral pelvic translation, loss of spinal neutral, or loss of general postural control. During transition to the opposite side, differentiate between mobility (ability to bring the knee to the chest without impairing plumb line alignment, myofascial restriction, or neural tension) and stability (ability to initiate movement and transition without pelvic translation).

If lumbopelvic stability is not preferred, then use of TATD breath can be discontinued and A-D breath can be resumed. This may be preferred when evaluating for fascial integrity and extensibility or when assessing for ilium gliding.

Exit   Bring the foot back to the floor. Repeat on the other side.

SRAs (static restorative approximations)

- Supported supine with bolster under knees and knee flexion 15–20 degrees

- Supported supine with lower extremities resting on padded chair

- If resting the torso over the quarter-fold blanket, the cervical spine retracts to facilitate plumb line alignment and arthrokinematic mobilization for preservation or restoration of the cervical lordosis.

DMs (dynamic modifications)

Bilateral knee-to-chest:

- Proprioceptive awareness

- Bilateral feet lift-off without loss of spinal neutral and with maintenance of TATD breath (advanced local lumbopelvic stability test)

- Complete release into spinal flexion, beneficial for those with spinal stenosis often responsible for posterior nerve impingement.

Single knee-to-chest:

- Blanket or hand support under lumbar spine to provide external support for maintenance of spinal neutral

- Use unilateral knee-to-chest only in those with impaired trunk control

- Place a thinly rolled blanket under the lumbar spine or cervical spine to support the lordosis in the absence of a quarter-fold blanket

- Use yoga couch.

TTCP (teaching and tactical cuing primer)

- The spine remains in neutral with movement of the lower quarter unless testing for posterior tilt ability.

- If the anterior superior iliac spines move asymmetrically during lifting or transition, differential diagnosis for trunk control (testing of TATD breath and canister/cylinder) and neural patterning is indicated.

Contraindications Second and third trimester pregnancy must modify and use hip flexion, abduction, and external rotation (FABER); COPD, vertigo, dizziness, nausea, GERD, FAI, asthma or allergies may preclude complete supine lying; excessive femoral anteversion or femoral retroversion, psoas or tensor fascia lata dominance and/or hypertrophy, internal snapping hip.

Hip telescoping and windshield wipers

Prerequisites Same as knee-to-chest.

TI (therapeutic intention)

- Hip osteokinematic FABER or flexion, adduction, and internal rotation (FADDIR)

- Hip arthrokinematic motion in posterior glide and anterior roll of femoral head in acetabulum

- Assess arthrokinematics of hip and shoulder — Same as knee-to-chest pose

- Screen for, and development of, movement strategy for arthrokinematic ilium gliding (Chapter 5)

- *Self-scour test* for femoral head tracking in acetabulum (Chapter 5)

- Myofascial mobility — Superficial back, spiral, posterior arm, lateral, and posterior functional lines/bands may be most implicated

- Pediatric *"sensory diet"* therapy. Deep-pressure proprioception through brushing followed by joint compressions (May-Benson, 2007) and possible influence on CSF "third circulation" flow (Cushing, 1927) for affecting posture, focus, and breathing via autonomic regulation (Whedon and Glassey, 2009) through sacral pressure or rocking

- Windshield wipers (Chapter 5) adds:

  - rotation, sidebending, and flexion segmental mobility in thoracolumbar spine

  - external oblique strategy (indicative of nonoptimal load transfer from the trunk to the pelvis and pelvic floor)

  - functional mobility for ADLs such as turning and reaching for objects or participating in recreational activities. Myofascial mobility in superficial back line, spiral line, arm lines, lateral line, posterior functional line, and deep front line may be most implicated

  - differential diagnosis of hip mobility versus thoracic and lumbosacral mobility impairment (Chapter 5).

SP (starting position) Knee-to-chest

Hip telescoping entry (see Figs 5.10–5.14):

Reaching behind the knee, passively move the head of the femur in the acetabulum through all available safe ranges of motion except hip extension. Can be performed unilaterally or bilaterally.

Windshield wipers entry (see Figs 5.19–5.24; Code 5.3):

In a hook lying position with the lateral borders of the feet at the outside edges of the mat, allow one knee to move toward the floor within natural limitations and comfort of the individual available in FADDIR. Allow the other knee to move toward FABER within the same parameters. Legs can perform the windshield wiper movement separately or simultaneously. Unilateral movement can identify available hip range while bilateral movement is used to identify movement impairment related to trunk control and neural patterning of synergistic trunk stabilizers and primary movers.

Exit Return to hook lying, preferably using TATD breath to facilitate safe return.

SRAs (static restorative approximations) Yoga couch or corpse with active assistive ROM (AAROM) (strap) or passive ROM (PROM) (by therapist).

DMs (dynamic modifications)

- Shorten ROM.

- Windshield wipers — Use blocks under the knees to avoid full FABER and FADDIR.

- Complete on yoga couch.

- Windshield wiper lateral articulation (Chapter 5) tests unilateral trunk motor patterning strategy, strength of transversus abdominis (TA), obliques, and fascial response on pose exit.

TTCP (teaching and tactical cuing primer)

- At the onset of movement, watch for ilium glide restriction(s), which would decrease available hip adduction and internal ROM and contribute to sacroiliac joint (SIJ) malalignment, quadratus lumborum splinting, or hip impingement.

- On transition in the pose, watch for loss of symmetrical TA recruitment and excessive external oblique recruitment, a nonoptimal movement strategy that increases pelvic floor pressure.

- Watch for symmetry in ribcage mobility, diaphragmatic excursion, hip ROM, and trunk rotation.

Contraindications Lumbar stenosis or fusion, total hip arthroplasty, acute postoperative hip preservation surgery, hip osteoarthritis, FAI, hip joint instability or labral insufficiency or injury; subspinal (hip) impingement, ischiofemoral impingement.

Supine arm spiral and supine arm floats

See Chapter 5 for assessment and instructions; see also Figs 5.29, 5.30 and 5.31–5.33.

Happy baby pose (Ananda balasana [ah-nahn-duh bah-lah-sahn]) (Fig. 8.5)

Prerequisites Same as knee-to-chest plus FMA column (1) 1, 2, 4.

TI (therapeutic intention)

- Hip osteokinematic hip FABER

- Hip arthrokinematic motion in posterior glide and anterior roll of femoral head in acetabulum

- Assess arthrokinematics of hip and shoulder — Same as knee-to-chest pose

- Sacral counternutation (if not performed in yoga couch)

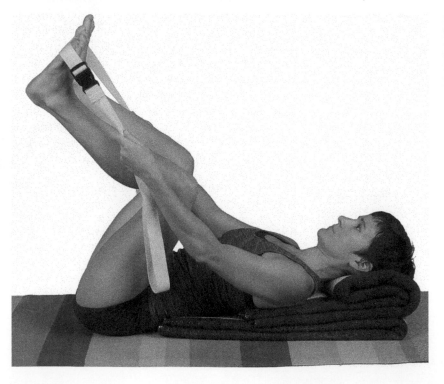

Figure 8.5
Happy baby, modified on yoga couch with strap (see also Fig. 5.16)

- Spinal neutral hip FABER (if performed in yoga couch with strap)

- Scapulothoracic tactile input for proprioception, motor control, and stabilization

- Postural control in and outside of spinal neutral

- Pediatric *"sensory diet"* therapy and CSF influence (see previous posture)

- Hip impingement screen (unilateral or bilateral). If excessive anterior tilt is present with groin pain, differentially diagnose FAI. Correction of spinal alignment that does not decrease hip impingement should be further evaluated or referred out

- Myofascial tensile force — Superficial back, possible lateral, spiral, posterior arm, and functional lines/bands may be most affected.

SP (starting position) For compromised postural awareness needing tactile input for postural control — Supine lying on yoga couch. For no contraindications to spinal flexion and bilateral sacral counternutation — Supine lying.

Entry From hook lying, lift one knee into the chest using deep abdominal breathing (not TATD breath). Repeat on opposite side. Grasp the medial arches of the feet, the lateral edges of the feet, or use a strap on the balls of the feet. Experiment with hip FABER ROM in and out of spinal neutral. The upper extremities resist scapular protraction, internal rotation or winging, and anterior rotation or tipping by engaging the serratus anterior and lower trapezius, as well as the external rotators of the shoulder (teres minor and infraspinatus).

Exit Release the legs and lower them to the floor one at a time.

SRAs (static restorative approximations)/DMs (dynamic modifications)

- Unilateral happy baby

- Sidelying happy baby (fetal position)

- Supported reclined tree

- Supported reclined cobbler's

- Strap-assisted reclined half lotus

- Corpse with imagery.

TTCP (teaching and tactical cuing primer)

- Breathe into the hip and lower spine using three- or four-part breath.

- For beginner students, create safe stability in the pose. Flexibility is secondary.

- For advanced students, play with pelvic lift off (mini-plow pose) without yoga couch.

Contraindications Intra-articular hip injury or hip dysplasia; acute back pain, acute disc derangement or bulge; compromised spinal curves or lack of postural awareness should use yoga couch; hip joint instability or labral insufficiency or injury; subspinal (hip) impingement, FAI, SIJ instability.

Bridge "lock" (Setu bandha [seh-too bahn-duh]) and two-foot (Dvipada pitham [devwee pah-duh peeth-uhm]) (Figs 8.6 and 8.7)

Bridge is a non-articulating (used for those with spinal flexion contraindications) posture that does not use shoulder external rotation. The glenohumeral joints extend and the forearms pronate. The arms actively reach toward the toes to encourage neural mobilization via brachial plexus tension.

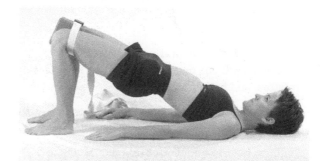

Figure 8.6

Bridge, modified with block and strap (see also Fig. 5.36 for modification on blankets, which is typically used as an adjunct to Fig. 8.6)

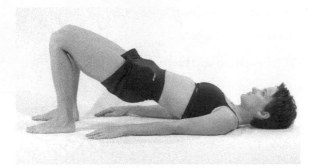

Figure 8.7
Bridge, full

Two-foot (see Figs 5.37–5.42) is an articulating (segmental articulation in spinal flexion that tests spinal thoracic and lumbar segment mobility) posture that allows for slight external rotation of the glenohumeral joint and pectoralis lengthening with inferior distraction of the shoulders and increased anterior line myofascial mobilization.

Bridge is a prerequisite for two-foot. Two-foot is a prerequisite for half-upward-facing bow pose

Prerequisites Same as knee-to-chest plus:

- FMA column (1); (3) 1, 3 only

- Ability to control pelvic translation or rocking in frontal or sagittal planes during an alternate heel lift while maintaining TATD breath in spinal neutral.

TI (therapeutic intention)

- Gateway pose for neural patterning and dissociation of the gluteus maximus (GMAX), hip external rotators, and hamstrings isolation as hip extenders

- Form closure of hip (femoral head in acetabulum and humeral head in glenohumeral joint)

- Gateway pose to spinal extension and shoulderstand

- Assess arthrokinematics of the shoulder — Roll and glide should occur in the same direction as the convex surface (humeral head) is fixed and the concave surface (glenoid fossa) is moving. Arthrokinematics of the hip — Roll and glide should occur in the opposite direction as the convex surface (femoral

head) is moving and the concave surface (acetabulum) is fixed

- Gravity-assisted and *"sump pump"* action of muscular and fascial connections to the pelvic floor for venous and lymphatic aid in pelvic congestion management. Pelvic congestion syndrome can be characterized by feelings of fullness in the legs or urinary tract symptoms caused by varicosities in the trigone, low back pain (LBP), nausea, bloating, and vulvar varicosities on physical examination often accompanied by varicosities of the rectum, anus, perineum, buttocks or lower extremities (Gupta, 2015)

- Facilitation of functional mobility (bridge) — Musculoskeletal balance for smooth ambulation or bed mobility transitions. (Two-foot) — Counteraction of restriction in the anterior arm lines that would impede simple ADL completion such as putting a bra on or tucking in a shirt

- Lumbopelvic neuromuscular education and stabilization

- Osteokinematic and arthrokinematic spinal segmental mobility (two-foot)

- Postural education and awareness

- Iliopsoas length

- Locks proprioception and neuromuscular patterning

- Inversion presents unique input for feeling diaphragm descent in a gravity-dependent, rather than typically gravity-assisted, position that can ease teaching diaphragmatic utilization

- Shoulder complex and forearm osteokinematic ROM (two-foot posture) in glenohumeral extension and external rotation (two-foot), forearm pronation, scapular depression, and medial rotation

- Myofascial tensile force — Superficial front, anterior arm, functional, and deep front lines/bands may be most affected.

SP (starting position) Supine lying in hook lying.

Entry to bridge:

From hook lying, the feet are hip width (from the true hip and not the lateral edges of the soft tissue of the pelvis). Lift the spine as a unit with no spinal segmental articulation, keeping the feet under the knees and knees hip width without cervical spine loading (which would only use the quadriceps and not the hamstrings).

Entry to two-foot posture:

From hook lying, lift one vertebra at a time, starting with the sacrum, until the shoulders, arms, and feet bear the body weight. Mildly extend the thoracic spine to roll the shoulders slightly under the body toward one another.

TS (thoracic spine) — Avoid cervical spine compression by maintaining a knee flexion (hamstring use) moment. The spine remains in neutral save a slight thoracic extension moment and pectoralis lengthening. Screen the cervical spine, neck, and shoulders for myofascial or neural tension, checking the nuchal ligament and the paraspinals in the posterior cervical spine.

UEs (upper extremities) — Remain in contact with the floor but externally rotate and extend the glenohumeral joints to progress toward half-upward-facing bow pose by interlacing the fingers together.

LEs (lower extremities) — The knees do not splay and the gluteals do not dominate the hip extension moment in absence of deep hip rotators and TATD breath. If iliotibial band, iliopsoas, or patellar tracking is an issue, or if hip external rotators demonstrate poor recruitment or endurance then the integrity of the posture will quickly degrade, causing the knees to splay and the gluteals to force hip extension in absence of TATD breath and hip form closure.

Exit

Bridge:

Return to hook lying moving the spine as a unit.

Two-foot:

Articulate the spine from the thoracic spine down to the sacrum, one vertebra at a time.

For both postures, create a traction moment at the spine via hamstrings action as knee flexors and hip extenders.

SRAs (static restorative approximations)

- Pelvic tilt or clock

- Supine blanket or bolster supported thoracic spine extender

- Ball-assist.

DMs (dynamic modifications)

- Blankets under the shoulders and spine but never under the head or neck to maintain cervical lordosis integrity

- For therapeutic reversal of excessive kyphosis, 1–2 blankets (quarter or tri-fold) may be placed under the shoulders and thoracic spine. However, if the thoracic spine is too rigid, a cervical extension moment may be created, which will require secondary blanket placement under the head until thoracic kyphosis is normalized, if possible

- Strap the knees at the distal femur to prevent excessive hip abduction and external rotation

- Strap the knees at the distal femur with a block to encourage anterior superior iliac spine (ASIS) approximation, hip adductor involvement, and freedom of SIJ accommodation to movement

- For osteoporosis, lift the spine all at once as in an unbendable tree trunk, instead of segmentally moving the vertebrae. Place a quarter-fold blanket under the trunk, not the head.

TTCP (teaching and tactical cuing primer)

- Manual cuing for thoracic spine — Place the hands under the inferior lower half of the scapula and lift the trunk to roll the shoulders under in order to progress the posture toward half upward-facing bow

- Manual cuing for iliac crest or SIJ decompression — Narrow ASIS and broaden posterior superior iliac spines (PSIS)

- Articulation — Palpate for segmental mobility of each vertebra during entry and exit from pose

- Turn off the GMAX in order to prevent full nutation and premature locking of the pelvis, especially in those with SIJ obliquity or dysfunction

- Use the GMAX to facilitate gross spinal extension and/or form closure of the hip joint after hamstring and quadriceps co-contraction have been demonstrated in absence of gluteal domination

- Employ use of the hip external rotators for synergistic lumbopelvic strength building

- Avoid weight-bearing through the head and neck as it can cause breath-holding, neck pain, or neurovascular headaches.

Contraindications No spinal flexion segmental articulation is performed with osteoporosis or osteopenia of the spine or spinal fusions. Instead, bridge (no segmental articulation) is performed. Excessive thoracic kyphosis may need several blankets in order to modify pose; SIJ dysfunction (torsion or rotation) should recruit the hamstrings (with its direct relationship in stability provision to the SIJ via the sacrotuberous ligament) in favor of the GMAX until alignment issues are resolved, after which, reintroduction of the GMAX is resumed. If the femoral head is anterior and contributing to impingement symptoms, the anterior tibialis and quadriceps are engaged to diminish psoas contribution (to anterior joint loading). Extension-based pain disorders of hip or spine; hip or shoulder anterior instability, acid reflux (fire/water imbalance). The GMAX may also be used as primarily a stabilizer in those with debility (under-recruitment or weakness of the GMAX) or maladaptive positioning of the femoral head in the acetabulum.

Reclined supported tree pose (Supta salamba vrkasana [soup-tuh sah-lahm-buh vrick-shah-suhn]) (Figs 8.8–8.10)

Prerequisites Same as yoga couch plus:

- Craig test/femoral version screen.

TI (therapeutic intention)

- Hip osteokinematic ROM – FABER and potential arthrokinematic motion in posterior glide if sandbag is used

- Assess arthrokinematics of the shoulder and hip — Roll and glide should occur in all planes of motion in opposite directions when the concave surface (glenoid fossa and acetabulum) is fixed and the convex surface (humeral and femoral head) is moving

- Manage round ligament pain in pregnancy and PMS-type cramping and pelvic pain

- Myofascial tensile force — Superficial front, anterior arm, spiral, anterior functional, and deep front lines/bands may be most implicated

- Pectoral group lengthening, depending on arm position chosen

- Contralateral (straight leg) iliopsoas extensibility

- Ipsilateral (bent leg) adductor extensibility

Props 1–2 blocks, 1–2 blankets.

SP (starting position) Supine; supine on yoga couch.

Entry Flex the right knee to place the foot flat. Use a block to support the right leg in FABER. The spine remains in neutral with plumb line alignment from the cervical spine to pelvis if using the yoga couch. If lying in supine, full plumb line alignment is maintained. The legs are supported at all times with blocks or blankets. Hip FABER action should not place torque moment(s) at the spine or knees.

Exit Transition out of this pose by helping the legs up to hook lying and log-rolling to the side, returning to seated meditation. Restorative postures can be held several minutes. Repeat on the other side.

SRAs (static restorative approximations)

The SRA for tree.

- Yoga couch

- Place extra blankets on top of the blocks under the knees.

DMs (dynamic modifications)

- Add additional blankets over the supporting block, especially for those with fibromyalgia or point tenderness.

- Put the entire pose on an incline (yoga couch) for those with respiratory difficulties or pregnancy.

- Practice unilaterally with only one leg opening to the side at a time.

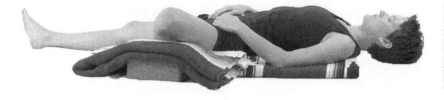

Figure 8.8
Reclined supported tree on quarter-fold blanket with block and blanket support under knee

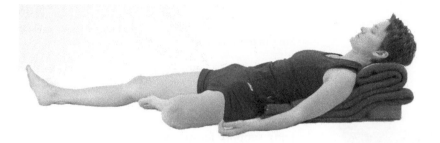

Figure 8.9
Reclined supported tree on high yoga couch

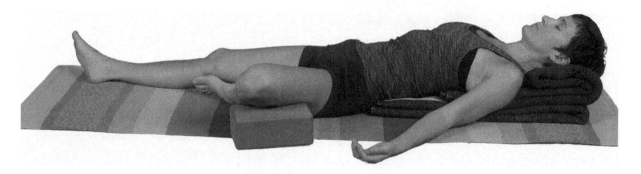

Figure 8.10
Reclined supported tree on low yoga couch with block support under knee

- Add a blanket under the head and neck if thoracic kyphosis creates cervical extension.

TTCP (teaching and tactical cuing primer)

- The student should be comfortable and pain-free. Continue to offer modifications until a pain free posture is found.

- Encourage depth of breath.

- Encourage remaining alert in restorative postures.

Contraindications   Pregnancy after first trimester and COPD or respiratory difficulties may need an incline of blankets against the wall, intra-articular hip pathology or congenital malformation of the hip or pelvis, such as excessive femoral anteversion or shallow acetabulum present in hip dysplasia.

Reclined supported cobbler's pose (Supta salamba baddha konasana [soop-tah sah-lahm-buh bah-duh kuh-nah-suhn]) (Figs 8.11 and 8.12)

Prerequisites   Same as reclined tree pose.

TI (therapeutic intention)

Same as reclined tree pose plus:

- Bilateral adductor extensibility

- Increased fascial extensibility.

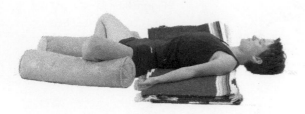

Figure 8.11
Reclined supported cobbler's on quarter-fold blanket with bolster support under knees

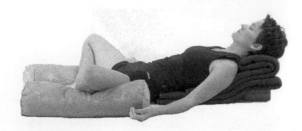

Figure 8.12
Reclined supported cobbler's on high yoga couch with bolster support under knees

Sandbags are generally not used bilaterally on hip joints in this pose.

Props   1–2 blocks, 1–2 blankets.

SP (starting position)   Supine in yoga couch.

Entry   Bring the soles of the feet together and allow the knees to rest out to the side. Place the blanket and/or block under each knee, supporting it near the hip joint.

TS (thoracic spine) — Maintain spinal curves via yoga couch as needed.

UEs (upper extremities) — The upper extremities rest at a 45-degree angle out from the sides with forearm supination, or they can rest in shoulder flexion/abduction or with the fingers interlaced and hands resting behind the head.

LEs (lower extremities) — Always support the legs with props, unless both knees can completely rest on the floor. The hip FABER is never a free-floating position owing to its high risk of pelvic, groin, hip, knee, or sacral injury.

Exit   Passively return the legs to hook lying with hand assist and remove the blocks to the left side. Logroll to the right side. Remain here for several breaths before returning to seated.

SRAs (static restorative approximations)

The SRA for cobbler's.

Same as reclined supported tree plus:

- Supported reclined tree pose.

DMs (dynamic modifications)

- Yoga couch (higher incline)
- Thoracic spine (1–2 blankets in tri-fold or quarter-fold) support for thoracic extension or cervical retraction, respectively)
- Small blanket roll under the low back, in the cervical lordosis, or under the knees for support.

TTCP (teaching and tactical cuing primer)

- As hip ROM improves via arthrokinematic gliding of the innominate over the inferior lateral angle of the sacrum, improved posterior glide of the hip, or improved tissue extensibility, move the supporting prop closer to the knee to allow for more opening of the hip.
- Use reclined postures on a gradient, gradually introducing leg movements that would involve the perineum, in order to facilitate pelvic relaxation for pelvic myalgia/vaginismus.

Contraindications   Second trimester and beyond pregnancy avoid supine lying, and asthma, vertigo, vestibular disorders, dizziness, or related conditions preventing supine lying should use yoga couch. SIJ dysfunction; intra-articular hip pathology or hip dysplasia; limiting osteoarthritis of the trunk or lower quarter.

Strap-assisted reclined half-lotus pose (Supta salamba ardha padmasana [soup-tuh sah-lahm-buh are-duh pad-mah-suhn]) (Fig. 8.13)

Prerequisites   Same as yoga couch plus:

- TATD breath (if stability preferred)

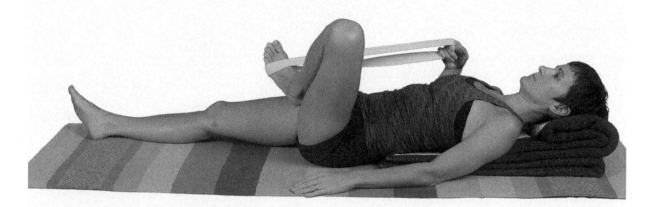

Figure 8.13
Strap-assisted reclined half-lotus

- Arm spiral

- Craig test/femoral version screen.

TI (therapeutic intention)

- SRA for postures requiring hip osteokinematic FABER

- Hip arthrokinematic posterior roll and anterior glide

- Assess arthrokinematics of the shoulder and hip — Moving into the pose — Roll and glide should occur in all planes of motion in opposite directions when the concave surface (glenoid fossa and acetabulum) is fixed and the convex surface (humeral and femoral head) is moving. Once in the pose — Arthrokinematic roll and glide in all planes of motion should occur in the same direction when the convex surface is fixed and the concave surface is moving. The upper shoulder will continue to function in an open chain, which means it will follow the roll and glide in opposite directions, unless it becomes fixed and the glenoid fossa moves over it

- Postural and lower quarter proprioceptive training

- Gentle visceral massage through hip FABER and trunk movement

- Both restorative and dynamic

- Myofascial tensile force — Superficial back, lateral, posterior spiral, posterior arm, functional, and lower torso and quarter portion of the deep front lines/bands may be most likely implicated

- Psoas, sartorious, rectus femoris, and tensor fascia lata downtraining (relaxation).

SP (starting position)   Supine lying or yoga couch.

Entry   Place a strap over the right midfoot and hold the strap with the left or right hand. Experiment with hip FABER and any combination of knee extension or flexion while maintaining ankle co-activation to hold neutral position of the foot, which helps keep the strap in place. Use of three-tier approach helps maintain spinal neutral for those who need tactile input for postural awareness and control. Maintenance of spinal neutral is not required but should be maintained under conscious effort as needed. Protect the hip by not *"strong-arming"* ROM via upper extremity force. Maintain the opposite (uninvolved) leg in co-activation for synergistic trunk support during active posture experimentation.

Exit   Release the leg slowly and repeat on the other side.

SRAs (static restorative approximations)

- Unilateral happy baby

- Sidelying happy baby (fetal position)

- Supported reclined tree

- Corpse with imagery.

DMs (dynamic modifications)   To increase upper extremity and lower extremity ROM simultaneously, hold the strap in the ipsilateral hand as the involved/strapped foot. Bring the contralateral arm into shoulder flexion and cradle the head with the arm. Pass the strap into the contralateral hand (left hand for right strapped foot) and rest in this position for several breaths.

TTCP (teaching and tactical cuing primer)

- Always cradle and reach under (rather than over) to minimize iliopsoas recruitment.

- Students tend to force this pose before their body is ready. Provide reminders to practice non-violently (*ahimsa*).

- If floor dwelling (sitting) is difficult, begin habituation to this posture by spending less time chair-dwelling and more time floor-dwelling with support.

Contraindications   Excessive tibial torsion or femoral anteversion; poor hip, knee, or ankle osteokinematic or athrokinematic ROM; aggression, intra-articular hip or knee joint pathology (meniscus or ligamentous insufficiency) or hip dysplasia; joint hypermobility/hypomobility or degeneration at the spine, hip, knee, or ankle; FAI, subspinal impingement (hip), or ischiofemoral impingement; internal or external snapping hip.

Half upward-facing bow/wheel pose (Ardha urdhva dhanurasana [r-duh oard-vuh duh-newh-ruh-suhn] and Salamba ardha urdhva dhanurasana) (Figs 8.14 and 8.15)

Prerequisites   Same as yoga couch plus:

- FMA column (1); (3) 1, 3, 4, 5

- Craig test/femoral version screen.

TI (therapeutic intention)

- Gateway pose to:

  - lumbopelvic neural patterning and motor control

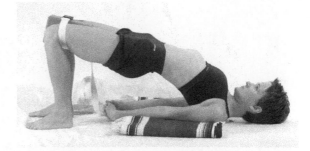

Figure 8.14
Half upward-facing bow with strap and block. Begin with the block on its low, flat side (not pictured), then turn to the narrow side to progress. The final progression is shown in this figure

  - gluteal dissociation from hamstrings as hip extenders

  - spinal extension postures

  - shoulderstand

- Both restorative and dynamic

- Osteokinematic ROM: spinal extension, glenohumeral extension, external rotation, and horizontal adduction; thoracic extension, lumbar extension with cervical lordosis (neutral) maintenance

- Assess arthrokinematics of the shoulder — Roll and glide should occur in the same direction as the convex surface (humeral head) is fixed and the concave surface (glenoid fossa) is moving. Arthrokinematics of the hip — Roll and glide should occur in the opposite direction as the convex surface (femoral head) is moving and the concave surface (acetabulum) is fixed until the end range of hip extension, wherein roll and glide may revert to moving in the same direction

- Arthrokinematic segmental spinal articulation and sacral nutation, counternutation, ilial gliding

- Pectoralis extensibility

- Lumbopelvic stabilization, proprioception and synergistic motor control

- Dissociation of GMAX from lumbopelvic prime agonists

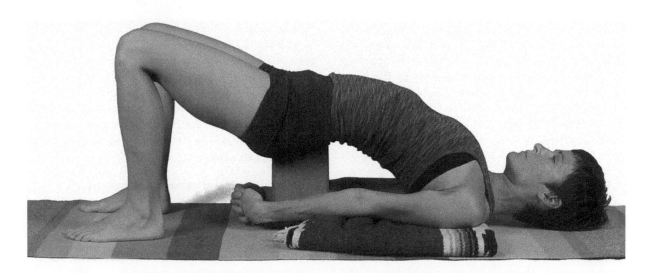

Figure 8.15
Half upward-facing bow, modified on quarter-fold blanket with block assist

- Lung expansion/alveolar ventilation via intercostal flexibility and ribcage mobility

- Lower extremity co-contraction

- Lung and congestion-clearing; allergy relief through gravity-assisted sinus drainage

- Endurance plus strength (power)

- Neural mobilization through combined glenohumeral inferior glide and brachial plexus mobilization

- Myofascial tensile force — Superficial front, anterior spiral, anterior arm, anterior functional, and deep front lines/bands may be most implicated

- Partial inversion presents unique input for feeling the diaphragm descent in a gravity-dependent, rather than typically gravity-assisted, position.

SP (starting position)   Supine hook lying.

Unsupported version

Entry   First, screen the cervical lordosis for integrity. If a loss of cervical lordosis is palpated, add a quarter-folded blanket under the spine (not under the head) to facilitate cervical retraction. Next, with palms pressing earthward at sides, feet hip width, with ankles directly under knees; segmentally lift the spine one segment/vertebra at a time until only the head, shoulders, and feet are on the mat. If possible, clasp the hands by interlacing the fingers. Lift one shoulder and tuck it under the body by encouraging pectoralis and anterior myofascial mobility, brachial plexus lengthening, and glenohumeral extension, external rotation, and horizontal adduction. Repeat on the opposite side. Dig the heels in and isometrically "draw" them toward the body in order to co-contract the quadriceps and hamstrings and disengage the GMAX.

Beginners can inhale into the pose. Experienced yogis exhale into the pose.

Exit   Exhale and release the hands, roll off the shoulders, and segmentally articulate the spine back to the mat facilitating the movement with isometric hamstring contraction and eccentric gluteal lengthening.

Supported version

Entry   Place a quarter-folded blanket under the spine but not under the head to encourage cervical retraction and cervical lordosis preservation. Segmentally articulate into bridge then two-foot. Place the flat, wide side of the block longitudinally under the sacrum (not shown). To progress, turn the block up on its narrow, thin side, also longitudinally (parallel to the trunk, not perpendicular). Lift the chest and tuck the shoulders as in the previous version. To progress further, clasp the hands and roll each shoulder under the body, one at a time. Release the hands, and place the block under the sacrum, turned up to its tallest position. The block-supported version should only be undertaken if the pelvis remains neutral. Spinal extension should come from the thoracic, not the lumbar spine.

Exit   As for the unsupported version, above.

TS (thoracic spine) — The cervical spine should not bear weight in this pose, just as in a shoulderstand. There should be a hollow under the cervical thoracic spine honoring the cervical lordosis with thoracic spine extension. The pelvis remains in relative neutral due to the dominant action of thoracic extension and pectoralis lengthening. Watch for premature sacral nutation, indicative of loss of normal lumbosacral reciprocity and mobility.

UEs (upper extremities) — Glenohumeral extension, external rotation, and horizontal adduction; elbow extension without hyperextension; wrists in neutral.

LEs (lower extremities) — Knees hip width apart; ankles under knees; the beginner may use a GMAX strategy alone to enter into bridge. The advanced patient can dissociate a hamstring (as hip extender) strategy from a gluteal strategy. If the GMAX and the hamstrings can be separately recruited on cue as hip extenders, neuromuscular control is generally better in the lumbopelvic region. If the two actions cannot be separated, risk for back, pelvic, hip, or sacroiliac pain or dysfunction is increased. The heels do not press away from the body creating a knee extension moment. Knee flexion and hip extension strategy is preferred to develop dissociative neural patterning in management of low back pain, SIJ dysfunction, or spinal segmental mobility or stability. Knee flexion, hip extension, and ankle dorsiflexion strategy are used to mediate psoas domination typically found in hip intra-articular injury (anterior labral tears).

Block-assisted version

Place half-folded blankets, lengthwise (or perpendicular to your body) under the shoulders and trunk only to create a supported, gentler backbend; the block running lengthwise with the body, press the sacrum into the body. The bodies of the lumbar vertebrae rest off of the block completely, and are extended as a secondary effect of the block placement under the sacrum. The lumbar spine should not feel compressed. This posture facilitates thoracic extension which, in its final form (upward-facing bow), utilizes full spinal extension.

SRAs (static restorative approximations)

- Pelvic tilt
- Supine blanket or bolster supported thoracic spine opener
- Ball-assisted backbends.

DMs (dynamic modifications)

- Blankets under shoulders and trunk (not under head). Two to three are usually required
- Strap-assist over distal thighs
- Block-assist between knees
- Block- plus strap-assist to develop higher-level neural patterning for lumbopelvic stabilization and pelvic floor health. If SIJ dysfunction (torsion or rotation), downtrain GMAX and recruit the hamstrings as the preferred hip extender until SIJ alignment has been corrected. Then GMAX can be reintroduced, in concert with synergistic stabilizer development
- Block-assisted supported version — Keep the block on its lowest, widest side for the easiest backbend.

TTCP (teaching and tactical cuing primer)

- Manual cuing for:
  - cervical spine protection — Traction and distraction force over the anterior thighs
  - sacroiliac protection and release — Approximation of the ASIS with the knees
  - thoracic spine extension
- To use or not to use the GMAX:

- turn off the GMAX for neural patterning training to teach freedom to find spinal neutral, manipulate the pelvis, release the pelvic floor when necessary, recruit the external rotators, and/or find sacral counternutation

- use the GMAX to improve hip stability, pelvic stability, and/or increase spinal extension. *Caveat:* If using the GMAX degrades spinal integrity by becoming a primary strategy over TATD breath, impairs the breath, or negatively affects the pelvic floor through tonic contraction or valsalva, then avoid GMAX as a primary mover

- Differential diagnosis of weak hip external rotators and their potential contribution to knee pain or back pain. Perform the posture with hip rotator involvement, to address patellofemoral pain syndrome (PFPS)

- Watch for five levels of cervical spine involvement (see previous list).

Contraindications Hyperacidity (fire/water elemental gastrointestinal inflammation); pregnancy; stenosis, spondylosis, spondylolisthesis, thoracic or lumbar fusion; SIJ, anterior shoulder, or anterior hip instability; ischiofemoral impingement; internal or external snapping hip; hip intra-articular injury.

Eastern-facing pose and tabletop (Purvottanasana [pour-vo-tah-nah-suhn])
(Figs 8.16–8.19)

Prerequisites Same as yoga couch plus:

- FMA column (1), (2) cobra only

- Craig test/femoral version screen

- Half upward-facing bow pose.

TI (therapeutic intention)

- Osteokinematic ROM: glenohumeral extension, internal or external rotation (depending on modification chosen); wrist extension, ankle plantarflexion

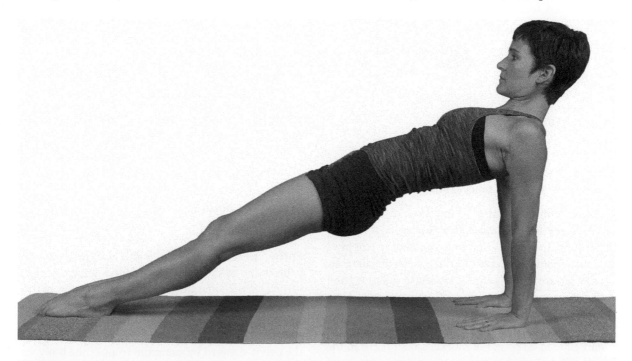

Figure 8.16
Eastern-facing, full

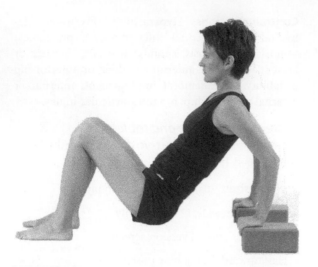

Figure 8.17
Tabletop, partial lift from blocks

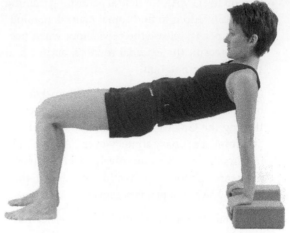

Figure 8.19
Tabletop, full lift from blocks

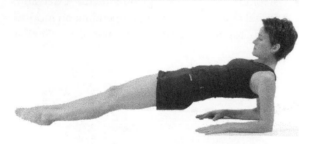

Figure 8.18
Eastern-facing, modified from forearms

- Arthrokinematic cervical spine and cranium, C1–C2 mobility; carpal and talus/calcaneal/tarsal gliding

- Assess arthrokinematics of the shoulder and hip — Placement of hands and feet in the pose and the hip on entry into the pose — Roll and glide should occur in all planes of motion in opposite directions when the concave surface (acetabulum and glenoid fossa) is fixed and the convex surface (femoral and humeral head) is moving. Entering the pose (for the shoulder and once the femur is fixed in the pose) — Arthrokinematic roll and glide in all planes of motion should occur in the same direction when the convex surface is fixed and the concave surface is moving

- Lumbopelvic awareness and postural control within spinal neutral

- Identification of excessive pelvic anterior tilt or femoral head positioning (anterior joint load) secondary to iliopsoas restriction

- Scapulothoracic stabilization via arm spiral

- Gentle iliopsoas extensibility

- Myofascial tensile force — Superficial front, anterior spiral, anterior arm, anterior functional, and deep front lines/bands may be most implicated.

SP (starting position)   Seated.

Modified (tabletop)

Entry   Knees are bent hip width and the hands are behind the body, palms down and fingers facing, turned to the side, or facing away from the pelvis, about 10 inches behind the pelvis. The feet are placed so that when the body is lifted the ankles are directly under the knees and hip width apart. On inhale, lift the pelvis skyward by using the front of the body via a TATD strategy. The cervical spine should remain in retraction in a mild chin lock.

Full (Eastern-facing)

Entry Bring the hands, fingers facing the body, about 10 inches behind the body. Place them, shoulder width, palms facing down. Draw the heels in 1–2 inches, slightly bending the knees. Lift the pelvis from the floor, bearing the weight only on the feet and hands. The cervical spine can adopt either of the following strategies: (1) (preferred strategy) chin remains in cervical retraction or mild chin lock or (2) (advanced) cervical retraction followed by cervical extension.

TS (thoracic spine) — Maintain spinal neutral; the trunk is only lifted parallel to the floor; cervical spine takes one of the two offered positions in the action section. Screen for psoas restriction indicated by presence of 10 degrees or more anterior tilt in the posture that is unable to be resolved with manual or verbal cuing.

UEs (upper extremities) — Glenohumeral extension; arm spiral with wrist extension.

LEs (lower extremities) — The hips are in zero degrees of extension or mild extension (less than 5 degrees) with full expression of pose; the knees are hip width and in zero degrees extension. The ankle is in full plantarflexion with the anterior tibialis on an active stretch.

Exit Exhale to return the pelvis to the floor, righting the cervical spine last via maintenance of the mild chin lock/cervical retraction.

SRAs (static restorative approximations)

- Supine over tri-fold blanket for mild reversal of thoracic kyphosis

- For identified asymmetry in the quadratus lumborum, functional or structural leg length discrepancy, or scoliosis, place the shortened side of the torso on stretch (facing up) over *"Ganesha-fold."*

DMs (dynamic modifications)

- Prop-assist — Blocks under hands
- Partial lift of pelvis from floor

- Supine non-articulating bridge
- Shoulders rotate to assume three different positions, depending on comfort of the shoulders and wrists:
  - fingers facing feet — Glenohumeral internal rotation
  - fingers facing laterally — Glenohumeral open-packed position
  - fingers facing posteriorly — Glenohumeral external rotation
- Forearm weight-bearing through both expressions of pose
- Three-legged table — Alternate lifting one leg at a time to target gluteus maximus and hip rotator cuff strength plus endurance (power).

Contraindications Wrist weakness, osteoarthritis, or immobility; lack of gluteal or scapulothoracic support may anteriorly load the joint and contribute to acetabular or glenoid labral injury, respectively.

Reclined supported hero pose (Supta salamba virasana [soup-tuh sah-lahm-buh vee-rah-suhn]) (Figs 8.20 and 8.21)

> **Code 8.3** (subscription code)
> Reclined supported hero

Prerequisites Same as yoga couch plus:

- FMA column 1 as needed; (3)
- Craig test/femoral version screen
- Half upward-facing bow
- Hero
- Optional: warrior I and/or half or full bow.

TI (therapeutic intention)

- Osteokinematic spinal neutral or pelvic posterior tilt (depending on depth of pose), hip internal rotation, knee flexion, ankle plantarflexion, shoulder extension

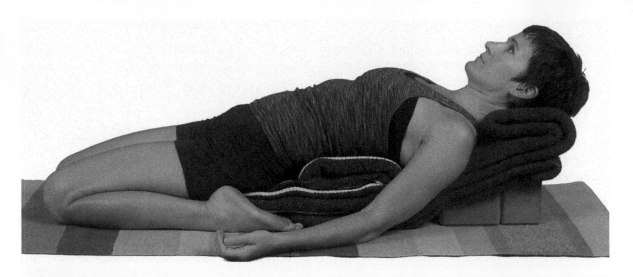

Figure 8.20
Reclined supported hero from high yoga couch

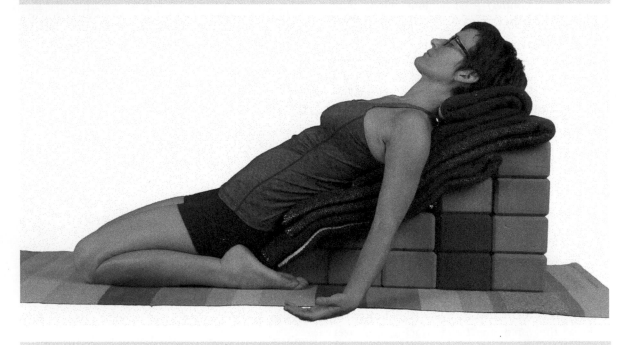

Figure 8.21
Reclined supported hero from higher yoga couch. Once the yoga couch exceeds a 45-degree angle, wall support may be needed to secure the blanket configuration so it does not topple

- Assess arthrokinematics of shoulder and hip — Overall, shoulder and hip arthrokinematics means roll and glide will occur in opposite direction when the concave surface (glenoid fossa and acetabulum) are fixed and the convex surface is moving (humeral and femoral head). Once the convex surfaces become fixed (in the final resting position), the concave surfaces may be adjusted, thus reversing the arthrokinematic chain of movement. Also assess sacral nutation (mild) or counternutation (full pose)

- Myofascial tensile force — Superficial front, anterior spiral, anterior arm, anterior functional, and deep front lines/bands may be most implicated

- Iliopsoas, rectus femoris, and pectoralis lengthening while in spinal neutral (mild) or posterior pelvic tilt (full pose)

- Soft tissue mobilization of acupressure/Marma points (if chosen to perform manually prior to entry in pose) of the gastrocnemius/soleus complex, beneficial for gastrointestinal motility

- Visceral mobilization

- Lower quarter circulation and lymphatic drainage via meditation with movement — Long, deep A-D breath paired with lower quarter mechanical compression via loaded knee flexion compression.

Props Multiple blocks and blankets (yoga couch-style).

SP (starting position) *Virasana with support as needed* (see Chapter 7 for instructions).

Entry (full expression) Exhale and bring the hands to the floor behind the trunk. Tuck the tailbone under to create a flat surface for the sacrum (counternutation). Bring the palms, fingers facing forward, to the heels and press the heels forward (if there is no contraindication to plantarflexion or anterior ankle glides). If possible bring the forearms to rest on the ground in line with the feet. Rest on the forearms. To continue, posteriorly tilt the pelvis and rest the trunk on the floor or, in the vast majority of populations, multiple three-tier folds. Document the number of three-tier folds and/or blocks needed to support the spinal curves in the pose and completely fill the space between the torso and the earth. Differentially diagnose myofascial restriction, diaphragmatic involvement of the periodontal ligaments, or dura mater neural tension through introduction of mild chin lock and shoulder flexion or elevation.

Final progression Perform arm floats and snow angels to differentially diagnose or screen for superficial and deep front line/band(s) or shoulder complex

ROM limitation(s). Glenohumeral joint flexion should not affect trunk positioning.

TS (thoracic spine) — The spine is in a posterior pelvic tilt, reversal of lumbar lordosis, and SIJ counternutation in the full pose. The modified, supported version allows for spinal neutral or SIJ nutation.

UEs (upper extremities) — The shoulders are allowed to rest in open-packed position with and without blanket support, although the yoga couch allows for easier pectoralis extensibility gains and/or myofascial release.

LEs (lower extremities) — The hips are in slight internal rotation. The majority of populations will not attain zero degrees of hip flexion. The knees are fully flexed and ankles plantarflexed in the full pose. Do not allow the knees to separate past hip width or lift during the pose, which would increase fibrocartilaginous or ligamentous injury risk due to asymmetrical or shear-force load transfer across joint lines.

Exit *To return:* bring the heels of the hands to the soles of the feet. Lift the chest and draw the shoulders open and back while maintaining a mild chin lock. Bring the forearms and elbows underneath to bear weight on them in order to press back up to modified hero. The head follows and rights itself in sitting and not before.

SRAs (static restorative approximations)

- Elevate the sitting surface with blocks/bolsters/blankets

- Chair sitting or sitting against wall

- *"Sleepy or kissing knees"* (Chapter 7).

DMs (dynamic modifications)

- Use yoga couch configuration with blocks between the heels to elevate the sitting service to protect the knees and spine. Hero and reclined hero performance are not encouraged in their full expression due to cartilaginous and ligamentous knee injury risk.

- Use a thinly rolled blanket under the axis of rotation in the ankle to avoid full plantarflexion where contraindicated, or with lateral anterior talofibular ligamentous laxity.

- Reclined hero is not taught with cervical extension due to vertebral artery insufficiency risk.

TTCP (teaching and tactical cuing primer)

- Spine support — When there are neck problems, keep a mild chin lock and eliminate dropping the neck into extension during all portions of the posture.

- Trunk support — Use blocks and blankets (2–4 of each), as shown below, to create a graduated surface on which to recline.

- Knee support — Loosen the skin over the knees (superficial front line myofascial release) by reaching over the anterior knee and drawing the skin of the knee cephalad. Add additional blankets to elevate the sitting surface and avoid full knee flexion.

- Ankle support — Use a thinly rolled blanket under the axis of rotation in the ankle to avoid neurovascular impediment, excessive anterolateral ligamentous instability, or to accommodate missing or uncomfortable end-ranges of plantarflexion.

Contraindications Degenerative joint disease or degenerative disc disease causing acute pain or neurovascular signs or symptoms; knee meniscus injuries and ligamentous injuries, severe osteoarthritis, not to be performed during pregnancy without props due to joint laxity, children in bone growth stage secondary to risk of femoral torsion; caution for "yoga foot drop" secondary to nerve compression of the common peroneal nerve as it traverses the fibular head; SIJ dysfunction; stenosis; intra-articular hip injuries, such as FAI or acetabular labral tears and congenital or acquired hip joint malformation such as dysplasia, which could include but is not limited to excessive femoral anteversion, femoral retroversion, shallow acetabulum, and/or acetabular version; SIJ asymmetry; stenosis; anterior disc derangement (acute); spondylolisthesis (acute).

Hand-to-big toe pose (Supta padangusthasana [soup-tuh pah-duhn-goose-thu-suhn]) (Figs 8.22–8.24)

Prerequisites Same as yoga couch plus:.

- FMA column (1) and column (3) 1, 3

- Craig test/femoral version screen.

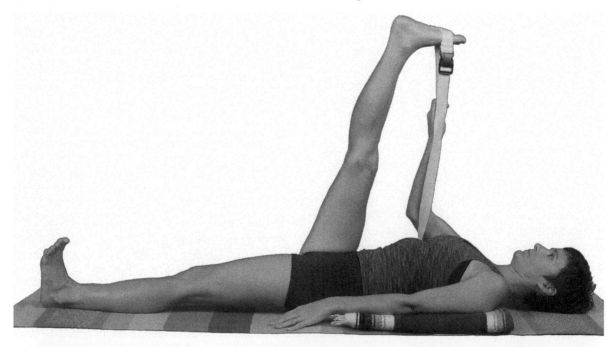

Figure 8.22

Hand-to-big toe, modified with quarter-fold blanket and strap

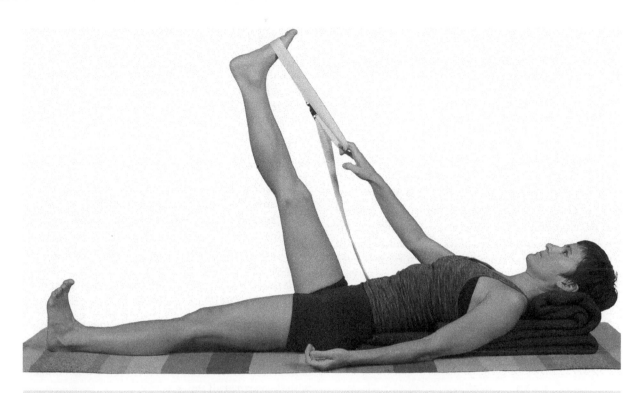

Figure 8.23
Hand-to-big toe, modified on yoga couch with strap

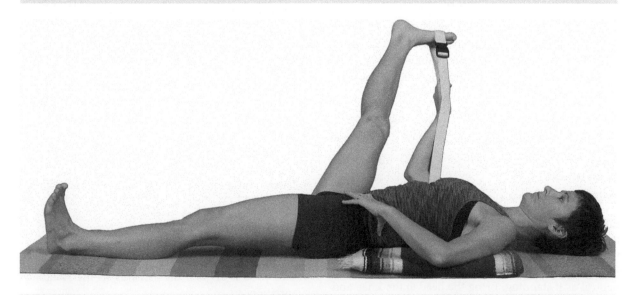

Figure 8.24
Hand-to-big toe, lateral variation modified with quarter-fold blanket and strap plus biofeedback for contralateral TATD breath via C-grip

TI (therapeutic intention)

- Gateway pose to standing postures, for balance, and postural awareness

- Osteokinematic hip flexion in spinal neutral; glenohumeral flexion

- Assess arthrokinematics of the shoulder and hip. Moving into the pose — Roll and glide should occur in all planes of motion in opposite directions when the concave surface (glenoid fossa and acetabulum) is fixed and the convex surface (humeral and femoral head) is moving. Once in the pose — Arthrokinematic roll and glide in all planes of motion should occur in the same direction when the convex surface is fixed and the concave surface is moving

- Hamstring extensibility (airborne leg)

- Hip flexor resting extensibility (ground leg)

- Dynamic lumbopelvic and scapulothoracic stabilization

- Restorative and dynamic pose

- Neural mobilization (sciatic nerve, peroneal nerve, and lateral branch of sciatic nerve)

- Myofascial tensile force — Superficial back, posterior back, posterior arm lines/bands may be most implicated; lateral variation: anterior, functional, lateral deep front, and spiral lines/bands may be most implicated

- Lateral variation: contralateral abdominal strengthening and myofascial targets as above

- See Chapter 5 (knee-to-chest series) for further assessment.

SP (starting position)   Supine.

Entry   Draw the right knee into the chest while maintaining spinal neutral. Grasp the big toe with the first two fingers of the right hand and straighten the knee. Keep the left leg grounded and active with the ankle in neutral as if standing. Bring the head to the knee and hold for 3–5 breaths maintaining spinal neutral. Flex the elbow to increase pose depth. Return to original hold and maintain.

Lateral variation

Bring the leg out to the side while keeping spinal neutral and bilateral ASIS facing skyward and level bilaterally. The ipsilateral shoulder that holds the airborne leg externally rotates with simultaneous elbow flexion in order to deepen hip abduction while targeting periscapular strengthening.

Exit   Return the leg to supine. Repeat on opposite side.

TS (thoracic spine) — Maintain spinal neutral in all variations unless spinal flexion is needed. If hip intra-articular injury is suspected, maintain spinal neutral since increased anterior pelvic plane on a sagittal axis that interrupts vertical alignment of the ASIS and pubic symphysis (an imaginary line drawn that connects them) increases hip impingement risk (Banerjee and McLean, 2011).

UEs (upper extremities) and LEs (lower extremities) — Remain engaged through the pose as if in standing. Shoulder alignment in the lateral variation is indicated above. Both shoulders remain in contact with the earth at all times.

SRAs (static restorative approximations)

- Knee–to-chest

- Supported strap-assist.

DMs (dynamic modifications)

- Place a quarter-fold blanket under the torso to externally maintain/support spinal neutral. The head and pelvis remain on either end of the blanket

- Hand-to-knee variation

- Lateral variation with head turn in contralateral direction

- Strap-assist.

TTCP (teaching and tactical cuing primer)

- This pose is aligned the same as in the standing variation.

- For strength and lumbopelvic stability, maintain spinal neutral throughout pose variations.

Contraindications   Acute low back pain; sciatica; active disc injury; positive slump test; FAI, subspinal impingement (hip), hip instability (posteriorly), internal or external snapping hip, psoas or tensor fascia lata dominance.

Upward-facing forward seated bend pose (Urdvha mukha paschimottanasana [urhd-vuh moo-kuh pahs-chee-moe-tuh-nuh-suhn]) (Figs 8.25–8.27)

Prerequisites   Same as yoga couch plus:

- FMA column 1 as needed, (3) 1, 3, 4, 5; (4) 1, 2, 3, 6
- Craig test/femoral version screen
- Half upward-facing bow
- Swan dive to forward standing bend
- Forward seated bend
- Boat pose.

TI (therapeutic intention)

- Gateway pose to shoulderstand
- Osteokinematic global trunk and extremity flexion
- Assess arthrokinematics of the shoulder and hip — Same as hand-to-big toe pose
- Visceral mobilization
- Lumbopelvic awareness and postural control outside of spinal neutral
- Locks strengthening
- Hamstring extensibility
- Neural mobilization of sciatic nerve and dura mater via flexion moment (slump test) in spine combined with full diaphragmatic excursion
- Myofascial tensile force — Superficial back, posterior spiral, arm, functional, and quadratus lumborum of deep front lines/bands may be most implicated

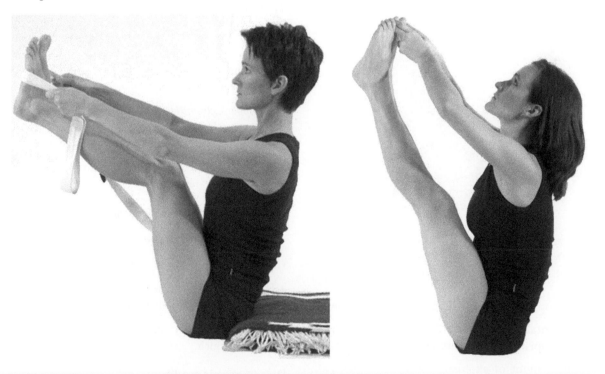

Figure 8.25
Upward-facing forward seated bend (phase 1), full upright and full upright modified with strap

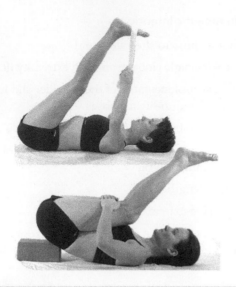

Figure 8.26
Upward-facing forward seated bend (phase 2), modified supine with strap and modified with block

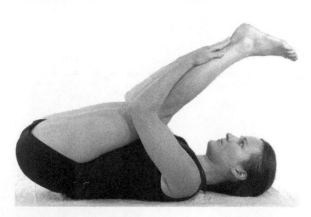

Figure 8.27
Upward-facing forward seated bend (phase 2), full supine

- Lumbopelvic power, strength, and motor control

- Segmental spinal mobilization, strengthening and proprioceptive awareness

- Management of extension-based low back pain in static restorative approximation form

- SIJ mobilization (with block as shown) for managing bilateral chronic nutation (the block should run

vertically with the body so it "fits" the apex of the sacrum, in order to facilitate counternutation).

SP (starting position)   Supine.

Entry (full expression)   Bend the knees and grasp the great toes with the first two fingers of each hand. Draw the knees straight and through finding a balance point on the ischial tuberosities and using TATD breath to maintain the balance point. Hold and breathe. Second, hold the sides of the legs and roll to supine lying. If rolling is too advanced, begin in supine lying.

For both versions: extend the knees as able and stabilize through light support at the backs of the calves while also keeping the sacrum close to the ground in counternutation.

Exit   With ease and slow control, return to supine lying with exhalation without arm support as able (internal pose support).

TS (thoracic spine) — Requires segmental spinal mobilization and stabilization for safe performance of pose. The cervical spine should remain in a neutral position, preserving the lordosis. The sacrum counternutates with lumbar flexion using a reciprocal motion strategy.

UEs (upper extremities) — Keep the upper extremities in contact with the floor with minimal scapular protraction and shoulder elevation on return from the posture.

LEs (lower extremities) — The knees are extended without hyperextension.

SRAs (static restorative approximations)

- Child's pose on yoga couch

- Supported knee-to-chest on yoga couch

- Supported forward seated bend (advanced) seated on blankets and using a therapy ball for trunk support

- Supported hand-to-big toe, modified with a strap on yoga couch.

DMs (dynamic modifications)

- Strap-assist with bent knees

- Leave the pelvis on the floor and use a strap

- Place a block under the pelvis to assist with weak lumbopelvic stabilizers and/or to mobilize a chronically bilateral nutated SIJ.

TTCP (teaching and tactical cuing primer)

- Full pose — An advanced pose, maintain extended knees and a long spine that minimizes spinal flexion

- Partial pose — This pose should precede seated upright versions (such as the third one in the SRA section) and standing upright versions. This pose is applicable for novices in its beginner form to assist with extension-based pain disorders.

Contraindications Acute sciatica, weak TATD, pelvic organ prolapse; inability to recruit pelvic floor and prevent valsalva or increased pressure on pelvic floor; pregnancy, posterior disc derangement, osteoporosis, osteopenia, torsion of the sacrum, COPD, posterior hip joint instability or labral insufficiency; FAI, subspinal impingement (hip), hip instability (posteriorly), internal or external snapping hip, psoas or tensor fascia lata dominance.

Upright extended foot pose (Urdhva prasarita padasana [erd-vuh prah-sarh-ree-tuh pah-dah-suhn]) (Figs 8.28–8.31)

Prerequisites Same as yoga couch plus:

- FMA column (1 as needed), (3), (4) 1, 2, 3, 6
- Craig test/femoral version screen
- Swan dive to forward standing bend
- Forward seated bend

- Boat pose
- Standing postures (for endurance).

TI (therapeutic intention)

- Lumbopelvic endurance and control (advanced) development and testing

- Lower extremity osteokinematic hip flexion (advanced)

- Assess arthrokinematics of the shoulder and hip — Same as hand-to-big toe pose

- Neural mobilization of dura mater and/or sciatic nerve (advanced)

- Scapulothoracic stabilization (advanced)

- Lock strengthening and awareness (advanced)

- Requires excellent hamstring length 90 degrees without loss of spinal neutral (advanced)

- Myofascial tensile force — Superficial back, and posterior spiral, functional, arm, and quadratus lumborum of the deep front lines/bands may be most implicated. In legs dropped (below 90 degrees hip flexion), this tensile force reverses to the anterior lines.

SP (starting position) (full expression) Supine with arms at sides.

Entry Lift the legs and arms simultaneously as a unit until the feet are straight over the pelvis (90 degrees of hip flexion) and dorsiflexed and the arms in full flexion above the head. Hold and breathe for 2 breaths.

> **Figure 8.28**
> Upward extended foot, full

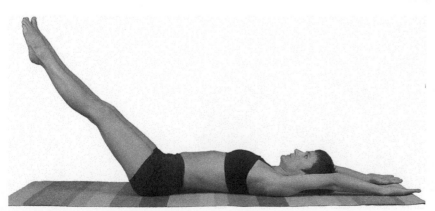

251

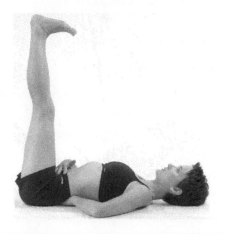

Figure 8.29
Upward extended foot, full with biofeedback for maintaining spinal neutral

Alternate:

Lift and lower the arms in stages 25 degrees, 45 degrees, 75 degrees, taking 1–5 breaths at each angle. The spine must maintain neutral position throughout the entire posture progression.

Exit   Inhale and return the arms and legs to the floor with arms to the sides and without allowing the head, neck, or shoulders to lift from the floor.

SRAs (static restorative approximations)

- Supine hook lying spinal neutral with TATD breath
- Legs-up-the-wall pose.

DMs (dynamic modifications)

- Beginners should bend the hips and knees to a 90/90 degree position and then slowly lower them
- Use a strap to minimize lumbopelvic load until strength and endurance improve. The strap can be placed around the balls of the feet
- Use a quarter-fold approach for spinal neutral maintenance
- Hook lying knee lift (FMA).

TTCP (teaching and tactical cuing primer)

- Self-manual assist — Place a hand or blood pressure cuff inflated to 40 mmHg under the lumbar

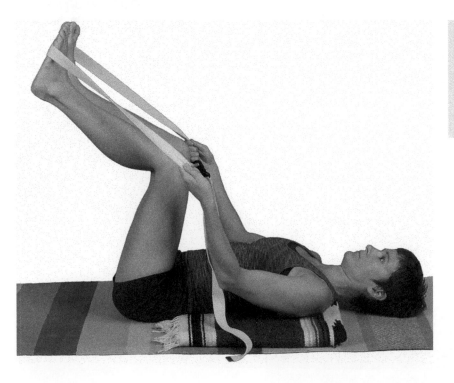

Figure 8.30
Upward extended foot, modified with quarter-fold blanket for biofeedback to maintain spinal neutral and strap for lumbopelvic control (bent knees)

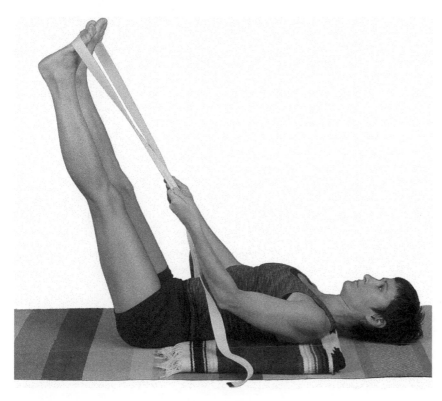

Figure 8.31
Upward extended foot, same as Fig. 8.29 but with extended knees

spine to maintain spinal neutral and provide feedback. The pressure in the cuff should not change as the legs move through space.

- Remove degrees of freedom via bending the knees to shorten the lever arm and reduce lumbopelvic load until lumbopelvic control and TATD strategy improves.

- Manual cues over the ribcage for oblique assist with TA and pelvic floor isolation (TATD breath).

Contraindications Inability to isolate the TATD without valsalva and maintenance of spinal neutral. Stenosis, spondylosis, spondylolisthesis, shoulder instability; spinal fusion, particularly cervical, pelvic organ prolapse, inability to recruit pelvic floor and prevent valsalva or increased pressure on pelvic floor; FAI, subspinal impingement (hip), hip instability (posteriorly), internal or external snapping hip, psoas or tensor fascia lata dominance or hypertrophy.

Review

The supine postures presented in this chapter cover dynamic and restorative movements. Level I postures cover FMA assessment and concomitant management, which means yoga, as a complementary adjunct in rehabilitation delivery, saves valuable clinic time that has historically been spent on separate evaluation and management. Level II postures cover additional options for supine postures, which include restoratives and advanced dynamic stabilization and mobilization postures. Note that most supine postures can be adapted to be restorative and/or dynamic in nature, depending on whether external or internal support is used. This makes supine postures equal to standing and seated postures for their utility and accessibility for all patient populations.

Postures in this chapter are foundational prone postures chosen for their diagnostic and therapeutic utility and accessibility for all patient populations. They are essential postures that create space for teaching functional breathing patterns, safe transitions, and for facilitating lumbopelvic and scapulothoracic balance and health, including enjoying the plethora of biopsychosocial benefits outlined in Table 3.9.

> **Outline**
>
> - Child's pose (FMA)
>   - A/P child's pose
>   - Lateral child's pose
>   - "Reach, roll, and rise"
> - Four-point (FMA)
>   - Cat/cow
>   - Neutral spine (FMA)
>   - Downward-facing dog preparation (FMA)
> - Plank (FMA)
> - Four-limbed staff, modified and full (advanced)
> - Locust
> - Cobra — Mini and maxi (FMA)
> - Sphinx
> - Upward-facing dog (advanced)
> - Bow
> - Pigeon
> - Review

Therapeutic benefits and general precautions and contraindications are listed in Table 3.9. Additional benefits and precautions are listed under each pose. See Table 9.1 for an overview of prone postures.

Child's pose and supported child's pose with lateral variation and "reach, roll, and rise" (Balasana and Salamba balasana [baa-lah-suhn]) (Figs 9.1–9.6)

> **Code 9.1** (subscription code)
> Child's pose
>

Prerequisites

- Orofacial and respiratory assessment
- FMA column (1); (3) 1–2
- Transversus abdominis-assisted thoraco-diaphragmatic (TATD) breath for transfer from supine-to-sit and vice versa or when the pose is used for stability training ("reach, roll, and rise" portion)
- Standing-to-floor transfer if performing from floor
- Craig test/femoral version screen
- Other yogic breath types in Chapter 4 are helpful but not required.

TI (therapeutic intention)

- Posterior ribcage expansion via long, deep breathing
- Scapulohumeral/thoracic proprioceptive feedback via tactile cuing
- Assessment of diaphragmatic symmetry during respiration and neuromuscular re-education for chest or paradoxical breathers
- Osteokinematic hip flexion, abduction, and external rotation (FABER) or flexion if knees are together (for visceral input and mobilization); knee flexion; lumbar reversal of lordosis and increased thoracic kyphosis; glenohumeral flexion and external rotation; possible elbow flexion if shoulder flexion is limited; ankle plantarflexion

Table 9.1
Prone yoga postures

Pose	Figure	QR code
Child's pose • Anterior/ posterior • Lateral • Reach, roll, and rise	Figs 9.1–9.6	Code 9.1
Four-point • Cat/cow • Neutral spine • Downward- facing dog Preparation	Figs 9.7– 9.18	Code 9.2
Plank	Figs 9.19–9.21	
Four-limbed staff	Figs 9.22–9.24	
Locust	Figs 9.25–9.28	Code 9.3
Cobra	Figs 5.27–5.28	Code 9.4
Sphinx	Fig. 9.29	
Upward-facing dog	Fig. 9.30	
Bow	Figs 9.31–9.36	
Pigeon	Figs 9.37–9.40	Code 9.5

- Posterior glide symmetry assessment of the ischial tuberosities

- Arthrokinematics of the shoulder and hip — Moving into the pose — Roll and glide will occur in all planes of motion in opposite directions when the concave surface (glenoid fossa and acetabulum) is fixed and the convex surface (humeral and femoral head) is moving. Once in the pose — Arthrokinematic roll and glide in all planes of motion will occur in the same direction when the convex surface is fixed and the concave surface is moving

- Psychoemotional-social protection — Position for grief, trauma, exhaustion, or a victim of violent crime

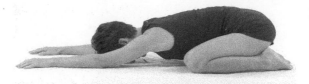

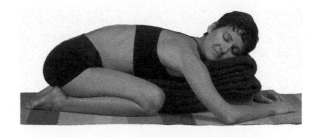

Figure 9.1
Child's pose, full

Figure 9.2
Child's pose, supported with high yoga couch

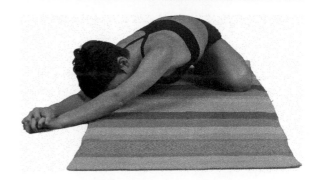

Figure 9.3
Child's pose, lateral with glenohumeral joint and tissue traction

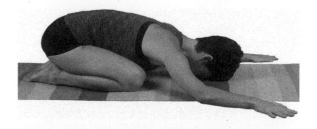

Figure 9.4
Child's reach (full) in resting scaption

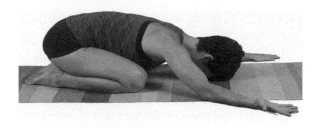

Figure 9.5
Child's roll (full) in scaption with forearm supination

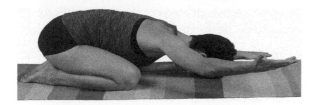

Figure 9.6
Child's rise (full) in dynamic scaption

- "Reach, roll, and rise" — Scapulothoracic stabilization

- Perineal tensile force if heels are separated

- A/P child's pose myofascial tensile force — Superficial back (trunk, head, neck portions), spiral (if asymmetry in arm range of motion (ROM), or length/tension of arm and trunk fascia exists), anterior and posterior arm, posterior functional (if asymmetry of posture exists), and deep front (lower quarter, diaphragm) lines/bands may be most implicated

- Lateral child's pose myofascial tensile force — Superficial back (trunk, head, neck portions), lateral, spiral, arms as above, functional (anterior if arm or shoulder asymmetry exists, posterior in general), and deep front (lower quarter, diaphragm, quadratus lumborum, psoas, iliacus, cervical spine and head) lines/bands may be most implicated

- "Reach, roll, and rise" myofascial tensile force — As in A/P but increase arm, functional, spiral, and deep front lines/bands involvement may be likely seen.

SP (starting position) Kneeling on floor or from thunderbolt.

Props Yoga couch, inverted plus blocks, bolsters, wedges, or a combination. Alternately, use a rectangular bolster or blocks to elevate the sitting surface or resting (trunk) surface, or both.

Entry

Option 1 — Spread the knees to allow the trunk to rest between the knees. The toes may or may not touch here. Lower the chest toward the floor onto a yoga couch or a combination of props in order to elevate the pose to a restorative one.

Option 2 — Leave the knees together to create a spinal flexion moment and facilitate visceral mobilization via introduction of compression via the lower extremities or with manual therapy or tactile input from the upper extremities.

Full child's pose — Sit back toward the heels and rest the forehead to the floor. The arms (1) fully flex and rest on the floor, or (2) abduct and the elbows flex for trunk if shoulder complex or lower quarter mobility is limited.

Lateral child's pose — Sidebend the trunk into a right crescent using the hands to "walk." Rest into child's pose by interlacing the right fingers over the left fingers. Exert a traction force in the right sidebending direction. The spine also slightly right rotates. After 5–10 breaths, release and repeat on the opposite side.

"Reach, roll, and rise" — From child's pose, find plumb line alignment from the head to the torso (avoid cervical spine shear and excessive thoracic kyphosis, which could contribute to internal shoulder impingement). Take prone scaption at the following angles:*

- "Reach" — Prone scaption at 100 degrees, "roll"-/thumb up/supination position, "rise" – lift arm to recruit the:

  - infraspinatus at approximately 39% MVIC

  - teres minor at approximately 44% MVIC

  - supraspinatus and deltoid at approximately 82% MVIC

  - posterior deltoid at approximately 88% MVIC (Escamilla et al., 2009).

- "Reach" — Prone scaption at 135 degrees, "roll" / thumb up/supination position, "rise" – lift arm to recruit the:

  - upper trapezius at approximately 79% MVIC

  - middle trapezius at approximately 100% MVIC

  - lower trapezius at approximately 97% MVIC

  - serratus anterior at approximately 43% MVIC (Escamilla et al., 2009).

Note: small weights or Theraband tubing could be added to increase MVIC/recruitment. Allow the palm to rise no more than 6–8 inches from the floor. Note input of the aforementioned muscles. An absence of this movement is a positive test for weakness, inhibition (through fascial, muscular, or joint restriction) and/or indication that arthrokinematic joint mobility testing should be completed at the four joints of the shoulder complex.

Repeat on the opposite side. Never perform the pose bilaterally simultaneously due to the cervical spine shear force moment it provokes, including isometric neck flexion moment. See Chapter 4 for more assessment techniques.

TS (thoracic spine) — Avoid cervical spine shear by not forcing the forehead to rest on the floor. Use props, such as a blanket or block, to support the cervical spine in plumb line alignment. Avoid a dominant flexion moment in the spine to complete the pose if lack of postural awareness and control is present.

UEs (upper extremities) — The shoulders are relaxed, not rigid or held tightly. Glenohumeral joint flexion occurs up to, but not past, 180 degrees. If impingement is a concern, flex the elbows and eliminate shoulder flexion. Substitute shoulder horizontal abduction. Avoid using the upper trapezius as a primary movement strategy. See dynamic modifications.

LEs (lower extremities) — The ankles rest without excessive inversion and forefoot supination if lateral ankle instability is an issue. See dynamic modifications.

Exit   Inhale to lift the trunk and return to thunderbolt or kneeling. Inhale to prepare to move and exhale to use a TATD breath to assist a safe return.

SRAs (static restorative approximations) and DMs (dynamic modifications)

- Use extra blankets or blocks to elevate the trunk higher and reduce the need for shoulder elevation.

- Place a block and/or block and blankets under the forehead to support cervical lordosis.

- Knee flexion restriction — Use evenly folded blankets at the distal calf (never proximally placed as that can create arthrokinematic joint gapping/distraction at the knee which could lead to cruciate ligament instability), under the buttocks and over the ankles.

- Ankle plantarflexion restriction or lateral ankle instability or frequent lateral ankle sprains — Place a thin blanket roll under the axis of rotation in the ankle.

- Treat as a restorative pose (active rest) rather than a dynamic one (increasing hip flexion and spinal mobility).

- Partner hip iliopsoas or rectus femoris biofeedback, soft tissue mobilization, and/or thoracolumbar or crossed line myofascial release.

- For lateral child's pose, use sidelying over "Ganesha-fold" (see Fig. 7.32).

- For "reach, roll, and rise" — Use guided imagery to elicit lower trapezius activation if the arm cannot clear the floor. Substitute wall "push-up plus" or use less shoulder flexion.

TTCP (teaching and tactical cuing primer)

- Place the hands on the posterior ribs for tactile input to back breathe between the ribs and feel the expansion of the intercostal muscles.

- Place the heels of the hands on the base of the sacrum or ilia with slight caudally directed pressure to create energetic or physical elongation the spine.

- This pose is effective for teaching relaxed abdominal and "back breathing."

Contraindications   Third trimester or larger abdomens may need more space between the knees and the torso and floor; those with osteoporosis and those with osteopenia can perform the pose safely in the absence of spinal flexion and with preservation of spinal curves; those with osteoarthritis should avoid full knee flexion and instead sit on an elevated surface that does not require full knee flexion; hip intra-articular injury, excessive femoral anteversion; femoroacetabular impingement (FAI), subspinal impingement (hip), hip instability (posteriorly), internal or external snapping hip, psoas or tensor fascia lata dominance or hypertrophy.

Hands and knees/four-point

(Figs 9.7–9.18)

Code 9.2 (subscription code)
Four-point

Prerequisites

- Orofacial and respiratory assessment
- FMA column (1), (3)

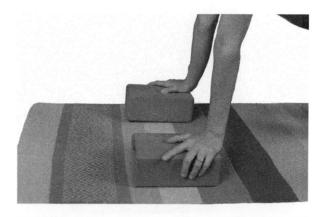

Figure 9.9
Four-point, modified on blocks with cascading fingers

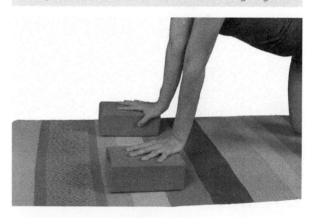

Figure 9.10
Four-point modified on blocks with cascading thumbs

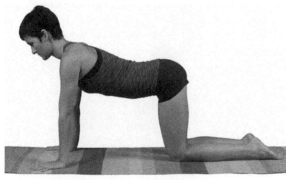

Figure 9.7
Four-point, full

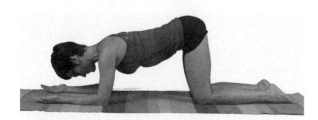

Figure 9.8
Four-point, modified on forearms in arm spiral moment

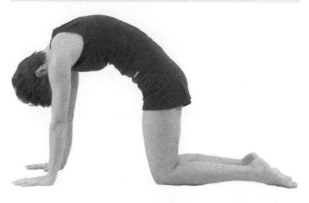

Figure 9.11
Cat, full with arm spiral

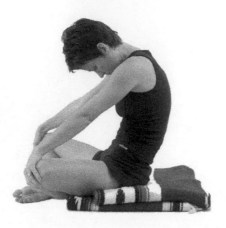

Figure 9.12
Cat, seated on scaffolded quarter-fold blankets in easy seated pose

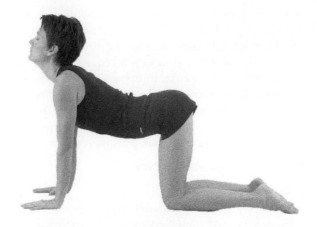

Figure 9.14
Cow, full with arm spiral

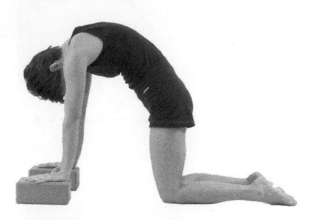

Figure 9.13
Cat, modified on blocks with cascading thumbs

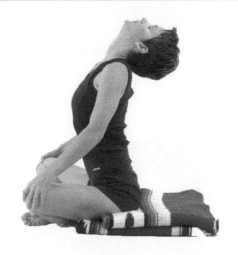

Figure 9.15
Cow, seated on scaffolded quarter-fold blankets in easy seated pose

- Standing to floor transfer if performing from floor

- Other yogic breath types in Chapter 4 are helpful but not required.

TI (therapeutic intention)

- Preparation for lumbopelvic and scapulothoracic stabilization

- Osteokinematic ROM: shoulder, hip, knee, and toe flexion; glenohumeral joint external rotation; scapular depression, internal rotation (IR), medial rotation; wrist and toe extension, forearm pronation, ankle dorsiflexion and plantarflexion

- Arthrokinematic spinal neutral

- Closed kinetic chain recruitment for the upper and lower quarter for global and local stabilization

- Biofeedback for force couple recruitment for scapulohumeral rhythm

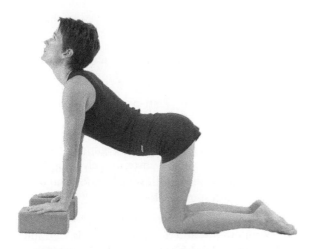

Figure 9.16
Cow, modified on blocks with cascading thumbs

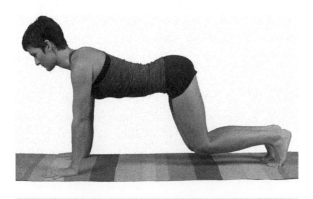

Figure 9.17
Downward-facing dog preparation, full with arm spiral

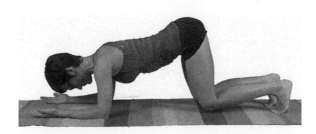

Figure 9.18
Downward-facing dog preparation modified on forearms

- All fascial lines are relevant. Lack of mobility, resilience, or appropriate response from any part of the fascial meridians would be visible in four-point.

SP (starting position)   Hands and knees or forearms and knees or seated in chair or on floor.

Entry   Place the hands under the shoulders with the arms in an arm spiral. Abduct the fingers to engage the intrinsic musculature of the hand. Bring the knees under the hips at hip width. Inhale to find spinal neutral. Exhale and engage TATD breath.

TS (thoracic spine) — The spine is in neutral or plumb line alignment from head to the hip. Common tendencies are posterior tilt guarding or gluteal gripping, which increase injury risk via destabilizing open-packed mechanisms (sacroiliac joint (SIJ) counternutation and lumbar lordosis reversal). Lack of proprioceptive awareness in the spine usually presents with loss of spinal neutral and cervical shear.

UEs (upper extremities) — Maintain arm spiral. Weakness or lack of proprioceptive awareness in the upper extremities usually causes elbow flexion, and scapular protraction and dyskinesis.

LEs (lower extremities) — Maintain hip over knee alignment.

Exit   This is a transition posture into other postures.

SRAs (static restorative approximations) and DMs (dynamic modifications)

- Four-point pose can be completed in seated with hands against a wall or holding the back of a chair.

- Four-point pose can be completed from the forearms, to eliminate elbow and wrist extension. If performed from the forearms, supinate them to encourage scapulothoracic biofeedback and co-activation of the posterior thoracic scapular stabilizers.

Contraindications   Rheumatoid arthritis, wrist weakness or limitation, upper or lower quarter injury or instability, FAI, psoas or tensor fascia lata dominance or hypertrophy in absence of trunk or hip stability. Non-weight-bearing substitutions such as chair-sitting or aquatic yoga can be performed.

Geriatric patient populations who cannot complete a floor-to-standing transfer can begin on a plinth or seated in a chair or using an assistive device.

Cat/cow (Marjaryasana/Bitilasana [mahr-jahr-eeh-yah-suhn/biht-eel-ah-suhn]) (Figs 9.11–9.16)

Prerequisites   Same as four-point plus FMA column 2.

TI (therapeutic intention)

- Spinal segmental mobility

- Assess arthrokinematics of the shoulder and hip — Moving into the pose — Roll and glide should occur in all planes of motion in opposite directions when the concave surface (glenoid fossa and acetabulum) is fixed and the convex surface (humeral head and femoral head) is moving. Once in the pose and performing cat/cow — Arthrokinematic roll and glide in all planes of motion should occur in the same direction when the convex surface is fixed and the concave surface is moving

- Upgrade nutrient transport via mechanically-induced solute diffusion through end plates to the intervertebral disc healing with a concomitant increase in intradiscal pressure via alternating and repetitive end-range movement in flexion and extension (Key, 2013) afforded with cat and cow movements

- Gross gastrointestinal motility and visceral mobilization

- *Cat variation* — Myofascial tensile force — Superficial back (trunk, head, neck), posterior spiral, posterior arm, posterior functional, and deep front lines/bands via diaphragm may be most involved

- *Cow variation* — Myofascial tensile force — Superficial front, anterior spiral, anterior arm, anterior functional, and deep front lines/bands may be most involved

- *"Wag-the-dog" variation* — Ipsilateral (lengthened side) myofascial tensile force — Superficial back, lateral, spiral, functional, and deep front lines/bands may be most involved

- Multiplanar segmental mobility in thoracolumbar spine and "thoracic ring shift", a phrase coined by physiotherapist Diane Lee, assessment (see Chapter 5; "hula hoop" variation)

- Marriage of the exhale to flexion and inhale to extension of the spine

- Elongation of the breath as a result of slowed movement.

SP (starting position)   Four-point/hands and knees.

Entry

Cat — Exhale and flex the spine beginning with the tucking of the coccyx and posterior pelvic tilt. Move up the kinematic chain with spinal flexion and complete cat cervical spine flexion.

Cow — Inhale and initiate spinal extension with the coccyx, followed by anterior tilt of the pelvis. Continue up the chain and finish with cervical spine extension.

TS (thoracic spine) — (Cat) — Full spinal flexion and SIJ counternutation; (Cow) — full spinal extension and SIJ nutation.

UEs (upper extremities) — Maintain arm spiral throughout cat/cow, with shoulders over wrists, unless a modification is used.

Exit   Return to four-point.

SRAs (static restorative approximations)

- Cat — Supported child's pose or prone over "Ganesha-fold" (see Fig. 7.32)

- Cow — Supine over tri-fold blankets for thoracic extension; supine over "accordion fold" (see Fig. G.4).

DMs (dynamic modifications)

- Supine hook lying pelvic tilts, clock or mini-cat/cow

- Seated cat/cow

- Standing cat/cow

- "Wag-the-dog" variation — Side-to-side elongation of the waist and lateral raphe by looking toward the pelvis bilaterally

- "Hula hoop" variation — Combine sidebending, flexion, and spinal extension by creating a "jumping rope" type motion with the trunk. The motion is similar to the movement required to use a hula-hoop

- Cat/cow at wall or with chair-assist

- Blocks under hands as in hands and knees/four-point with downward-facing dog preparation.

TTCP (teaching and tactical cuing primer) The heart and chest remain open and not collapsed (shortening the pectoralis with scapular protraction as a dominant strategy rather than use of spinal flexion) throughout both ranges of motion (cat/cow).

Contraindications As in four point, and also including:

Cat — Osteopenia, osteoporosis of spine; degenerative disc or lumbar disease; cervical or lumbar fusion.

Cow — Stenosis, spondylosis, spondylolisthesis; cervical or lumbar fusion; FAI, subspinal impingement (hip), hip instability.

Downward-facing dog preparation (Adho mukha svanasana [ahdho-mook-ahh shvah-nah-suhn]) (Figs 9.17 and 9.18)

Prerequisites Same as four-point plus FMA column 2, (4) 1–2

TI (therapeutic intention)

- Downward-facing dog preparation is an FMA gateway pose and a prerequisite for downward-facing dog

- Mobilization with movement and meditation with movement (in Moon salute)

- Scapulohumeral rhythm and screening for scapular winging or tipping

- Osteokinematic ROM: hip, shoulder, and toe flexion wrist and toe extension; glenohumeral joint external rotation, forearm pronation, ankle dorsiflexion and plantarflexion

- Isometric isolation of, and segmental spinal stabilization of lumbopelvic spine using TATD breath and knee lift

- Postural proprioception and awareness — Screen for dorsal vagus or visceral response, which would be noted if the external obliques dominate the attempted lumbopelvic strategy with subsequent increased intra-abdominal pressure that increases inferior pelvic floor pressure and creates a lower abdominal "pooch"

- Screen for thoracic spine ring shift (nonoptimal isolated or group lateral shifting or rotation of a thoracic vertebral segment or ribcage)

- All myofascial lines are relevant. Lack of mobility, resilience, or appropriate response from any part of the fascial meridians would be visible in downward-facing dog preparation.

SP (starting position) Four-point neutral spine position.

Entry Exhale and engage TATD breath. Exhale and lift the knees 1–2 inches off the floor and hold for 5 breaths.

TS (thoracic spine) — Maintain plumb line alignment, spinal neutral, and TATD breath throughout the transition and holding phase(s). See Chapter 4 for more assessment techniques.

UEs (upper extremities) — Maintain arm spiral. The scapulothoracic "joint" works toward medial rotation of the scapula at the inferior angle via lower trapezius action and the force couple provided by the serratus anterior and the upper trapezius. However, scapulothoracic stabilization is not dominated by upper trapezius recruitment. Approximation of the scapulae at the chest wall happens with shoulder depression, medial rotation and slight retraction (retraction is not a dominant strategy). The elbows maintain zero degrees without hyperextension. The wrist and forearms require 90 degrees or more of wrist extension, which is beyond clinical normative values. As a result, blocks can be used or a forearm strategy can be substituted for the wrist extension.

LEs (lower extremities) — Knees remain under hips at hip width.

Exit Lower to mat after 5 breaths.

SRAs (static restorative approximations)

- Supine hook lying TATD
- Supine hook lying knee lift
- Prone lying TATD breath.

DMs (dynamic modifications)

- For wrist restriction or pain, place blocks under hands and let either (1) fingers or (2) thumbs cascade over the edges, depending on which has the most restriction or pain

- Gradually progress time spent in this pose for women who may have weak wrists or for men who may have restricted shoulders or a weak rotator cuff

- Progression — "downward-facing dog preparation glide".

TTCP (teaching and tactical cuing primer) Typical substitutions like trunk or spinal flexion will occur when lack of postural awareness or control is present.

Contraindications Rheumatoid arthritis, wrist weakness or limitation, upper or lower quarter injury or instability, FAI, psoas or tensor fascia lata dominance or hypertrophy in absence of trunk or hip stability.

Plank (Phalakasana [pah-lah-kah-suhn])
(Figs 9.19–9.21)

Prerequisites Same as four-point plus FMA column 4, (5), downward-facing dog preparation, *"reach, roll, rise"* or prone variation.

TI (therapeutic intention)

- Calibration pose — A transitional pose that can determine placement of the hands and feet in

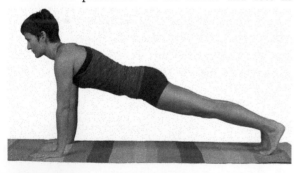

Figure 9.19
Plank, full with arm spiral

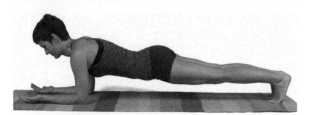

Figure 9.20
Plank, modified on forearms with arm spiral moment

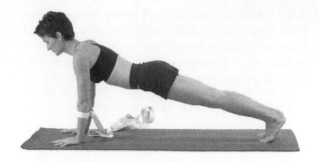

Figure 9.21
Plank, strap to bind forearms below extensor muscle mass with arm spiral

downward-facing dog. Transition to and from plank should not require a change in hand or foot position when moving to downward-facing dog

- Gateway pose for all upper extremity weight-bearing postures and for four-limbed staff

- Postural awareness in prone for plumb line alignment and proprioceptive input for postural control

- Assess arthrokinematics of the shoulder — Roll and glide should occur in the opposite direction as the convex surface (humeral head) is moving and the concave surface (glenoid fossa) is fixed (if there is adequate scapular stability)

- Spinal alignment assessment (thoracolumbar)

- Closed kinetic chain strength (upper/lower quarter)

- Scapulohumeral rhythm and screening for scapular winging or tipping

- All myofascial lines are relevant. Lack of mobility, resilience, or appropriate response from any part of the fascial meridians would be visible in plank

- "Push-up plus" — Concentric serratus anterior contraction with abduction and lateral rotation of scapula with scapular depression; return of "plus" is eccentric training with adduction and medial rotation to decelerate scapula. In those who cannot perform a concentric push up at 55 degrees flow flexion (the ideal angle for serratus anterior engagement), the serratus anterior can also, but less effectively, be used (San Juan et al., 2015).

SP (starting position)   Downward-facing dog preparation (beginner/intermediate) or downward-facing dog (advanced).

Entry   Inhale from downward-facing dog preparation or downward-facing dog into a plumb-line plank with knees off the floor, standing on hands and toes.

UEs (upper extremities) — Screen for scapular winging or tipping. The hands are a minimum of shoulder width to avoid shoulder impingement. Correct alignment in plank is a position where the shoulders are over the wrists and the arms are in arm spiral.

LEs (lower extremities) — Separate the feet enough to allow the heels to tap (as in Dorothy tapping her heels together in *The Wizard of Oz*) and then return to their original position, about 6 inches of distance between the feet. The ankles are neutral (neither dorsiflexed nor plantarflexed) to allow for maximum degrees of freedom and efficiency in transition and posture performance.

Exit   Exhale and return to downward-facing dog preparation or downward-facing dog.

SRAs (static restorative approximations)

- Supine mountain
- Mountain at wall.

DMs (dynamic modifications)

- Knees or forearms plank
- Side plank — Balance unilaterally on forearm or extended wrist
- Strap-assisted plank — Bind the elbows 2–3 inches below the elbow and isometrically perform arm spiral, pressing the arms into the strap bilaterally
- Plank at wall
- "Push-up plus" — Adding controlled scapular abduction and lateral rotation with protraction and slow return or descent to plumb line alignment to target serratus anterior
- Three-legged plank — Alternating lifting the legs, one at a time, to target gluteus maximus (GMAX) and hip rotator cuff (RTC) strengthen and/or

endurance (the combination of which represents power).

TTCP (teaching and tactical cuing primer)

- Externally stabilize the posture through manual assist at the pelvis.
- Give the spine and breath priority.

Contraindications   Any condition where weight-bearing through the upper quarter or lower quarter is contraindicated such as, but not limited to, a compromised glenoid or acetabular labrum; shoulder tendinopathy; osteoarthritis, rheumatoid arthritis, acute Achilles tendonitis; acute back pain.

Four-limbed staff, modified and full (Chataranga dandasana (chah-tah-rangah dan-dah-suhn]))

(Figs 9.22–9.24)

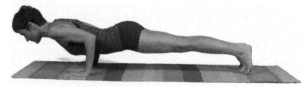

Figure 9.22
Four-limbed staff, full

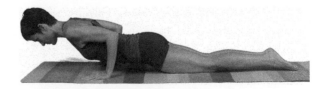

Figure 9.23
Four-limbed staff, modified from knees

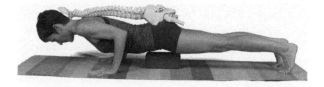

Figure 9.24
Four-limbed staff, reverse with skeleton

Prerequisites Same as four-point plus FMA column (2) cobra, (4), (5)

TI (therapeutic intention)

- Gateway pose to hand and arm balances and inversions

- Lumbopelvic stabilization (advanced)

- Scapular stabilization (advanced)

- Total body power (endurance plus strength)

- All myofascial lines are relevant. Lack of mobility, resilience, or appropriate response from any part of the fascial meridians would be visible in four-limbed staff.

SP (starting position) Prone lying. Transitioning from plank down introduces excessive degrees of freedom that increase injury risk and allow for high-risk compensatory patterns to be too easily used. The prone lying entry point with mirror biofeedback is a "best fit" for clinical safety and efficacy.

Knee position

Entry

1. Place a block under the pubic symphysis and pelvis. Pre-position the upper body so that the humerus of each arm is parallel to the floor and the forearm is perpendicular to the floor.

2. Pre-fire the scapular stabilizers, biceps, triceps, gluteals, and hip rotator cuff (external rotators), including lifting the knees from the floor to pre-fire the quadriceps and hamstrings (co-contraction). Avoid "butter shoulders" or being "boneless" (sinking into the shoulders like a toddler with a tantrum who doesn't want to be picked up). This action requires lifting the trunk to a parallel position with the floor.

3. Engage TATD breath prior to lifting the pelvis off the block 1–2 inches or enough to generate adequate load transfer to challenge the upper quarter and torso to stabilize the body from the knees up.

Full position

Entry Follow the directions in 1 and 2 but perform the posture from the forefoot and hands instead of from the knees and hands by doing the following:

1. Engage the quadriceps and hamstrings by lifting the knees from the floor.

2. Now return to step 3 with the knees clearing the floor. The scapula should not protract and the upper trapezius should not be a dominant strategy for pose completion.

TS (thoracic spine) — Maintain plumb line alignment, spinal neutral, and TATD breath. No spinal movement takes place.

UEs (upper extremities) — Maintain arm spiral. Keep hands under shoulders. The scapula is held dynamically on the chest wall without winging or tipping.

LEs (lower extremities) — Co-contraction throughout; the feet are together about 6 inches apart as described in plank.

Exit Lower to the floor, press back up into plank, or transition into upward-facing dog on inhalation.

SRAs (static restorative approximations)

- Supine mountain — Rest in supine for body awareness and postural training with the feet against the wall for autogenic biofeedback for co-activation to create joint stability

- Standing mountain — Autogenic feedback for co-activation to create joint stability.

DMs (dynamic modifications)

- Downward-facing dog preparation with/without bent elbows

- Reverse four-limbed staff is encouraged over the descending phase of the pose for clinical safety and efficacy. If the pose cannot be stabilized or preformed from its eccentric (reverse) position, then safe descent from plank to the floor is compromised

- Supine ceiling punch

- Supine arm floats

- Four-point weight shift and elbow bend

- Arm spiral

- Place a block under the pelvis to practice dropping to this parallel position with the upper arms.

TTCP (teaching and tactical cuing primer)

- This pose is more like a sequence of postures than a single pose.

- Watch for trunk excessive lumbar lordosis, thoracic kyphosis, or scapular dyskinesis.

- Manual assist — Provide external support at the pelvis at bilateral anterior superior iliac spines to enter/exit.

Contraindications Shoulder complex and hip instability, active rotator cuff impingement or weakness, lumbopelvic weakness; hernia; pregnancy.

Locust (Salabasana [cha-luh-bah-suhn])
(Figs 9.25–9.28)

Code 9.3 (subscription code)
Locust

Prerequisites Same as four-point plus FMA column (2) cobra, (4) 1–4.

TI (therapeutic intention)

- Gateway pose to spinal extension

- Osteokinematic spinal extension, hip extension, ankle plantarflexion, glenohumeral joint external rotation and extension

- Lumbopelvic awareness and postural control outside of spinal neutral

- Assess arthrokinematics of the hip and shoulder — Roll and glide should occur in all planes of motion in opposite directions when the concave surface (acetabulum and glenoid fossa) is fixed and the convex surface (femoral and humeral head) is moving

- Posterior trunk extensor musculature endurance is correlated with hip extensor strength (Ambegaonkar et al., 2014)

- Co-contraction of lower quarter

- Dissociation of GMAX from hamstring/quadriceps co-contraction

- To test endurance, also known as the McGill (Amgedaonkar et al., 2014) or Sorenson (Demoulin et al., 2016) trunk extensor test when performed from a plinth with the lower extremities secured by straps, the trunk is extended in locust pose at a height

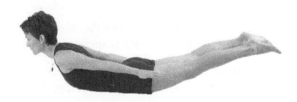

Figure 9.25
Locust, full

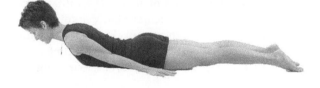

Figure 9.27
Locust, step 2

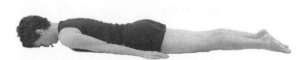

Figure 9.26
Locust, step 1

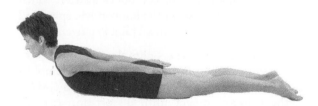

Figure 9.28
Locust, step 3

maintainable by the patient. Place the hands by the back or at the sides. The test is timed until the patient can no longer hold position. A period of 90–240 seconds, not to exceed 5 minutes (Demoulin et al., 2016), is an acceptable range in a healthy athletic population

- Respiratory diaphragmatic isolation for concentric and eccentric resistive training (strength and endurance) in hold phase of posture

- Myofascial tensile force — Superficial front, spiral (if asymmetry exists), anterior arm, anterior functional, and the deep front lines/bands may be most implicated.

SP (starting position)   Prone.

Entry   With the arms at the sides, palms facing down, press the palms earthward to externally rotate the glenohumeral joint. Depress, medially rotate, and mildly retract the scapulae. Co-contract the lower extremities to lift the knees from the floor. Clear the head and chest from the floor. Maintain neutral cervical spine. Lift the thighs and feet from the floor with hip and knee extension. Finally, lift the hands and allow the arms to hover above the earth, reaching to the toes. Maintain for several breaths to isolate the diaphragm and feel the rocking sensation that isolation brings.

TS (thoracic spine) — Maintain TATD breath. Avoid abdominal ballooning to facilitate lift. Maintain cervical spine neutral through a small chin nod. Maintain mobility of the sacroiliac joint (SIJ) by avoiding only using the GMAX as a primary and/or solo movement strategy.

UEs (upper extremities) — Glenohumeral joint flexion is usually not taught in this pose secondary to the long lever arm of the upper quarter, which places increased stress on the lumbopelvic spine and increases risk of glenohumeral joint impingement.

LEs (lower extremities) — Employ deep hip rotators as synergists to TATD breath. If SIJ hypomobility dysfunction is present, avoid using the GMAX as the primary mover until dissociation (neuromuscular isolation of hamstrings as hip extender versus GMAX) can be taught and SIJ dysfunction corrected, since the GMAX can increase SIJ compression (force closure).

Exit   Exhale to return to starting position.

SRAs (static restorative approximations)

- Prone lying with guided imagery

- Prone lying over "Ganesha-fold."

DMs (dynamic modifications)

- Eliminate the arm or leg-lift and complete isometrically.

- Eliminate glenohumeral external rotation.

- Prone over reverse yoga couch.

TTCP (teaching and tactical cuing primer)

- With gross instability or basic motor patterning problems (i.e. hamstring dominance or inability to isolate GMAX), the GMAX is used to facilitate primary force closure.

- Watch for premature SIJ nutation that could be indicative of SIJ or neural patterning dysfunction.

- The heels do not touch. Turn the heels away from each other (hip internal rotation) to dial down GMAX recruitment as needed.

- Manual lumbar spine traction via lower extremity manual traction.

- Manual cuing — Hold the anterior shoulder with the palms of the hands to offer gentle spinal extension.

Contraindications   Pregnancy; stenosis, spondylosis, spondylolisthesis, lumbar fusion; hyperacidity (pitta gastrointestinal inflammation); caution with GERD; hip intra-articular injury such as labral tear; anterior hip or shoulder instability, SIJ dysfunction.

Cobra and Sphinx (Bhujangasana [boo-jahn-gah-suhn])

(see Figs 5.27 and 5.28)

Code 9.4 (subscription code)

Cobra

Prerequisites   Same as four-point plus:

- FMA column (2) cobra only, (4) 1–4
- Locust (at least upper trunk portion if patient is too aggressive with arm press).

TI (therapeutic intention)

- Gateway pose for spinal and hip extension; in cobra, shoulder extension
- Spinal segmental articulation in extension
- Assess arthrokinematics of the shoulder — Roll and glide should occur in the opposite direction as the convex surface (humeral head) is moving and the concave surface (glenoid fossa) is fixed (if there is adequate scapular stability). In sphinx or once in cobra, the humeral head may remain fixed, thereby causing roll and glide to occur in the same direction
- Lumbopelvic awareness and postural control outside of spinal neutral
- Scapulothoracic proprioception and stabilization to improve scapulohumeral rhythm via closed kinetic chain strength training
- Screen for SIJ dysfunction in prone and spinal extension (Chapter 5)
- Dissociation of GMAX from hamstring/quadriceps co-contraction
- Respiratory diaphragmatic isolation for concentric and eccentric resistive training (strength and endurance) in hold phase of posture
- Myofascial tensile force — Superficial front, spiral (if asymmetry exists), anterior arm, anterior functional, and deep front lines/bands may be most commonly involved
- Visceral mobilization for gastrointestinal motility.

SP (starting position)   Prone lying.

Entry

Option 1 — Without the hands, retract the cervical spine (mild *jalandhara bandha*). Lift the knees from the floor to co-contract the quadriceps and hamstrings and employ the hamstrings as hip extenders without GMAX employment. Continue to lift the upper torso without use of the hands and maintain cervical retraction without spinal extension. The arms remain by the side and the hands clear the floor.

Option 2 — Once option 1 is mastered, provide additional spinal extension through a gentle press-up using the hands.

The pelvis should remain on the floor in cobra.

Progression   Once options 1 and 2 are mastered and cobra can be performed without the GMAX and if any found hypomobility SIJ has been resolved, the GMAX can be added to the action for postural support.

Sphinx — Once options 1 and 2 have been mastered, progress to a forearm prop in the absence of myofascial restriction, involuntary gluteal gripping, and with initiation and maintenance of TATD breath (Fig. 9.29).

TS (thoracic spine) — Extension with voluntary control over the lower quarter and hip so the gluteals, hamstrings, and quadriceps can be isolated on demand. No shearing of the lumbar spine should be noted. TATD breath is employed during dynamic execution of the posture to facilitate postural control and safety to prevent lumbar shearing and provide internal support.

UEs (upper extremities) — Glenohumeral joint extension with scapulothoracic depression, medial rotation, and mild retraction. Flex the elbows and approximate the arms at the thorax.

LEs (lower extremities) — The hips mildly extend and the knees lift from the floor to co-activate the quadriceps and hamstrings, which facilitates neural patterning for higher-level trunk control. The ankles are plantarflexed.

Exit   Return to prone lying.

SRAs (static restorative approximations)

- Prone lying with imagery
- Sphinx — Prone on elbows without TATD breath

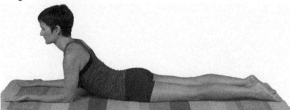

Figure 9.29
Sphinx

- Supine lying over tri-fold blankets to encourage thoracic extension

- Block-supported half-upward-facing bow.

DMs (dynamic modifications)

- Bridge

- Two-foot.

TTCP (teaching and tactical cuing primer)

- Manual SIJ counternutation

- Manual lumbar spine traction via lower extremity manual traction

- Manual pectoralis mobilization and biofeedback for upper quarter alignment to avoid shoulder impingement.

Contraindications Acute stenosis, spondylolisthesis, tonic plantarflexion from spasticity or other neurological impairment; after second trimester and/or high-risk pregnancy; anterior shoulder and/or hip instability, or SIJ dysfunction; inability to dissociate GMAX from hamstrings, especially in populations with pre-existing lumbosacral pain; lumbar fusion.

Upward-facing dog (Urdhva mukha svanasana [erd-vuh moo-kuh shvahn-nah-suhn]) (Fig. 9.30)

Prerequisites Same as four-point plus:

- All FMA columns

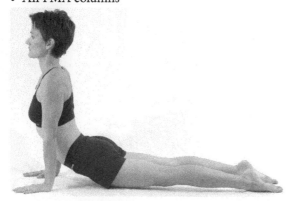

Figure 9.30
Upward-facing dog, full

- Locust

- Screen for hip instability.

TI (therapeutic intention)

- Advanced gateway pose to hand and arm balance and inversions

- Advanced spinal extension

- Prerequisites: plank or for advanced progression, four-limbed staff

- Assess arthrokinematics of the shoulder and hip— Moving into the pose — Roll and glide should occur in the opposite direction as the convex surface (humeral or femoral head) is moving and the concave surface (glenoid fossa or acetabulum) is fixed (if there is adequate scapular stability). Once in the pose — The humeral or femoral head may remain fixed, thereby causing roll and glide to occur in the same direction in both the shoulder and hip

- Lumbopelvic stabilization in a large neutral zone outside of spinal neutral

- Deeper myofascial tensile force — Superficial and deep front, and anterior functional and arm lines or bands may be most implicated

- Total body power.

SP (starting position) Plank (beginner) or four-limbed staff.

Entry

Beginner — Drop from plank through thoracic extension first followed by lumbar and SIJ extension and nutation last.

Advanced — Press up from four-limbed staff into upward-facing dog posture without allowing the humerus to translate anteriorly, the scapula to protract, or the shoulders to collapse and create excessive upper trapezius contraction or thoracic kyphosis. The knees clear the floor with the same co-activation effort as in cobra.

TS (thoracic spine) — The spine is supported with TATD breath. The muscles of the neck and face should not be strained. The GMAX is not fully contracted in the presence of SIJ hypomobility dysfunction or if the GMAX is a primary driver for trunk stability in absence of other synergist use.

UEs (upper extremities) — Provide support while remaining in arm spiral without elbow hyperextension.

LEs (lower extremities) — Co-contraction of the quadriceps and hamstrings without GMAX contraction (if wanting hamstring and hip rotator isolation or if there is presence of SIJ malalignment or pain) or vice versa. Maintenance of the six individual yogic locks will lend the most support in the posture (Chapter 4).

Exit Press back to downward-facing dog or for a very advanced progression return to four-limbed staff and then back to downward-facing dog.

SRAs (static restorative approximations)

- Prone lying

- Supported cobra

- Supported Sphinx.

DMs (dynamic modifications)

- *Beginner* — Leave the ASIS, pelvis, and lower extremities in contact with the earth as in cobra.

- *Advanced*

  - Turn the toes under and stand on them for a variation that assists with increased spinal extension and sacral nutation

  - Weight shift in the upper extremities to screen for unilateral shoulder impairment or develop unilateral proprioception and shoulder control

  - Shrug and roll ("milk") the shoulders superiorly and posteriorly and maintain the posture beyond five breaths.

TTCP (teaching and tactical cuing primer)

- The heart remains brightly open via a beginner entry point of fostering form and force closure in the shoulder complex.

- Initiate movement from the strength of TATD breath.

- The spine receives priority.

Contraindications Stenosis of the spine, spondylolisthesis, TATD weakness, SIJ dysfunction; acute back pain; anterior hip joint instability.

Bow (Dhanurasana [dah-newh-ruh-suhn])
(Figs 9.31–9.36)

Prerequisites Same as upward-facing dog.

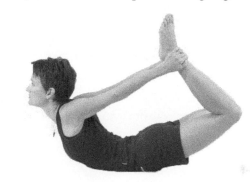

Figure 9.31
Bow, full bilateral

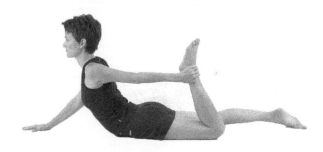

Figure 9.32
Bow, full unilateral

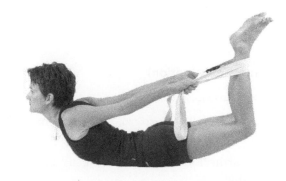

Figure 9.33
Bow, modified bilateral with strap

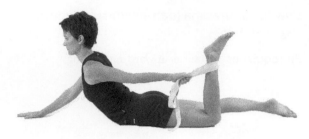

Figure 9.34
Bow, modified unilateral with strap

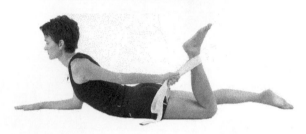

Figure 9.35
Bow, modified unilateral with strap from Sphinx

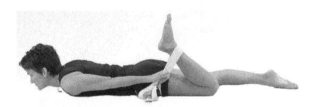

Figure 9.36
Bow, modified unilateral with strap from prone

TI (therapeutic intention)

- Gateway pose to spinal extension

- Osteokinematic ROM: spinal, hip extension; knee flexion, ankle plantarflexion or dorsiflexion

- Assess arthrokinematics — Same as upward-facing dog pose

- Pectoralis group extensibility

- Diaphragmatic isolation and strengthening

- Visceral mobilization

- Gastrointestinal motility

- Myofascial tensile force — Superficial front, spiral (if asymmetry exists), anterior arm, anterior functional, and the deep front lines/bands are most likely implicated, including the hip flexor and abdominal group.

SP (starting position)   Prone.

Entry   Bend the knees and grasp both ankles (not the forefoot) from the outside of the ankle. Inhale and lift the thoracic spine, shoulders, chest, and head (in that order). Lift the upper thighs simultaneously and press the feet into the hands.

Alternate pose — Grasp one ankle and only perform a one-sided bow pose. Use the arm not holding the ankle to perform a press-up on the mat. As the spine extends the bottom, the weight-bearing arm moves closer to the ipsilateral shoulder.

TS (thoracic spine) — Spinal extension without putting the sacrum in a close-packed (locked) position.

UEs (upper extremities) — Shoulders in full extension, wrist in neutral.

LEs (lower extremities) — Keep the knees in line with the hips, not allowing the gluteals to force hip extension. Lift via TATD breath, saving gluteal-driven extension for the final, more advanced version of the posture.

Exit   Exhale to lower and return to prone. Repeat on opposite side if performing one sided/unilateral bow.

SRAs (static restorative approximations)

- Pelvic tilting

- Supported block assisted half upward-facing bow

- Chair supported shoulderstand

- Ball-assist.

DMs (dynamic modifications)

- Ball-assist

- Unilateral bow

- Partner-assist
- Strap/yoga belt around ankles.

TTCP (teaching and tactical cuing primer) Manual cuing for spinal extension — Anterior shoulder hold as in locus manual cuing assist (palms face outward to hold strap).

Contraindications Hyperacidity (fire/water gastro-intestinal inflammation); pregnancy; stenosis, spondylosis, spondylolisthesis, lumbar fusion; anterior hip or shoulder instability; ischiofemoral impingement.

Pigeon pose variation (Ekapada rajakapotasana [ehkah-pah-duh rah-jah kah-poh tah-suhn]) (Figs 9.37–9.40)

> **Code 9.5** (subscription code)
> Pigeon

Prerequisites Same as upward-facing dog plus Craig test/femoral version screen.

TI (therapeutic intention)

- Osteokinematic ROM in all planes, spinal flexion or extension, glenohumeral joint flexion or extension, knee flexion, and/or ankle plantarflexion
- Iliopsoas, quadriceps, quadratus lumborum, and hip external rotator extensibility
- Asymmetrical posture to treat unilateral SIJ hypomobility
- Assess arthrokinematics — Same as upward facing dog pose

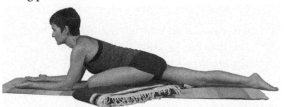

Figure 9.37
Pigeon, full modified on tri-fold blankets resting down in spinal flexion

- All myofascial lines are implicated due to asymmetrical nature of the pose, especially functional, spiral, and the deep front lines/bands.

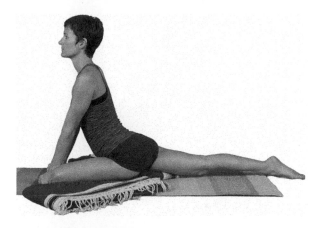

Figure 9.38
Pigeon, full modified up on tri-fold blankets bilaterally in spinal extension

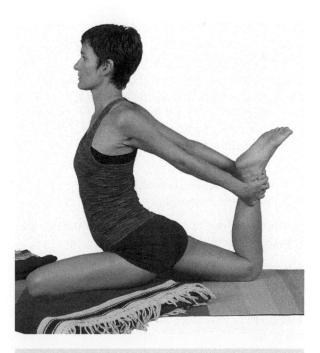

Figure 9.39
Pigeon, full modified up on tri-fold blankets in spinal extension with bound knee flexion

273

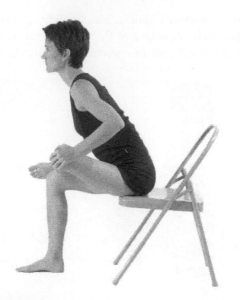

Figure 9.40
Pigeon, modified from chair

SP (starting position)   Four-point.

Entry   Bend the right knee and foot and place it so that the right heel rests near the groin. The right knee and hip rest on the floor or on tri-fold blankets. Place the left leg straight behind the torso so the hip is in internal rotation. The left leg rests on the floor or on blankets so the patella can clear the floor if chondromalacia patella is an issue or if the anterior hip cannot reach the floor.

Option 1 — Rest the trunk on the floor in prone with the elbows bent or straight.

Option 2 — Press up so the torso is over the pelvis in spinal extension.

TS (thoracic spine) — SIJ symmetry should be maintained in spinal flexion (option 1) or spinal extension (option 2).

UEs (upper extremities) — Use arm spiral to support the pose.

Exit   Carefully press up to the hands and knees while simultaneously pulling the right knee out from under the body. Repeat on the left side.

SRAs (static restorative approximations)

- Partial pose — Only perform the beginning entry point into the pose where the spine and trunk rests on the floor, supported by blankets and/or bolsters

- Supported reclined tree

- Supported reclined half-lotus.

DMs (dynamic modifications)

- Blanket-, bolster-, and/or block-assist — If either the hip or the knee cannot rest entirely on the floor, place a folded blanket under each hip to relieve any pressure through the lower quarter. If the back (straight) leg knee is not comfortable contacting the floor, place a blanket under the distal femur (not the knee) to relieve patellar compression. The majority of populations should use blanket assist. All populations with identified hip intra-articular injury, hip instability, knee instability, or femoroacetabular impingement should use blankets or perform SRAs (static restorative approximations).

- Remain in the supported prone position until the hips and spine are ready to progress.

- Flex the back knee to progress into the pose, grasping the ankle with the arms.

TTCP (teaching and tactical cuing primer)

- Assess and treat chronic SIJ nutation before using this pose.

- Spinal extension is a thoracic extension strategy with lumbar lordosis being secondary.

- Use TATD breath and the locks to maintain safety in the posture.

- Rotate the back hip into internal rotation to allow for a neutral but extended spine and to align the pelvis symmetrically to avoid asymmetrical forces on the SIJ.

Contraindications   Stenosis of the spine (only in extended backbend version), knee or hip replacements (need chair version); prior knee surgery or meniscus-related injuries in knee; consideration of hip pathology or osteokinematic limitations such as dysplasia, which could include but is not limited to excessive femoral anteversion (for front leg), femoral retroversion (for back leg), shallow acetabulum, and/or acetabular version; FAI, subspinal (hip) impingement, ischiofemoral impingement.

Review

The prone postures presented in this chapter offer many variations and modifications to teach movement, postural awareness and control in spinal neutral, flexion, and extension. The geriatric, injured, or traumatized population often lose the ability to lie prone, which can often evoke a sympathetic (fight or flight) or dorsal vagus nerve response (freeze) wherein they feel as if they are somewhat immobilized without a feeling of safety (as in trauma) or the position causes pain due to loss of kinematic motion (typically geriatric etiology) or tissue extensibility (as in injured states) issues. In any of these situations, however, there is inherently a loss of the individual's ability to adapt to imposed stresses. Return to Chapter 5 as needed to review the critical components of assessment in the section on helicopter analysis (optimal kinematics, efficient motor patterns, ability to adapt to imposed stressors, and tissue extensibility and sensorimotor integration), which can greatly aid in postural analysis in the prone position.

> *"Never solve a problem from its original perspective."*
>
> Charles Thompson

Postures in this chapter are considered either semi- or partial inversions and were chosen for their accessibility and adaptability to a broad range of patient populations. Semi-inversions are introduced as prerequisites for the inversions shoulderstand and headstand. Semi-inversions emphasize spinal unloading (gravity minimized) first, followed by spinal loading (gravity-dependent) postures second. Postures should be practiced in the order they are presented to achieve spinal segmental mobility, stability, and protection, and to cultivate general strength and endurance (power) of the lumbopelvic and scapulothoracic regions. Semi-inversions can provide safe progression toward full inversions and are gateway postures to accomplish shoulderstand and headstand.

Outline

- Pre-screening
  - Threading-the-needle
  - Legs-up-the-wall
  - Downward-facing dog
    - Tri-dog (asymmetrical/symmetrical)
    - Flipping-the-dog
    - Fire hydrant dog
    - X-dog
    - Figure-eight dog
  - Transition and preparation for headstand
    - Caterpillar
    - Dolphin dive

- Introductory rationale for the evolution of inversions
- Argument for non-weight-bearing headstands and non-axial loading shoulderstands
- Review

Therapeutic benefits and general precautions and contraindications are listed in Table 3.9. Additional benefits and precautions are listed under each pose. See Table 10.1 for an overview of semi-inverted postures.

> Precept Four: Medical Therapeutic Yoga emphasizes biopsychosocial stability as a primary focus with mobility as a secondary focus. Neurophysiologically, the spine receives priority over the extremities during stabilization, which is especially important during semi-inversion postures.

Pre-screening: cervical spine lordosis

Prior to semi-inversions or inversion practice, and to determine safest course of action in posture prescription and progression, evaluate the resting position of the cervical spine in supine. Entry, maintenance, and exit out of (1) bridge, (2) two-foot, or for advanced practitioners, (3) block-assisted half upward-facing bow are included in this assessment.

SP (starting position) Supine hook lying.

1. Cervical spine resting lordosis — Evaluate the resting position of the cervical spine in supine hook lying. Note a flattened, reversed, lateral shift, or absent cervical lordosis via palpation of the cervical vertebral spinous processes.

2. Evidence of flattened, reversed, or absent cervical lordosis or indication of dura mater tension or tethering (as noted in a change in neurological sensation anywhere along spinal nerve distribution C2–S2) or tonically recruited cervical paraspinals and related

Table 10.1

Semi-inversions

Pose	Figure
Pre-screening	
Threading-the-needle	Figs 10.1–10.6
Legs-up-the-wall	Figs 10.7–10.9
Downward-facing dog	Figs 10.10–10.16
• Knee extension	
• Knee flexion	
• Tri-dog	
• Flipping-the-dog	
• Fire hydrant dog	
• X-dog	
• Figure-eight dog	
Transition and preparation for headstand	
Caterpillar	Figs 10.17–10.19
Dolphin dive	Figs 10.20 and 10.21

fascia (most likely the superficial back and deep front lines/bands) is an indication that the pose is too advanced and should be downgraded (via removal of degrees of freedom) or substituted with other therapeutic movement to restore cervical health. Reversed or absent cervical lordosis is an absolute contraindication to performing shoulderstand.

3. Monitor the status of the cervical lordosis and surrounding musculature during a component-by-component entry into bridge, as in the functional movement assessment (FMA) algorithm (Chapter 5). If bridge can be successfully completed as outlined in Chapter 5, progress to two-foot as in the FMA. Once two-foot has been mastered with maintenance of cervical spine, dura mater, muscular/fascia, and movement strategy integrity, progress to block-assisted upward-facing bow, monitoring the same biomechanical and soft tissue standards.

4. In block-assisted half upward-facing bow — Palpate the spinous processes of the lower cervical vertebrae and make sure that a hollow can be felt between the neck and the floor to ensure that the shoulders, not C7, are bearing the weight.

5. Stop at the first sign of tonic contraction or loss of cervical lordosis and maintain the pose integrity without loss of lordosis or "standing" on C7.

6. If there is loss of cervical lordosis, add 1–2 quarter-fold blankets under the shoulders (not under the head) in hook lying. Address therapeutic restoration of lordosis through addition of seated, standing, or supine mild chin lock.

7. Simultaneously screen for neural tension and myofascial restriction from the FMA (Chapter 5).

Threading-the-needle (Parsva balasana [pahrshva buh-lah-suhn]) (Figs 10.1–10.6)

Prerequisites

• Orofascial and respiratory assessment

• FMA column 1

• Transversus abdominis-assisted thoracodiaphragmatic (TATD) breath for transfer from supine to sit and vice versa or when the pose is used for stability training ("*Reach, roll, and rise*" portion)

• Standing-to-floor transfer if performing from floor

• Craig test/femoral version screen

• Other yogic breath types in Chapter 4 are helpful but not required.

TI (therapeutic intention)

• The only posture which offers unloaded, gravity-assisted spinal rotation in spinal neutral

• Restorative pose

• Assess arthrokinematics of shoulder and hip — Moving into the pose — Roll and glide should occur in the opposite direction as the convex surface (humeral or femoral head) is moving and the concave surface (glenoid fossa or acetabulum) is fixed (if there is adequate scapular stability). Once in the pose — The humeral or femoral head may

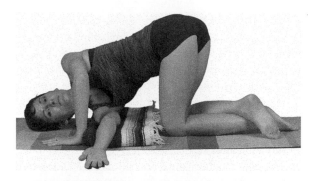

Figure 10.1
Threading-the-needle, modified on tri-fold blanket with supportive arm in arm spiral moment and crossed ankles to diminish hip impingement

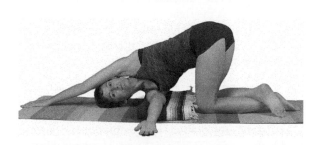

Figure 10.2
Threading-the-needle, modified on tri-fold blanket with shoulder flexion and crossed ankles

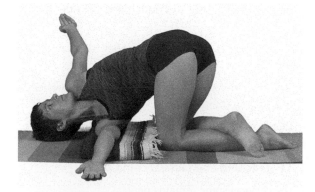

Figure 10.3
Threading-the-needle, modified on tri-fold blanket with shoulder horizontal abduction and crossed ankles

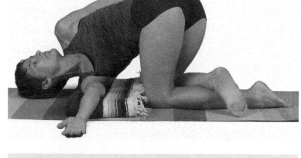

Figure 10.4
Threading-the-needle, modified on tri-fold blanket with shoulder internal rotation and horizontal adduction and crossed ankles

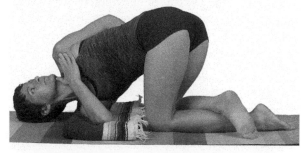

Figure 10.5
Threading-the-needle, modified on tri-fold blanket with shoulder internal rotation and horizontal adduction with contralateral "two-finger approach" biofeedback with crossed ankles

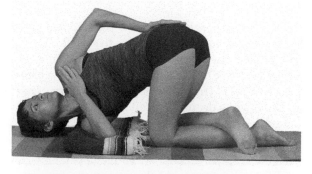

Figure 10.6
Threading-the-needle, modified on tri-fold blanket with lumbar traction moment and contralateral "two-finger approach" with crossed ankles

remain fixed (except for the bottom arm), thereby causing roll and glide to occur in the same direction in both the shoulder and hip

- Thoracic segmental T2–T8 rotation, some rotation and extension

- Posterior shoulder capsule, rhomboid, middle trapezius mobility and scapular protraction

- Serratus anterior biofeedback

- Respiration and breath awareness for posterior ribcage expansion during inhalation, supported to improve trunk stability via full, symmetrical use of the respiratory diaphragm (Kolar et al., 2012)

- Piston action descent of the thoracic (eccentric lengthening), respiratory (concentric contraction), and pelvic diaphragms (eccentric lengthening) acting in concert against gravity with inhalation

- Myofascial tensile force — Superficial back line and lateral raphe, as well as oppositional arm and functional lines/bands may be most affected. When the top arm abducts and/or adducts with extension, superficial and/or deep front line mobility can be accessed

- Posterior peritoneal fascia mobilization when combined with deep abdominal breathing and accentuated by using three-part breath.

SP (starting position) Four-point posture in declined yoga couch or tri-fold blankets stacked one or two high.

Entry With the spine in neutral (cervical and lumbar), rotate the mid-thoracic spine to the left. The left arm supports the torso while the right arm is threaded through the "eye" of the left arm's support. Use a blanket stack (1–2) to maintain cervical spine neutral (rest the shoulder on the blanket and the head on the floor) and prevent reversal of lumbar lordosis.

TS (thoracic spine) — The cervical and lumbar spine remains in spinal neutral while the upper thoracic spine extends and the mid-thoracic spine rotates.

UEs (upper extremities) — The left arm may remain in a weight-bearing position to provide support, or in one of the following positions: (1) lift the left hand from the floor into the air, palm facing out in the same direction

as the body is rotating to keep the shoulder in open-packed position; (2) place the left arm behind the trunk in glenohumeral joint extension, internal rotation, and horizontal adduction; (3) rest the top arm over the head with palm down on the floor; (4) rest the top arm in 90 degrees flexion on the floor to support the trunk in the pose. The right arm remains in scapular protraction and the elbow remains extended or flexed to provide additional light biofeedback for left glenohumeral joint external rotation, horizontal abduction, and 90 degrees flexion, facilitating upper thoracic extension and mid-thoracic rotation and deepening the myofascial experience via increased depth of breathing concomitant with superficial and/or deep front line elongation.

LEs (lower extremities) — For hip impingement or limited flexion, adduction, and internal rotation (FADDIR), cross the right ankle over the left to allow for right hip flexion, abduction, and external rotation (FABER) when rotating left. Otherwise, the ankles remain uncrossed.

Exit Press up using the weight-bearing arm to return to four-point. Repeat on the other side.

SRAs (static restorative approximations) Supine windshield wipers (Chapter 5) with/without blocks under knees to protect iliolumbar ligaments and posterior tissues if rotational articulation is lost in thoracic segments or arthrokinematics are lost in the sacrum or ilia.

DMs (dynamic modifications)

- See upper and lower extremity options in the Entry section.

- Use a blanket for padding under the knees as needed.

- Substitute dynamic windshield wipers with lateral articulation (Chapter 5).

- Tactile or manual cuing can be added to facilitate spinal decompression or thoracic rotation.

TTCP (teaching and tactical cuing primer)

- The cervical spine remains neutral.

- Isolate the posterior capsule and rotator cuff without a positive Hawkins–Kennedy impingement sign.

- The spine should feel elongated and decompressed.

Contraindications Osteoporosis precautions for spinal flexion and/or hip internal rotation; knee pain or injury; femoroacetabular or glenohumeral impingement; subspinal impingement (hip), hip instability, hip intra-articular injury, psoas dominance or hypertrophy; glaucoma, hypertension, acromioclavicular joint separation.

Legs-up-the-wall pose (**Viparita karani [vee-puh-ree-tuh kah-rahn-ee])** (Figs 10.7–10.9)

Prerequisites   Same as threading-the-needle.

TI (therapeutic intention)

- Restorative

- Assess arthrokinematics of shoulder and hip — Moving into the pose — Roll and glide should occur in the opposite direction as the convex surface (humeral or femoral head) is moving and the concave surface (glenoid fossa or acetabulum) is fixed (if there is adequate scapular stability). Once in the pose — The femoral head may remain fixed, thereby causing roll and glide to occur in the same direction in the hip

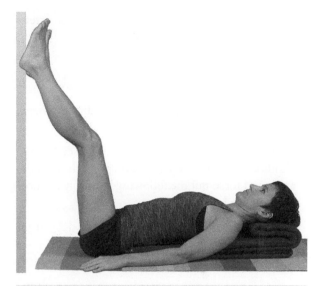

Figure 10.8
Legs up the wall, modified on inclined yoga couch

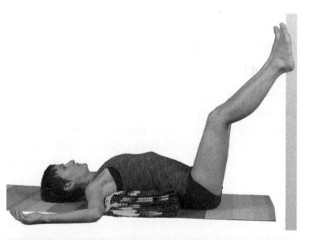

Figure 10.9
Legs up the wall, modified thoracic extension opener

- Pelvic organ prolapse (use inverted yoga couch)
- Turn breech babies (use inverted yoga couch)
- Manage pelvic pain
- Sciatic nerve and dura mater mobility
- Lumbar traction and/or hip posterior/inferior glide (via manual therapy)

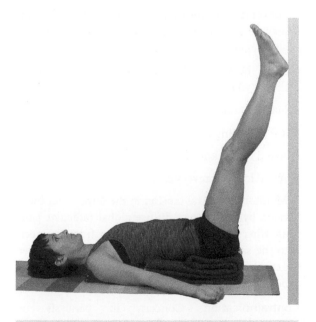

Figure 10.7
Legs up the wall, modified on inverted yoga couch

- Spinal osteokinematic segmental mobility in extension (thoracic extension opener)

- Nausea relief (use inclined yoga couch)

- Hamstring extensibility

- Lower quarter circulation, lymphatic drainage, edema management

- Myofascial tensile force — All myofascial lines/bands are relevant, depending on positioning of the arms and torso but the following lines may be most often involved:

  - thoracic extension – superficial and deep front lines

  - hip flexion – superficial back line

  - inclined yoga couch – superficial back line

  - inverted yoga couch – to a lesser degree, superficial back line

  - added shoulder flexion or abduction – superficial, deep front, and anterior arm lines.

Props 1–2 blankets, strap, block.

SP (starting position) Mat perpendicular to a wall. Blankets in yoga couch or quarter-fold approach, depending on therapeutic intent. Stack either (1) at wall or (2) 12–18 inches away from the wall, depending on hamstring length and presence of any neural tension in the sciatic nerve, or myofascial restriction in the back lines.

Entry From right sidelying in either of the two options listed above, transfer into supine by logrolling onto the blankets. Rest atop the blankets via:

Option 1 — Thoracic extension opener: with tri-fold (shorter torsos) or quarter-fold blankets (for normal to longer torsos) resting perpendicular to mat. Encourages thoracic extension and deep front line fascial lengthening; facilitates intercostal length, symmetrical and full descent of the respiratory diaphragm; baroreceptor reactivity via long, deep abdominal breathing. The pelvis rests into a *"well"* created by the blankets being 12–24 inches away from the wall, depending on hamstring length and pelvic height.

Option 2 — Inverted yoga couch restoration: the pelvis rests on top of the yoga couch with the lower quarter and pelvis higher than the heart to increase semi-inversion effects. The yoga couch's top tier supports the pelvis, the second tier supports the torso and ribcage, the third (lowest) tier supports the upper torso and spine, and the head rests on the floor.

Option 3 — Inclined yoga couch restoration: the pelvis rests on the floor and the rest of the body is supported by a traditional yoga couch. This option works well for those with asthma, respiratory difficulties, allergies, vertigo, dizziness, or for pregnant women.

Exit Slide the legs down the wall into a modified knee-to-chest. Rest here for several breaths before returning to sidelying (use left sidelying for pregnant women or those with gastrointestinal distress). After several more breaths, return to seated through a safe transfer.

SRAs (static restorative approximations)

- Corpse with feet against wall or resting in chair

- Yoga couch with legs resting in chair.

DMs (dynamic modifications)

- For cervical lordosis maintenance — A blanket roll may be needed under the neck at the lordosis or with remarkable thoracic kyphosis.

- Strap the knees together with a block separating them 2–3 inches proximal to the femoral condyles.

- Place a sandbag on the feet for a grounding effect.

TTCP (teaching and tactical cuing primer)

- Avoid forced knee extension or hyperextension.

- Avoid lordosis reversal.

- Monitor for neural tension in the dura mater indicated by presence of diffuse global radicular pain anywhere along the spinal column from the neck to the sacrum. Any adverse sciatic or dura mater neural tension that causes sensory deficits should be differentially diagnosed.

Contraindications Concern in paralysis or neuropathy populations who may have venous insufficiency or spinal cord autonomic compromise; victims of sexual assault or abuse.

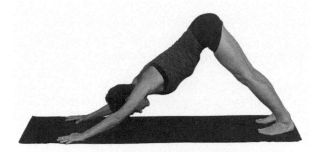

Figure 10.10
Downward-facing dog, knee extension

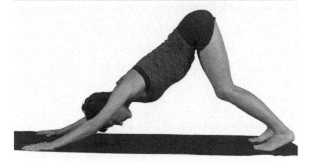

Figure 10.11
Downward-facing dog, knee flexion

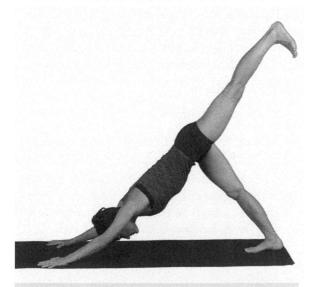

Figure 10.12
Downward-facing dog, tri-dog (neutral)

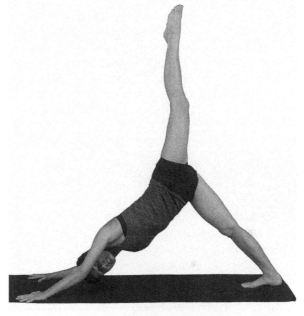

Figure 10.13
Downward-facing dog, flipping-the-dog (this pose is only shown with a partial flip since the full flip is only used for higher-level athletic populations)

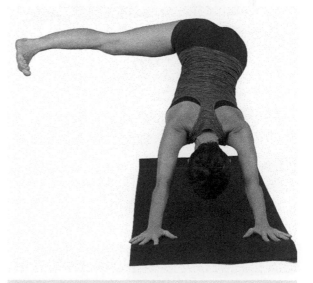

Figure 10.14
Downward-facing dog, fire hydrant

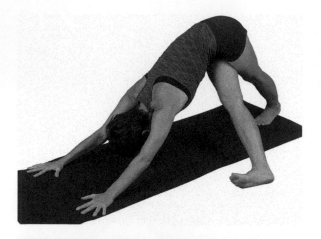

Figure 10.15
Downward-facing dog, X-dog

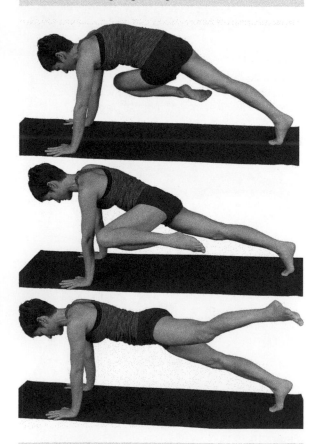

Figure 10.16
Downward-facing dog, figure-eight composite

Downward-facing dog pose with variations **(Adho mukha svanasana [ahdho-mook-ahh shvah-nah-suhn])** (Figs 10.10–10.16)

Prerequisites Same as threading-the-needle plus downward-facing dog preparation. Downward-facing dog preparation is an absolute prerequisite for downward-facing dog. Downward-facing dog is probably the most commonly misused yoga posture. It is typically too advanced for early stage rehabilitation or novice wellness populations.

TI (therapeutic intention)

- Osteokinematic range of motion (ROM): glenohumeral joint flexion, external rotation, forearm pronation (arm spiral), finger abduction, hip flexion, knee extension and flexion (to approximately 15 degrees only), ankle dorsiflexion

- Glenohumeral scaption (for those with joint capsule or range of motion restriction)

- Assess arthrokinematics of shoulder and hip — Moving into the pose — Roll and glide should occur in the opposite direction as the convex surface (humeral or femoral head) is moving and the concave surface (glenoid fossa or acetabulum) is fixed (if there is adequate scapular stability). Once in the pose — The femoral head may remain fixed, thereby causing roll and glide to occur in the same direction in the hip

- Hamstring extensibility

- Neurovascular gliding of posterior structures

- Foot proprioception for alignment in the forefoot, midfoot, and rearfoot

- Myofascial tensile force — All myofascial lines are relevant (superficial and deep front, arm, functional, and superficial back lines and lateral raphe; see variations for more detail)

- Global power (strength + endurance)

- Variations:

  - Tri-dog — Advanced lower quarter unilateral isolation open kinetic chain (airborne leg) gluteus maximus (GMAX) and hamstring strength and endurance; closed kinetic chain (earth-bound leg) bone mass, hip external rotator cuff (RTC) strength for pose stability, dynamic balance; advanced gastrocnemius (straight knee) or soleus tensile force (flexed knee)

- Flipping-the-dog — Myofascial tensile force. Superficial and deep front and contralateral arm line, spiral, and functional lines/bands most commonly implicated; open kinetic chain (airborne leg) femoral head ROM in the acetabulum; quadriceps length; GMAX and hamstring isotonics, spinal rotation, extension, ankle plantarflexion and anterior tibialis length; closed kinetic chain (earthbound leg) advanced stabilization of trunk, pelvis, and unilateral lower quarter strength and endurance (power)

- Fire hydrant dog — Open kinetic chain (airborne leg) gluteus medius, gluteus minimus, and hip external rotator isolation in an active insufficiency range (maximal overlap of sarcomeres), GMAX power, global lower quarter co-contraction, balance; closed kinetic chain (earthbound leg) – see flipping the dog; myofascial tensile force – upper quarter – functional and spiral lines (connecting points between the arm lines to the contralateral lower quarter) and contralateral arm line; lower quarter – perineal tension, superficial back, functional, spiral, and deep front lines most likely affected

- X-dog (crossed leg) — Iliotibial band and hamstring length; hip rotator length; if ankle plantarflexion is desired: peroneal branch of the sciatic nerve neural mobility and peroneal lengthening, otherwise the ankle is kept in neutral; hip flexion and adduction. Myofascial tensile force — Lateral, spiral posterior arm posterior functional, and deep front lines most likely implicated

- Figure-eight dog — Power (strength + endurance) of the lower quarter; dynamic stability outside of spinal neutral; open kinetic chain hip ROM in all planes (airborne leg); advanced TATD power outside of neutral; all myofascial lines relevant due to dynamic nature of posture.

SP (starting position) Downward-facing dog preparation pose.

Entry From downward-facing dog preparation, continue to lift slowly toward child's pose and move toward knee extension (without hyperextension) and shoulder flexion (without hyperflexion). Maintain spinal curves and TATD breath. The feet must be adjusted backwards away from the hands when moving from downward-facing dog preparation to downward-facing dog in order for downward-facing dog to be the correct height for load transfer and equal distribution through the upper and lower quarter. The correct "height" for downward-facing dog is one where, in plank, the hands are under the shoulders and the ankles are in neutral.

TS (thoracic spine) — Maintain spinal neutral throughout plank to downward-facing dog and entry to exit transitions. During all transitions, watch for stability in TATD breath as is evident through monitoring trunk stability and tissue response. For example, during open kinetic chain (i.e., three-legged dog) to closed kinetic chain (regular downward-facing dog) when the left leg is planted and the right leg is airborne, watch for a drop or unlocking of the sacroiliac joint on the left, which may signal ipsilateral abdominal weakness or inhibition, possibly due to myofascial impairment. During dynamic movements, such as transitions, unilateral weakness of TATD breath may be observed during contralateral lower extremity movement (i.e., during fire hydrant downward-facing dog). Other downward-facing dog variations include training outside of spinal neutral.

UEs (upper extremities) — Maintain arm spiral and an "unbroken wrist."

Arm spiral: The anterior elbow is not capable of facing forward in the posture, but the energetic quality of arm spiral provides proper load transfer from the wrist to the shoulder complex through activation of periscapular stabilizers and glenohumeral external rotators.

"Unbroken wrist": The wrist maintains a normal osteokinematic neutral ROM of approximately 10 degrees wrist extension. If joint capsule restriction and/or loss of 180 degrees of shoulder flexion are present, the arms must be placed wider than shoulder width at a scaption angle. Also note the head will not align with the arms (aka *"ringing the bell"*) secondary to absence of full glenohumeral joint flexion.

LEs (lower extremities) — Hip flexion strategy creates safety for the spine in this pose and creates an upside down "V" shape, rather than using a spinal curve reversal strategy (lumbar kyphosis and thoracic lordosis). Minimize unnecessary, extraneous movements in this pose by keeping the feet the same distance apart at all times during downward-facing dog, plank, and cobra. Maintain midfoot arch integrity and rearfoot subtalar neutral (no eversion or inversion) in the presence of dorsiflexion or plantarflexion. Co-activate antigravity musculature of the legs for joint stability. Downward-facing dog prescription should include both knees extended and knees in flexion (10–15 degrees) to address gastrocnemius and the soleus length separately, respectively. Compromise of the spinal curves should not occur in order to straighten the knees.

Exit   Inhale to return to four-point position or transition into a lunge or child's pose, depending on therapeutic intent.

Variation options

1. Three-legged downward-facing dog: symmetrical and asymmetrical

   • Symmetrical three-legged downward-facing dog ("tri-dog") — From downward-facing dog, move the left foot over to a centered location to create a tripod stance. The right foot lifts from the floor and the hip moves into neutral. Look down at the right patella and anterior superior iliac spine (ASIS) to keep the pelvis in neutral spine alignment. Dorsiflex the right ankle to facilitate co-contraction up the kinetic chain and support TATD breath. Hold for 5–10 breaths. Isolate the hip RTC to support TATD breath. Lower the right leg back down and repeat on the left side.

   • Asymmetrical three-legged downward-facing dog ("flipping-the-dog") — From tri-dog, lift the right leg and pelvis to rotate the spine, "opening" the downward-facing dog to the right. Plantarflex the right ankle and, after 3–5 breaths with an extended knee and neutral hip, work toward hip and knee extension, one degree of freedom at a time. The effect feels like "flipping-the-dog" and moving

almost toward an upward-facing bow, which is possible but is only done with optimal kinematics and motor patterning in the shoulder complex. After 3–5 more breaths, return to downward-facing dog via tri-dog, and repeat on the left side.

2. Hip abduction/adduction

   • Hip abduction ("fire hydrant") — From downward-facing dog, shift the weight into the left foot and begin to lift the right leg into hip abduction. The hip is in FABER in order to align the right leg parallel with the earth. The right ankle is dorsiflexed. The left hip is in closed kinetic chain abduction, flexion moment to allow the right leg to achieve parallel position. After 5–10 breaths, repeat on the other side or continue through to "X-dog."

   • Hip adduction ("X-dog") — From "fire hydrant" bring the right leg down and through into flexion and adduction. The foot position is determined by hamstring and iliotibial band length but is placed to isolate both if possible. Typical placement for isolation of the iliotibial band requires the right foot to be located at the halfway mark between the left hand and foot, on the left side of the mat. The foot can be placed in neutral position or plantarflexion, depending on therapeutic intent. If ankle instability is present, avoid ankle plantarflexion.

3. Figure-eight — From tri-dog, draw an "8" shape with the right leg, using all available ROM in the hip joint and moving from downward-facing dog to plank and back again to create the figure-eight shape. Repeat 5–10 times slowly and in each direction (clockwise and counterclockwise), emphasizing global development of power (endurance + strength) and careful open kinetic chain ROM in the airborne hip. Repeat on the opposite side.

SRAs (static restorative approximations)

• Supine spinal neutral with TATD breath

• Supine spinal neutral on yoga couch with TATD breath.

DMs (dynamic modifications)

- Downward-facing dog preparation
- Hands on the edges of the blocks with either (1) fingers cascading on outside of block to protect the fingers or (2) thumbs cascading onto inside of block to protect thumbs
- Hands turn out to 45-degree angle to protect the glenohumeral joint by assuming more gleno-humeral external rotation
- Perform from forearms
- Bend knees to give the spine priority when/if the hamstring length is compromised to less than 90 degrees hip flexion/straight leg raise
- Perform with rearfoot and midfoot supported with a tri-fold blanket to maintain neutral or support an injured, recovering, or fragile Achilles tendon
- Perform with hands against the wall, widening the thumb web spaces
- Strap assist — Bind the arms below the elbow joint just on or below the extensor muscle mass
- Strap plus block assist without cervical spine axial load. Strap the arms together as in strap-assist but add a block for non-axial loading biofeedback (via forehead contact) to keep the cervical spine in neutral. This block position only works with 180 degrees of glenohumeral joint flexion and excellent scapular kinesis
- Segmental spinal mobility progression or "slinky" — Move like a slinky, or a wave rolling into the shore, to focus on reciprocal segmental mobilization of the spine.

TTCP (teaching and tactical cuing primer)

- The fingers remain as wide and open as the mind
- "Ringing the bell" cervical spine check — See FMA
- Manual cuing of lumbar spine — Distraction/traction of the lumbar spine via hand placement over the ilia with or without stepping on the students' hands
- Manual cuing of thoracic spine — Approximation of the inferior angles of the scapula to the chest wall with concomitant widening of the shoulders into external rotation
- Manual cuing — Shoulder release via external rotation of the glenohumeral joints with forearm pronation (arm spiral)
- Maintain power in the lower quarter from the GMAX and deep hip rotators for femoral head positioning and in the upper quarter from the serratus anterior and lower trapezii
- Maintain pliability and responsiveness of the three diaphragms (thoracic, respiratory, and pelvic) by employing just enough TATD breath to maintain safety in the pose
- Depression of the shoulders toward the pelvis may reveal mobility restriction in the posterior capsule affecting the scapula which would present as excessive and early protraction of the scapula in downward-facing dog secondary to attempted glenohumeral joint flexion and/or nonoptimal strategy of the deltoid to dominate glenohumeral flexion action. The resulting affective input would likely be painful secondary to the glenohumeral joint impingement of the rotator cuff as it travels through a compromised coracoacromial arch space.

Contraindications Global debility involving weak TATD; RTC injury or impingement; wrist weakness or injury, osteoarthritis, or rheumatoid arthritis; Achilles tendonitis or active heel spurs; immediate postpartum; glaucoma; hypertension; menstruation; degenerative disc disease, degenerative joint disease; acute low back pain; intra-articular hip injury, FAI, subspinal (hip) impingement, anterior shoulder or global hip instability, shallow acetabulum, hip dysplasia; femoral retroversion may need to toe-out.

Transition and preparation for headstand

Modified dolphin dive (caterpillar) (Astang pranam [ahsh-tahng prah-nuhm])
(Figs 10.17–10.19)

Prerequisites Same as downward-facing dog.

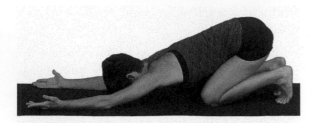

Figure 10.17
Dolphin dive modified (caterpillar) from forearms in arm spiral moment, step 1

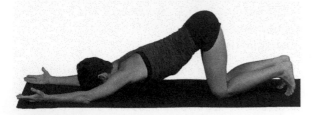

Figure 10.18
Dolphin dive modified (caterpillar), step 2

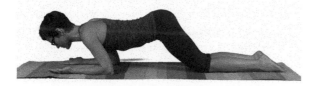

Figure 10.19
Dolphin dive modified (caterpillar), step 3

TI (therapeutic intention)

- Lumbopelvic control and power (intermediate)

- Scapulothoracic control and power (intermediate)

- Segmental spinal articulation and mobility (advanced)

- Assess arthrokinematics of the shoulder and hip — Modified dolphin dive is a complex movement that requires real-time dynamic postural readjustment. This means roll and glide could shift between opposite direction and same direction movements, particularly in beginners who may not be able to stabilize the scapula and pelvis when moving through the dive. Additionally, even with excellent stabilization, the scapula and pelvis will need to shift posturally to accommodate the dynamic movement, more so in the pelvis

- Introspective for self-diagnosis of spinal segmental restriction as well as rotator cuff and scapulo-humeral power (strength + endurance)

- Global power

- Myofascial tensile force — All myofascial lines are relevant. Lack of mobility, resilience, or appropriate response from any part of the fascial meridians would be visible in mountain.

SP (starting position) Downward-facing dog.

Entry Inhale and bring the knees to the floor as close to the toes as possible with maximal ankle and toe dorsiflexion. Exhale and bring the chin and chest toward the floor close to or between the hands and close to the feet. With a cobra-like motion and in a single exhale, fluidly dive the chin and chest barely above the floor until in prone lying without scapular protraction and compromise of the coracoacromial arch space.

TS (thoracic spine) — Segmental articulation into spinal extension in C2–C7, T9–T12, and L1–S2 occurs in the full expression of the pose. T2–T8 does extend but less than T9–T12 (Neumann, 2010). Modified expression for those with contraindications for segmental spinal mobilization into extension can occur by performing from forearms with no spinal mobilization in order to safely transfer to the floor and maintain shoulder complex integrity.

UEs (upper extremities) — Prevent scapular protraction or elbow winging (glenohumeral joint internal rotation, aka "*chicken winging*"). The elbows approximate the ribcage. The wrists experience full extension if performed from the hands. Maintain finger abduction. If weight-bearing through the wrists is not possible, perform from the forearms.

LEs (lower extremities) — Keep the feet and tibia on the ground.

Exit The next inhale progresses to cobra.

SRAs (static restorative approximations)

- Guided imagery

- Supine lying yoga couch with TATD breath

- Supine lying knee-to-chest
- Supine hook lying pelvic tilts and/or pelvic clock.

DMs (dynamic modifications)

- Supine hook lying anterior/posterior (A/P) two-foot (articulating)
- For shoulder complex and trunk weakness or lack of proprioception perform from forearms
- For osteoporosis or segmental spinal mobility contraindications, perform without spinal articulation as needed
- For upper and lower extremity modifications see individual sections.

TTCP (teaching and tactical cuing primer)

- Avoid using momentum to reach the floor. Collapsing or moving quickly to prone lying indicates a lack of motor control/neural patterning.
- Bring the knees as close to the toes as possible during the "entry-inhale" action. This provides more space for spinal articulation and isolates the soleus in a semi-unloaded way, a unique offering of this pose.

Contraindications   Same as downward-facing dog plus stenosis, spondylosis, spondylolisthesis, cervical or lumbar spinal fusion.

Dolphin dive (Astang pranam [ash-tahng prah-nuhm], *advanced variation*) (Figs 10.20 and 10.21)

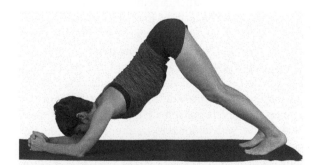

Figure 10.20
Dolphin dive, step 1

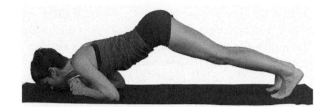

Figure 10.21
Dolphin dive, step 2

Prerequisites   Same as downward-facing dog plus caterpillar if not contraindicated.

TI (therapeutic intention)

- Gateway posture to all inversions
- Upper body power (advanced)
- Lower body power (advanced)
- Lumbopelvic control and power (advanced)
- Scapulothoracic control and power (advanced)
- Segmental spinal articulation and mobility (beginner)
- Segmental spinal control (advanced)
- Assess arthrokinematics of the shoulder and hip — Moving through the dive — Roll and glide should occur in all planes of motion in opposite directions when the concave surface (glenoid fossa and acetabulum) is fixed and the convex surface (humeral and femoral head) is moving. In the absence of scapular or pelvic stability, these movements could reverse, complicating the pose. However, overall, full dolphin dive is a less complex movement than modified dolphin dive/caterpillar, which makes both postures valuable for different reasons
- Introspective for self-diagnosis of spinal segmental restriction as well as rotator cuff and scapulohumeral power (strength + endurance)
- Myofascial tensile force — All myofascial lines are relevant. Lack of mobility, resilience, or appropriate response from any part of the fascial meridians would be visible in mountain.

SP (starting position)   Downward-facing dog.

Entry   From downward-facing dog bring the elbows, one at a time, to the ground in a controlled fashion without compromising the postural integrity of downward-facing dog. Press back up to the hands again one at a time. Lower bilateral elbows simultaneously and return to downward-facing dog. Repeat 3 times. Rest in child's pose. Clasp the hands, leaving the palms open, cup-like. The elbows are shoulder-width apart. Press back up to downward-facing dog. On exhale, lower the chin to the floor in front of the hands.

TS (thoracic spine) — Maintain spinal neutral and TATD breath throughout the pose.

UEs (upper extremities) — Employ scapular stabilizers to avoid over-recruitment of the upper trapezius as a primary mover.

LEs (lower extremities) — Extension without hyperextension of the knees as posterior tissues afford; ankles in dorsiflexion but subtalar neutral.

Exit Inhale and press back into downward-facing dog. Repeat 5 times. Rest in child's pose and release the triceps via elbow flexion so the hands rest on the upper trapezius.

SRAs (static restorative approximations) See previous posture.

DMs (dynamic modifications)

- Perform from downward-facing dog preparation.

- Perform from four-point — Lower chin between the hands (not in front of) to approximately 30 degrees below horizontal (parallel with the earth). Return to four-point. Repeat 5 times.

- Substitute caterpillar.

TTCP (teaching and tactical cuing primer)

- Do not collapse the shoulders toward the ears ("butter shoulders" or "boneless").

- Co-contract lower extremity musculature for stability.

- Employ yogic locks.

- Do not drop the body into plank. Maintain downward-facing dog shape.

Contraindications Same as downward-facing dog.

Introductory rationale for the evolution of inversions

The classic inversions taught in yoga today are the shoulderstand and headstand, known as the "queen" and "king" of yoga postures, respectively. However, the traditional headstand and shoulderstand contradict the natural purpose of the head and cervical spine, which leads to an evolved approach to use of these capstone postures.

The argument for non-weight-bearing headstands (*Sirsasana [sheer-sha-suhn]*)
(Figs 10.22 and 10.23)

Traditional teaching supports axial bearing of weight through the cervical spine during a headstand. However, the following argument establishes a basis for evolving the historical practice of axial loading of the cervical spine.

The average human head weighs anywhere from 11 to 15 pounds. The atlas and axis, as well as C3–C7, are meant to support the 11–15-pound head. The cervical vertebrae and ligamentous structure, which is slack under compressive force (Foreman and Croft, 2001; Yoganandan et al., 2001), also serve to protect the "delicate neural structures" (Panjabi et al., 1998, p. 11) while allowing for a wide range of motion. The caveat is that the cervical spine must be stable to perform these functions, since injuries to this area can have serious consequences.

The cervical region of the spine is the most mobile and delicate of the entire spine. The atlanto-occipital joint may offer many degrees of freedom, but it also must protect the delicate spinal cord and vertebral arteries. There is a rather large neutral zone, up to 50% larger than is available at the lower cervical spine (Goel et al., 1988; Norkin and Levangie, 1992), with C1–C2 demonstrating 75% of its movement in the neutral zone (Panjabi et al., 1998). Because of this large neutral zone and due to the laxity of the joint capsules, the cervical musculature must provide much (about 80%) of the stability in the cervical spine (Goel et al., 1988; Panjabi et al., 1998), with about 20%, or about 50 N, being the critical compressive load limit on the osteoligamentous cervical spine (Panjabi et al., 1988). These muscles are the suboccipital group, the multifidus, interspinalis, semispinalis capitis, and semispinalis cervicis (Nolan and Sherk, 1988). Without the presence of these

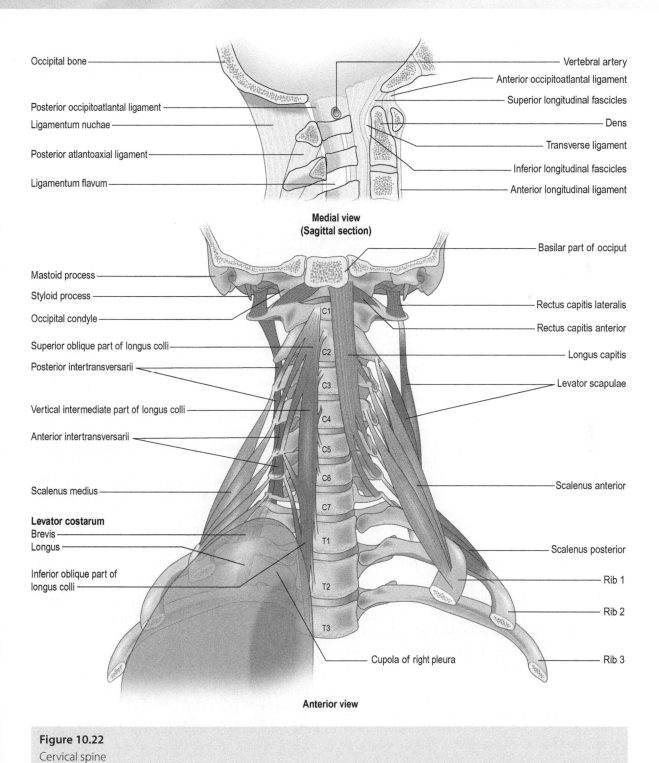

Occipital bone

Posterior occipitoatlantal ligament

Ligamentum nuchae

Posterior atlantoaxial ligament

Ligamentum flavum

Vertebral artery

Anterior occipitoatlantal ligament

Superior longitudinal fascicles

Dens

Transverse ligament

Inferior longitudinal fascicles

Anterior longitudinal ligament

**Medial view
(Sagittal section)**

Mastoid process

Styloid process

Occipital condyle

Superior oblique part of longus colli

Posterior intertransversarii

Vertical intermediate part of longus colli

Anterior intertransversarii

Scalenus medius

Levator costarum
Brevis
Longus

Inferior oblique part of
longus colli

Basilar part of occiput

Rectus capitis lateralis

Rectus capitis anterior

Longus capitis

Levator scapulae

Scalenus anterior

Scalenus posterior

Rib 1

Rib 2

Rib 3

C1
C2
C3
C4
C5
C6
C7
T1
T2
T3

Cupola of right pleura

Anterior view

Figure 10.22
Cervical spine

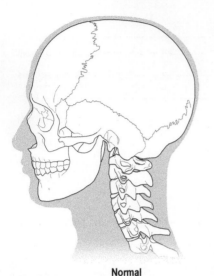

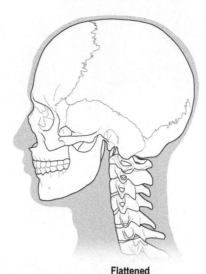

Figure 10.23
Cervical spine: loss of lordosis

Normal

Flattened

muscles, or in the absence of well-developed musculature and spinal alignment, the stability of the cervical complex in the upright position would be considerably compromised. Further, load-carrying capacity of the cervical spine is remarkably reduced (in vivo 20–40 N critical load caused collapse) when the compressive load is vertical (as occurs in a traditional headstand) rather than tangentially (following the curve) oriented (in vivo 250 N without instability) through the cervical spine (Patwardhan et al., 2000). Note this study was done on cervical spines with ideal lordosis and spinal alignment. Critical load capacity would diminish then, being inversely proportional to internal shear force or other bending moments, for example, in the average population in whom forward head posture and poor postural alignment are common.

Further, there are no discs between C1 and C2. During a traditional performance of a weight-bearing headstand the weight of the entire body is borne through C1–C2 to the articular facets of the axis. Any compressive or axial load would be dispersed through C1–C2 and the discs and facet joints below. Any degeneration, such as occurs as a result of natural aging (Brinjikji et al., 2015), would place the discs at risk of end plate failure, and the comorbidity of postural malalignment, such as forward head (cervical spine shear), or flattened lordosis, can place the cervical spine at higher risk for injuries such as disc compression and nerve root compression with or without extrusion.

Ligaments are also uniaxial in nature and designed to carry loads only in the direction their fibers run (Foreman and Croft, 2002), which means they are like "rubber bands," resisting tensile strength and collapsing under compressive loading. Disc degeneration is a common condition associated with aging (Brinjikki et al., 2015), and when in a degenerative state, those discs display less viscoelasticity, and offer less shock attenuation and load distribution (White and Panjabi, 1990), with significant increases in intradiscal pressure. Further, under rapid loading conditions, such as traditional axial weight-bearing inversion, there is an increased risk of injury secondary to increasing peak rupture stress (White and Panjabi, 1990). Other arguments which support non-weight-bearing (axial loading or cervical spine loading) inversions include the following:

- Axial loading conditions in the head and neck suggest a predisposition for degenerative diseases (Mehnert et al., 2005).

- Repetitive flexion–extension motions with low magnitude compressive forces have been shown to be an effective mechanism for causing disc herniations (Drake et al., 2005).

- Shear forces present in the cervical spine (such as are commonly present in a majority of the population, often seen via forward head posture) combined with flexion or axial compression further increase cervical injury risk.

- Axial compression of the cervical spine during sports is associated with a buckling effect on the cervical spine (Swartz et al., 2005).

- The mandible is a linking point between the originations and the insertions of the muscles of the cervical spine. Any contraction of the cervical spine musculature has a direct effect, if not completely understood, on the temporomandibular joint (TMJ). Anterior shearing or forward flexion of the neck closes down the space available in the TMJ and can create compression or chronic negative forces on the TMJ. This observation makes cervical spine problems and TMJ problems likely to occur concomitantly. For this reason, the weight-bearing headstand can have longstanding adverse effects on the TMJ and cervical spine that have not yet been considered.

- If a person is allowed to perform a full weight-bearing headstand they are missing a vital opportunity for shoulder complex stability development, which is critical for upper quarter longevity.

For all of the reasons stated, non-weight-bearing headstands, including forearm balances, are the preferred method for inversion posture prescription. The non-weight-bearing headstand is easily and safely taught to those with active shoulder pain in order to help rehabilitate the rotator cuff, and relatively difficult to achieve in other yoga postures for those in pain. The non-weight-bearing headstand, with its plethora of benefits, is a solution that allows for discarding of the traditional weight-bearing headstand, with its known and unknown dangers. The headstand is performed with no axial loading and with maximum weight-bearing through the shoulders and forearms, with control of the pose provided by the lumbopelvic region. In this way, non-weight-bearing headstands can be modified to allow everyone to enjoy the benefits it offers.

The argument for non-axial loading shoulderstands (*Salamba sarvangasana,* *[sah-lahm-buh sahr-vuhn-gah-suhn]*)

Traditional teaching supports stretching the cervical spine in extreme flexion during shoulderstand (Coulter, 2001). But as in headstand, the shoulderstand should be performed with no cervical weight-bearing and should provide proper support, such as via multiple blankets, under the shoulders to prevent complete reversal of the cervical curve.

The high prevalence of back pain (Freburger et al., 2009) and neck pain, cited as a major international public health problem (Fejer et al., 2006), in the general population precludes most populations from practicing headstand or shoulderstand; however, they can be practiced in the modified ways introduced in this chapter.

In orthopaedic rehabilitation, the majority of therapists spend the majority of their time treating low back and neck pain, educating patients on proper posture, ergonomics, and alignment of the spine, usually due to a reversal of the spinal curves. Postures that encourage a chronic reversal of curves, such as the traditional shoulderstands, do not serve the more than 84% of people who will at some point experience back pain (Freburger et al., 2009). For this reason, modified and full shoulderstand should be taught with mindful preservation of the cervical lordosis and avoidance of cervical lordosis reversal with concomitant cervical loading. Full shoulderstand is an advanced posture rarely appropriate for the general population.

If a patient has reversal of lordosis in a resting, supine position, then shoulderstand is absolutely contraindicated. Restoration and maintenance of the functional cervical lordosis without myofascial tension or dura mater tethering should be first priority in allowing a patient to progress toward shoulderstand.

Chapter 11 offers suggestions of both gender neutral and gender-sensitive sequences to prepare for the practice of inversions. Use of this chapter and Chapter 11 will prepare the individual for progression into full inversions, chiefly headstand and shoulderstand.

Review

The semi-inversion postures offered in this chapter are meant to serve as prerequisites to progression into full inversion, chiefly non-weight-bearing or axial load-ing headstand and shoulderstand. Because inversions offer so many systemic benefits, and because they are both advanced postures, practice of these semi-inver-sions should take place over a period of months or years in order to progress safely and therapeutically into full inversions. Finally, both semi-inversions and inversions should consider gender-sensitive contexts, offering individualized programs that are dependent on typical known gender strengths and weaknesses.

This chapter outlines photographic and tabular instructions for the Sun and Moon salutation series plus sample prescriptions based on three common orthopaedic pathophysiologies, two of which are discussed in case study format. The three themed prescriptions consider concomitant systemic comorbidities frequently found in the general adult population. Finally, two general sequences, in addition to two gender-sensitive sequences, provide prerequisites for patient preparation in safe nonaxial loading inversions (headstand and shoulderstand).

Outline

- FITT principle
- Sun and Moon salutation sequences
- Case studies and sequences
- Safe inversion progression prerequisites
- Gender-sensitive sequences
- Review

The FITT principle

The "FITT" in the FITT principle stands for frequency, intensity, time, and type (specificity) (ACSM, 2014). The recent addition of volume (V) and progression (P) produces the acronym FITT-VP.

The FITT principle

- Frequency
- Intensity
- Time
- Type

Yoga, when combined with exercise and rehabilitative science, has the potential to address all the factors outlined below, in addition to its biopsychosocial (BPS) benefits. The US Department of Health and Human Services issued their first recommendations on physical activity, which include the following (USHHS, 2008):

- *Children and adolescents* — Children need moderate to vigorous intensity physical activity for a minimum of 60 minutes every day of the week, with vigorous activity occurring at least 3 days of the week. Muscle and bone strengthening activity should happen, as part of the overall 60 minutes, at least 3 days a week.

- *Adults* — Adults need at least 150 minutes of moderate intensity aerobic exercise or 75 minutes of vigorous intensity aerobic exercise per week. Each episode of activity should be at least 10 minutes in duration. For increased health benefits, increase activity to 300 minutes (5 hours) of moderate or 150 minutes of vigorous aerobic activity per week. Muscle and bone strengthening exercises should also be performed on all major muscle groups a minimum of 2 days per week. Although not detailed in the report, maximizing strength development should generally include 8–12 repetitions of each exercise, resulting in a volitional fatigue.

- Children or adults with disabilities should engage in regular physical activity according to their abilities in order to avoid inactivity.

Sun and Moon salutation sequences

A sequence is a series of postures that can flow one after another with or without stopping. The Sun and Moon salutation sequences provide quintessential postural sequences from which a combination of standing, seated, prone, and supine postures can be selected for infusion with the salutation(s), based on therapeutic need.

Sun salutation historically serves to greet the day (hence "Sun") and can be combined with individual spiritual belief system practices. The most common one practiced in Christianity, for example, would be setting the Sun salute to the Lord's Prayer. However, any prayer, and/or unspoken (*mantra*) or spoken (*mantram*) inspirational phrase can be used during completion of the series.

Moon salutation is a hybrid creation of Sun salutation that is most appropriate when extreme postural changes (for example, repeated floor to standing transfers) are contraindicated or not necessary or desired. Conditions where the Moon salute is most often clinically appropriate include pregnancy (for example, where there is nausea), dizziness (caused by orthostatic hypotension or vestibular issues, for example), debility or fatigue (for example, when there is lack of independence or concerns over safety with floor to standing transfers), or other musculo-skeletal (MS) or neuromuscular (NM) pathophysiology. Photographic and tabular representation of the Sun and Moon salutations can be seen in Figs 11.1 and 11.2.

Note: The functional movement assessment (FMA) (Chapter 5) scaffolds the essential Sun salutation into an adaptation called Moon salutation, after which it breaks down the components of Moon salutation into individual parts. The individual postures and breath in the FMA together create the sum or whole of the salutation series, which can be considered a cornerstone of basic Medical Therapeutic Yoga (MTY) practice.

Case studies and sequences

The following sequences are presented in order of epidemiological orthopaedic frequency in the general population, while also recognizing the most common comorbidities for each condition. These include functional gastrointestinal disorders, osteoarthritis, type II diabetes mellitus, cardiovascular disease, obesity, and depression (AHNN, 2011). Remaining conditions that round out the top 20, and which can also be affected by yoga, include back pain, anxiety, allergic rhinitis, reflux esophagitis, respiratory problems, hypothyroidism, fibromyalgia, malaise and fatigue, pain in joints, acute laryngopharyngitis, acute maxillary sinusitis, acute bronchitis, and asthma (AHNN, 2011). Common

orthopaedic diagnoses are, in order of prevalence, back pain, knee pain, and shoulder injury:

1. Lumbopelvic pain: nonspecific back pain

2. Knee pain: patellofemoral pain and iliotibial band syndrome

3. Shoulder pain: rotator cuff tear and impingement.

Nonspecific back pain

Code 11.1 (free code)
More resources on back pain management

More than 84% of people will experience low back pain (LBP) at some point in their lives (Carey et al., 2009; Freburger et al., 2009), with the common cold being the only condition seen more often by primary care practitioners. LBP is a major cause of disability and absence from work (Balague et al., 2012), with more than 75% of work-related back injuries stemming from poor posture and mechanics. Back pain is described as an "epidemic" that is expected to increase substantially over the coming decades (Freburger et al., 2009) (Fig. 11.3).

But despite established clinical guidelines supporting the early use of physical therapy in best care practices for LBP management, referrals for conservative care remain unchanged since 1990. In a large retrospective study, the physical therapy referral rate was a paltry 20% (Mafi et al., 2013). Narcotic prescriptions, referrals for diagnostic tests, and other physician referrals all increased while patient quality of care and back pain outcomes decreased. This study is not the first to reveal the discordant care of LBP (Carey et al., 2009; Fritz et al., 2012).

The World Health Organization and the American Physical Therapy Association cite several risk factors for LBP, including work (manual labor, heavy lifting, operating heavy equipment, prolonged postures), leisure, individual (pregnancy, hypertension, poor lifestyle choices), and psychological factors, with psychological factors playing a larger role than physical factors (WHO, 2003; Delitto et al., 2012). Those psychological

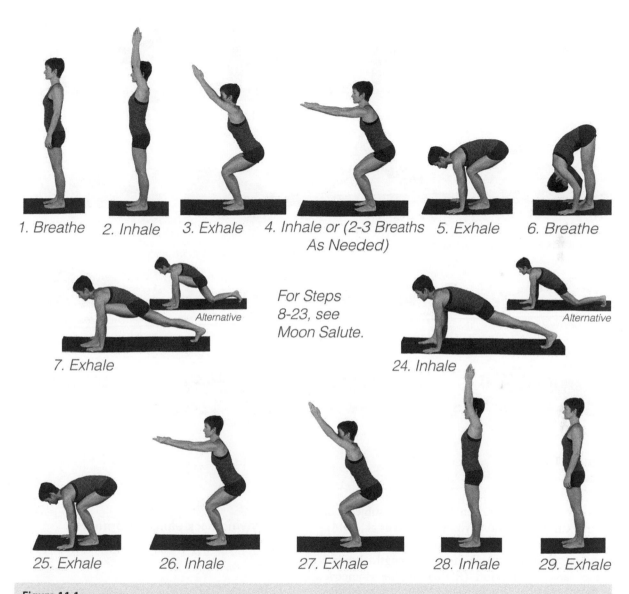

1. Breathe   2. Inhale   3. Exhale   4. Inhale or (2-3 Breaths As Needed)   5. Exhale   6. Breathe

Alternative

For Steps 8-23, see Moon Salute.

Alternative

7. Exhale   24. Inhale

25. Exhale   26. Inhale   27. Exhale   28. Inhale   29. Exhale

Figure 11.1
Sun salutation sequence with breathing pattern

factors include job dissatisfaction, sleep disturbances, fear of pain (chronic pain), depression, and stress.

Treatments for LBP vary widely and typically overuse medication and narcotics while under-using exercise and other helpful adjunct treatments such as treating depression, for example (Carey et al., 2009). Confirmed non-risk factors for LBP include diagnostic testing, for example magnetic resonance imaging (MRI) or myelography indicating degenerative changes such as degenerative joint disease, spinal canal narrowing or degenerative disc disease, and disc herniation (Savage et al., 1997; WHO, 2003; Delitto et al., 2012). Up to 75% of asymptomatic patients show evidence of degenerative joint disease or degenerative disc disease with diagnostic imaging (Savage et al., 1997). The percentage surges to over

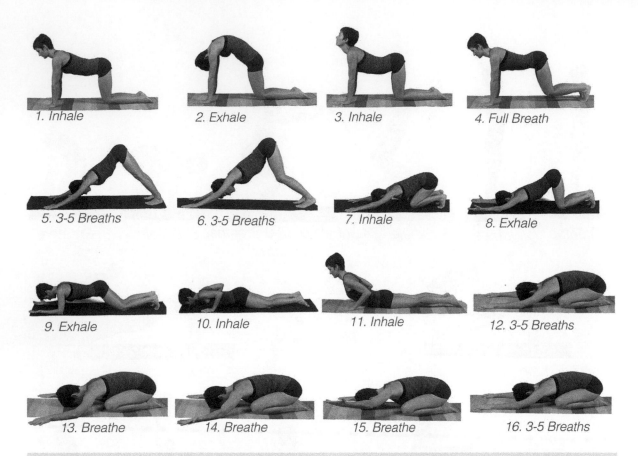

1. Inhale
2. Exhale
3. Inhale
4. Full Breath
5. 3-5 Breaths
6. 3-5 Breaths
7. Inhale
8. Exhale
9. Exhale
10. Inhale
11. Inhale
12. 3-5 Breaths
13. Breathe
14. Breathe
15. Breathe
16. 3-5 Breaths

Figure 11.2
Moon salutation sequence with breathing patterns

75% for disc degeneration in pain-free subjects in their sixth decade and beyond (Brinjiki et al., 2015). There is also inconclusive evidence for correlation between pain and trunk muscle strength, lumbar spine range of motion (ROM), and/or isometric endurance of trunk stabilizers (WHO, 2003; Delitto et al., 2012).

Improving back pain outcomes requires a shift in practice paradigm. The first action should help patients advocate for themselves. This requires education about self-care, as opposed to current practices, which send more than 75% of patients home with medications (Fritz et al., 2012). Second, care should be scientifically supported, which would limit the use of diagnostic imaging and avoid surgery (Balagué et al., 2012). Finally, since LBP does not resolve on its own (Hestbaek et al., 2003), the heaviest emphasis should

Improving back pain outcomes

Improving back pain outcomes requires a shift in practice paradigm

- Advocate for and use a biopsychosocial model of assessment and intervention, introduced in Chapter 2. The vector analysis used to complete the FMA, in Chapter 5, is a practical tool to apply both biomechanical and psychobiological assessment during breath and posture diagnostics and intervention

- Help patients self-advocate and practice self-care

- Care should be informed by best evidence practices

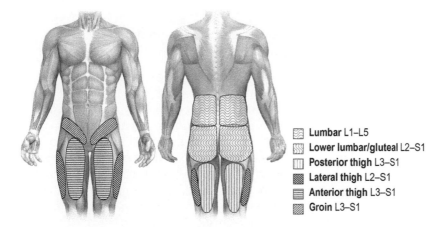

Figure 11.3

Distribution of common lumbar facet and general back pain (adapted in part from Gellhorn et al., 2013)

Lumbar L1–L5
Lower lumbar/gluteal L2–S1
Posterior thigh L3–S1
Lateral thigh L2–S1
Anterior thigh L3–S1
Groin L3–S1

- Heaviest emphasis should be on conservative intervention

- Early intervention, with attention to personal factors and environmental influences, is vital for optimizing outcomes.

be on conservative intervention. Delayed therapy for back pain is costly and associated with increased medical care for LBP later (Fritz et al., 2012). Overall, the consensus is that early intervention, with attention to personal factors and environmental influences, is vital for tackling the public health crisis of LBP.

Yoga for back pain research is limited in its scope and depth. Current studies segregate yoga from conservative rehabilitation, which limits the power of yoga's efficacy. They typically measure "usual or standard care" against yoga, rather than using an evidence-evolved approach that combines yoga with rehabilitation. Studies that disregard this powerful combination will not be able to address populations with complex LBP histories since most exclude anyone with a complex medical history or history of degenerative joint or disc disease, or other complicated LBP. Future studies should apply the evidence base in back pain rehabilitation to yoga principles to evolve the treatment, something that this chapter addresses. Future studies should also consider myofascial restriction, neural tension, and other complex issues such as visceral mobility or neuroendocrine regulation rather than clinging to outdated measures

such as range of motion or flexibility as biomarkers for back pain resolution.

The ideal research methodology would be a partnership-based BPS yogic approach that evolves yoga based on inclusion of medicine and allied health science. Level I/grade A evidence supports that early intervention in LBP with physical therapy reduces expense and offers the best overall chance of long-term successful management of LBP (Gellhorn et al., 2012). Therefore, it is plausible to deduce that yoga, with its gut–brain–body axis systemic benefits, combined with rehabilitation science can offer superior outcomes and patient satisfaction to yoga or therapy alone. This is especially true since yoga addresses comorbidities such as depression, panic, anxiety, systemic inflammation, and functional gastrointestinal disorders which are well known to influence LBP outcomes, as well as general orthopaedic outcomes such as shoulder, hip, and knee pain.

A full assessment prior to prescription of LBP is beyond the scope of this text (see Code 11.1 for additional resources). However, basic assessment should include the following seven qualitative and quantitative measures:

1. Centralization of symptoms and spinal mobility

2. Neural and fascial (including visceral) integrity and functional mobility

3. Joint function (spine and hip), integrity, and proprioception

4. Postural awareness and control

Chapter 11

5. Yogic locks assessment, including transversus abdominis, multifidus, thoracic, respiratory, and pelvic diaphragm functioning (the factors which together comprise transversus abdominis-assisted thoracodiaphragamtic (TATD) breath)

6. Endurance assessments

7. Psychometric outcome measures for pain, catastrophizing, disability, and functioning (Chapter 12).

Differential diagnosis should include screening for the following (list adapted in part from Delitto et al., 2012):

- Fascial or visceral adhesions related to previous abdominal, back, or pelvic surgery

- Back-related tumor that may be accompanied by unexplained weight loss, over age 50, history of cancer, constant pain not affected by activity, failure of conservative treatment within 30 days, no relief with rest, and night pain

- Cauda equina syndrome such as urine retention, fecal incontinence, saddle anesthesia, or sensory or motor deficits in L5–S1 areas

- Back-related infection such as recent infection (urinary tract infection, skin), drug abuser, immunosuppressive disorder, deep constant pain, increases with weight-bearing; fever, malaise, swelling

- Spinal compression fracture (fx) such as history of major trauma; over age 50; prolonged use of corticosteroids; point tenderness at site of fx; or increased pain with weight-bearing

- Abdominal aneurysm such as back, abdominal, or groin pain, presence of peripheral vascular disease or coronary artery disease and associated risk factors (over age 50, smoker, hypertension, diabetes mellitus); family history; non-Caucasian, female, abdominal girth greater than 100 cm; symptoms not related to movement stresses; palpation of abdominal aortic pulse.

Code 11.2 (free code)
Lateral knee drops

Nonspecific back pain postural progression

Use the functional movement assessment (FMA) columns 1–3 to assess postural control and awareness. Follow the biopsychosocial assessment guidelines (Chapter 2) and vector analysis (Chapter 5) for a complete biopsychosocial assessment that looks beyond biomechanical or soft tissue analysis. Pay particular attention to the patient's ability to identify, engage, and maintain transversus abdominis-assisted thoracodiaphragmatic (TATD) breath in:

- Anterior/posterior (A/P) and lateral spinal neutral

- A/P and lateral articulation

- Hook-lying knee lifts and lateral knee drops (lateral knee drops are not included in the FMA but are included in Code 11.2).

The remainder of the FMA can be followed as outlined in Chapter 5, using clinical reasoning and individual indications and contraindications to direct selection of the postures most appropriate for testing and intervention.

Other considerations for LBP management should include (Bunzli et al., 2011) patient education and counseling that addresses:

1. Activity pacing

2. Attention diversion

3. Cognitive restructuring

4. Goal setting

5. Graded exposure

6. Motivational enhancement therapy

7. Maintenance strategies

8. Problem-solving strategies.

Contraindications: Pregnant or postpartum women should see a women's health physical therapist for individualized programming. Acute, subacute, or chronic pain patients should follow the preceding schedule for management.

Acute care

Those with unilateral back, buttock, or thigh pain of less than 1 month that is movement-related should consider including manual therapy, therapeutic movement for the spine, and patient education for self-care concerning positive lifestyle choices (Delitto et al., 2012).

Yoga intervention can include restorative postures that offer passive restraint for those who do not have internal (TATD, etc.) support, such as postures from Chapter 8. Dynamic postures should address strength, endurance, and fascial integrity without pain, including respiratory training. The FMA provides a safe method for developing internal stability and awareness. Biomechanical and ergonomic training and neuromuscular re-education (re-ed) in mid-range positions, as well as temporary external devices for passive restraint (restorative yoga, belts, etc.) can assist with symptom reduction.

Subacute care

Back pain that persists for greater than 1 month can be considered subacute. Therapy should consider comorbidities such as poor lifestyle habits or nutrition and/or previous medical history that may affect long-range outcomes. Manual therapy should address identified deficits in the thoracic spine, ribs, lumbar spine, sacroiliac joint, and/or hip and should continue with therapeutic exercise and neuromuscular re-education for trunk and lumbopelvic strength and endurance. Self-care/home management and community or work reintegration training and pain management strategies (Delitto et al., 2012) can also be addressed in this phase.

LBP that is referred to the lower extremities may necessitate lumbar traction in order to centralize symptoms. Partner yoga practice can provide this manual therapy, as well as inclusion of postures which address lumbar extension and neural mobility.

Chronic care

Cognitive or affective tendencies as measured by psychoemotional outcome measures (see Chapter 12) are often notable in this population. Patient education should address depression, fear avoidance, and pain

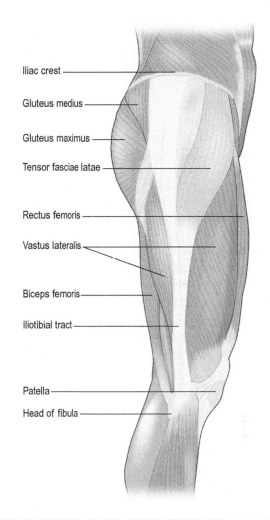

Figure 11.4

Iliotibial band syndrome (ITBS) anatomy

Labels: Iliac crest, Gluteus medius, Gluteus maximus, Tensor fasciae latae, Rectus femoris, Vastus lateralis, Biceps femoris, Iliotibial tract, Patella, Head of fibula

catastrophizing. Low intensity, prolonged aerobic exercise should also be included, with less emphasis on passive therapies and increased emphasis on self-management (Delitto et al., 2012).

Patellofemoral pain syndrome

Iliotibial band syndrome is the lead cause of distal lateral thigh/knee pain in athletes, with a reported incidence of 1.6–12% (Frederiscon et al., 2000; Lininger and Miller, 2009; Falvey et al., 2010; Lavine, 2010). Iliotibial band syndrome comprises 15% of all knee injuries and typically occurs secondary to repetitive motion (Lavine, 2010). Iliotibial band syndrome and patellofemoral syndrome often occur together (Fairclough et al., 2007). This sequence will be provided in a case study format.

The iliotibial band (ITB) is a tough, tendinous continuation of the tensor fasciae latae (TFL) and gluteus maximus (GMAX) that originates at the iliac crest and inserts on the lateral aspect of the tibia, fibular head, and patellar retinaculum (Messier et al., 1995) (Fig. 11.4). The iliotibial band has been found to be a uniformly lateral thickening of the circumferential TFL, firmly attached along the linea aspera (femur) from the greater trochanter up to and including the lateral femoral condyle (Falvey et al., 2010). Anatomy includes the iliac tubercle, GMAX, TFL, lateral patellar retinaculum, and patella (Sher et al., 2011).

Causative factors for iliotibial band syndrome are attributed to friction against the lateral femoral condyle and/or, due to its medial/lateral movement capability, compression of the highly vascularized and innervated layer of fat and connective tissue that separates the iliotibial band from the epicondyle (Fairclough et al., 2007). Chronic inflammation of the iliotibial band bursa is also a possible etiology (Strauss et al., 2011). There are many factors that contribute to these etiologies, including:

- Weak hip abductors (Fredericson et al., 2000; MacMahon et al., 2000; Noehren et al., 2007)
- Angle of knee flexion between 20 and 30 degrees during stance phase of activity (Noble, 1980; Orchard et al., 1996; Miller et al., 2007)
- Increased forces on landing, knee internal rotation, ipsilateral hamstring weakness
- Imbalance of the agonist/antagonist, genu recurvatum (Messier et al., 1995; Busseuil et al., 1998; Devan et al., 2004; Noehren et al., 2007)
- Genu varus (Lavine, 2010), and/or
- Inappropriate footwear, improper training, leg length discrepancy, running on sloped or banked running surfaces, excessive pronation or supination (eversion), large Q-angle/pelvic width, or excessive mileage increases (Fredericson and Wolf, 2005; Khaund and Flynn, 2005; Paluska, 2005)

- High-risk activities including running, rowing, soccer, field hockey, cycling, basketball (Devan et al., 2004; Lavine, 2010), yoga, gymnastics, and dance.

Iliotibial band syndrome usually presents as diffuse pain over the lateral aspect of the knee and typically begins as a general "achiness" but can progress into a sharp, more localized pain over the lateral structures (Khaund and Flynn, 2005). Proximal issues are a unique injury that should also be considered in patients with hip pain, and should consider imaging of both the hip and iliac tubercle, which is often excluded in diagnostic testing. Iliotibial band syndrome can also present as:

- Lateral thigh or knee pain and/or hip pain
- Increasing pain with activities such as cycling or running
- Patellar pain or tracking problems that can create medial knee pain
- Point tenderness over the iliotibial band insertion, proximal iliotibial band strain, and/or
- Positive Ober test, though it has failed to be validated (Cook and Hegedus, 2013) as a viable provocative test of poor hip control/neuromuscular function.

> **Biopsychosocial application in iliotibial band syndrome**
>
> **Physical**
> - Stress management
> - Barefoot yoga
> - Self-correction and self-Marma point massage
> - Shoe inserts and prescription.
>
> **Energetic/psychoemotional**
> - Breathwork
> - Address potential addiction issues
>   - Meditation
>   - Self-correction work in a flow series of higher level yoga postures

- Shift patient's focus in yoga from flexibility to stability (improving health literacy).

Intellectual

- Patient education: sport substitution
  - Sports psychology (identification of methods for cross-training)
  - Continued importance of anti-inflammatory nutrition in injury management and prevention.

Bliss/relational

- Determine preferred method of fitness participation (solo vs. group) and channel patient appropriately
- Shift thinking from yoga as only physical exercise to yoga as a lifestyle promoting self-care and self-reflection
- Encourage positive self-talk
- Explore deeper causative factors
- Foster common ground between belief system(s), self-care, and relationship health.

Management of iliotibial band syndrome must include evaluation of the biomechanics of muscle function during activity (Fairclough et al., 2007), which raises the importance of proper biomechanical alignment and co-contraction during yoga pose execution. Initial studies which claimed that iliotibial band syndrome was caused by a tight iliotibial band have been contradicted, and studies now seem to lend support to the idea that other factors are to blame for iliotibial band syndrome (Devan et al., 2004; Hamill et al., 2008), which supports the MTY theory that flexibility is a secondary or even tertiary benefit of yoga, behind stability. Designing a multifaceted program should include consideration of:

- Healing and prevention of re-injury, which depends on including meditation, yoga postures, postural awareness and proprioception, and variable movement speeds (depending on specificity of training)
- BPS application
- Massage or manual therapy techniques (Pedowitz, 2006) such as lower quarter Marma massage points,

trigger point therapy, strain/counterstrain, myofascial release, or neural mobilization combined with breathwork

- Education and identification of faulty movement patterns
- Closed kinetic chain postures, that is, sequencing/flow to target hip abduction/external rotation/extension strength (Prins and Van der Wurff, 2009), reduction of repetitive stress contributors with yoga program design, and use of restoratives for the acute phase.

Contraindications Running on uneven/sloped terrain, increased compression along the origin or insertion point of the iliotibial band, especially during the acute phase; overworking GMAX in yoga postures such as mountain, standing postures, and spinal extension postures.

Case study

Initial evaluation: A 25-year-old female runner runs 20–30 miles weekly; she does yoga for flexibility but complains of pain in the left knee (medial and lateral) which began 4 weeks ago. Pain in the kneecap now prevents maintaining fitness routine of running.

Past medical history: None that is remarkable or that affects healing prognosis or plan of care (POC).

Subjective report: Reports pain with running that increases during the first mile and forces cessation of running by the second mile. Feeling of stiffness and pain that migrates toward left low back, sacrum, hip, then knee. Type A (*pitta*) individual; eats organic and non-GMO diet; mostly vegetarian. Concerned about not being able to control stress or weight effectively if she is not running daily.

Objective measures: Point tender over distal insertion point of ITB; lateral tracking and overall loss of patellar mobility – little to no freedom in patellar mobility bilaterally; structural leg length discrepancy, right hypomobile SIJ; positive Ober, hip rotators 4-/5 with poor eccentric control bilaterally; manual muscle test (MMT) 4-/5; poor TATD breath.

Impression: Left ITBS and PF syndrome of insidious onset due to hip dysplasia and poor training regimen limiting fitness routine completion.

Acute care

Activity modification, rest/ice/compression/elevation (RICE), homeopathic anti-inflammatories, anti-inflammatory nutrition education, and strength training and manual therapy for ITB to facilitate proper tracking of the patella in the femoral groove. Tracking can be addressed through hamstring and quadriceps strength ratio balance and through tissue extensibility, joint mobility, and hip stability measures. Hip abduction, external rotation, and extension strength is of particular importance (Prins and Van der Wurff, 2009). Breathwork included: abdominodiphragmatic (A-D), TATD, three-part breath (*dirga*), and overcoming/victorious (*ujyaii*), which were also for pain and stress management, neuroendocrine regulation, and relaxation response.

Acute program

1. Moon salutation (progressing through the functional movement assessment), which includes transversus abdominis-assisted thoracodiaphragmatic (TATD) breath, arm spiral, downward-facing dog preparation (DDP), and downward-facing dog (DFD)

2. Gluteal/hamstring dissociation neuromuscular re-reduction (bridge, anterior/posterior (A/P) articulation)

3. Triangle (*trkonasana*)

4. Warrior series (*virabhadrasana I, II, and III*) – quadriceps/hamstring strength ratio balance, agonist/antagonist co-contraction; patellar tracking

5. Regional interdependence model work to address scapulohumeral rhythm, and thoracic and rib control and mobility in postures

6. Corpse (*savasana*).

Subacute care

Continue to facilitate proper patellar tracking through above postures and include specific cuing for hip abduction/GMAX training to reduce incidence and severity of ITBS (Fredericson and Wolf, 2005; Lininger and Miller, 2009), address tissue extensibility of TFL and GMAX (Messier et al., 1995; Paluska, 2005) and gait training and specificity of sport neuromuscular patterning (Frederickson and Wolf, 2005). Subacute treatment varies, and has in the past encouraged lengthening of the iliotibial tissue. However, conflicting evidence should prompt the therapist to come to his/her individual conclusions based on a full BPS assessment. Biomechanical analysis of yoga postures, as well as sport and activity analysis should be completed in order to identify risk factors for development, exacerbation, or prevention of ITBS.

Subacute program

1. Mountain to chair to squat – Mirror and visual input, tactile input, and manual resistance for biofeedback and hip abductor, extensor, and rotator strength

2. Standing/upright hand-to-big toe variations (*utthita padangusthasana*)

3. Reclined hand-to-big toe (*supta padangusthasana*), variations

4. Cultivate proprioceptive awareness and neuromuscular coordination during postures and gait (Fredericson and Wolf, 2005).

Advanced subacute progression

1. Revolved triangle (*parivrtta trkonasana*)

2. Pigeon, modified (*eka pada rajakapotasana*) – Modified with bent and straight back knee, flexed and extended heel

3. Half upward-facing bow (*ardha urdhva dhanurasana*)

4. Reduction in mileage by replacing running with high-level (aerobic, strength, endurance via FITT principle) yoga practice.

Post-test results (6 months)

- TATD breath within normal limits (WNL)

- No remaining point tenderness over distal insertion point of ITB

- Negative Ober

- TFL within functional limits (WFL)

- Hip internal/external rotation MMT 5/5, pain-free

- Patellar mobility still an issue; running was resumed; however, on 2-year follow-up the patient had finally decided to discontinue running and patellar mobility returned to WFL

- Differential diagnosis revealed hip dysplasia, presenting via excessive femoral anteversion, which is likely the chief underlying driver for the lack of normal patellar mobility and associated back and lower quarter pain

- Other concerns would be to replace running with an equivalent higher-level yoga conditioning program based on her dysplasia, regain remaining available patellar mobility and tissue extensibility as structural abnormalities allow, and address any further psychological issues surrounding her addictive tendencies (not wanting to give up running despite pain and loss of quality of life).

Rotator cuff tear and impingement (Fig. 11.5)

The third most common musculoskeletal complaint seen in orthopaedic or primary care sports medicine clinics, after back and knee pain, is shoulder pain (Croft, 1993; Glockner, 1995; Hudson, 2010). Approximately 36% of documented resistance training-related injuries and disorders occur at the shoulder complex (Kolber et al., 2010). With a peak incidence between ages 40 and 60, if left untreated, shoulder pain could result in: rotator cuff (RTC) tendonitis, tendinosis, or bursitis, impingement syndrome, sprain, strain or related structures, acromioclavicular joint separation, anterior or posterior instability or capsular laxity, superior labral anterior–posterior (SLAP) lesions, neck or upper back pain, or headaches. Acute or chronic shoulder pain may cause a feeling of internal "popping", sometimes audible, a feeling of instability, general pain (day and/or night), swelling or hemarthrosis (bleeding in the joint), limited range of motion, loss of strength, and an inability to complete activities of daily living (ADL).

Contributing factors to shoulder pain include age (greater than 40), repetitive activities and work that requires repetitive arm use, poor posture, and weak shoulder musculature. Shoulder pain falls into three categories (Krogsgaard et al., 2009):

1. Repetitive stress syndrome

2. Poor ergonomic set-up

3. Poor technique in sport, including yoga, execution.

The shoulder joint is made up of four joints: the glenohumeral, acromioclavicular, sternoclavicular, and scapulothoracic joints. Kinematic function of the shoulder depends on force couple action when the joints move in tandem. Dyskinesis occurs when there is an alteration in the normal motion of the scapula during scapulohumeral rhythm movements (Kibler and McMullen, 2003; Kibler et al., 2013) as a result of the inhibition or lack of activation patterns in scapular stabilizing muscles. Dynamic stabilization of the humerus during elevation depends on the load that the arm is lifting, since the proposed scapular:humeral ratio during shoulder elevation (2:1) widely varies during electromyographic (EMG) analysis of passive, load, and maximal loading of the glenohumeral joint (from 7.9:1 to 2.1:1 during passive elevation, 3.1:1 to 4.3:1 during active elevation, and 1.9:1 to 4.1:1 during heavy loading elevation) (McQuade and Smidt, 1998). Stability of the glenohumeral joint and the ability to elevate the arm above the head depends on the dynamic stabilization of the humerus by the scapular muscles. The scapula is responsible for orienting the glenoid for optimal load transfer through the four joints of the shoulder complex.

Anatomy and physiology

The muscles that connect the scapula to the chest wall and the humerus are known as periscapular stabilizers. They include the posterior deltoid, the upper,

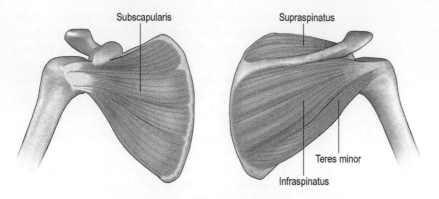

Subscapularis

Supraspinatus

Teres minor

Infraspinatus

Figure 11.5

Rotator cuff (RTC) anatomy and stages of RTC tears

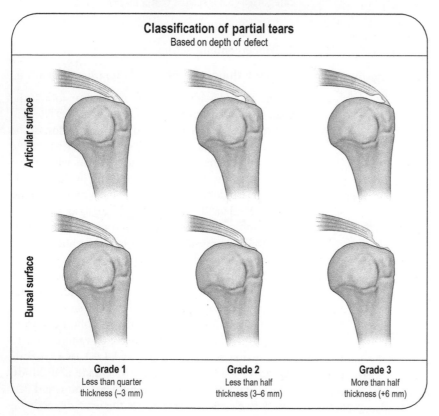

Classification of partial tears
Based on depth of defect

Articular surface

Bursal surface

Grade 1	Grade 2	Grade 3
Less than quarter thickness (–3 mm)	Less than half thickness (3–6 mm)	More than half thickness (+6 mm)

middle, and lower trapezii, rhomboids major and minor, levator scapula, serratus anterior, and the four muscles of the RTC. A total of 17 muscles attach or originate from the scapula (Terry and Chopp, 2000).

The supraspinatus acts as a stabilizer of the glenohumeral joint and provides a superior pull of the humeral head. The infraspinatus, subscapularis, and teres minor also act to stabilize the humeral head by providing lateral rotation via depression, thus acting as a dynamic fulcrum during abduction. Combined with the action of the deltoid in abducting the arm, the RTC provides a force couple and allows for perfect spinning of the humeral head in the glenoid fossa with minimal shear.

Compensatory patterns are common in RTC syndromes due to the lack of strength in the RTC and scapular stabilizers. With RTC deficits, a person will, in order to lift the arm above the head, utilize the upper trapezius muscle and shrug the shoulder. This repeated improper mechanical pattern can lead to compression of the RTC in the coracoacromial arch and impaction of the humeral head into the acromion due to lack of depression and lateral rotation from the force couple of the RTC muscles, the deltoid, and the scapular stabilizers. If left untreated it can manifest as cervical pain and dysfunction.

To prevent shoulder injury, follow the FMA (Chapter 5) to assess the spine, the arm and scapula in resting, moving, and functional positions. It is also important to evaluate posture, as increased thoracic kyphosis or vertebral segmental or myofascial mobility can reduce coracoacromial space by placing the scapula in a downward-anterior (sloping) position, which increases impingement risk. Cervical shearing moments due to abnormal postural alignment can also increase posterior compression and risk of nerve root impingement, which can also lead to referred shoulder pain.

Protrusion of more than one-third of the humeral head anterior to the acromion can place tensile stress on the anterior shoulder capsule and RTC and compressive stress on the posterior capsule and RTC. Short or restricted pectoralis group (major and minor) or associated (anterior or posterior) fascia can also reduce maneuverability of the RTC and decrease functional shoulder range of motion. Any winging (internal rotation) or tipping (flexion) of the scapula can also reveal a lack of neuromuscular patterning or motor control of the periscapular muscles. The scapular assistance test (SAT) and scapular repositioning test (SRT) can be used to optimize movement patterns and assess shoulder complex impairments (please refer to Chapter 5, p. 122, and Codes 5.5 and 5.6 for the SRT and SAT tests and instructions, respectively). Kinesiotape can be used to facilitate scapulohumeral rhythm and diminish scapular dyskinesis in the absence of therapeutic manual feedback. Finally, an assessment of the related joints, including the elbow, the torso and ribcage, can also reveal impairments that contribute to shoulder pain. Injury prevention and management should facilitate:

1. Optimal kinematics — This includes form closure (ideal alignment of the humeral head in the glenoid fossa and scapula on the chest wall) and force closure (motor control of the shoulder and periscapular musculature) to maximize coracoacromial arch space for passage of the RTC.

2. Efficient motor patterns — This includes neuromuscular patterning (timing and coordination of musculature) of the RTC, periscapular muscles, and global upper extremity musculature. Of the four RTC muscles, the supraspinatus is most often involved in RTC injuries.

3. Ability to adapt to imposed stresses — This includes consideration of physiological or psychoemotional response to imposed stress. Can the person maintain focus and a psychobiological "center"?

4. Tissue extensibility and sensorimotor integration — Deeper attention is given to neurovascular and/or myofascial trigger points (Lucas, 2007), resilience and response that most frequently includes the posterior capsule and RTC, and pectoralis major and minor and related fascia. Treating trigger points increases the pressure-pain threshold, decreases associated taut bands and can improve scapulohumeral rhythm.

Additional considerations for program prescription include proprioceptive activities *combined with* decision-making, closed kinetic chain postures such as inversions and flowing sequences, giving attention to transitions between yoga postures (which is often where injuries occur), and regional interdependence variables, such as attending to the cervical spine, core work, and related synergists (Isabel de-la-Llave-Rincón et al., 2011), thoracic mobility (Sueki et al., 2011), and elbow and wrist function (Lucado et al., 2010). In the acute phase of rehabilitation, avoid postures that include, but are not limited to, open kinetic chain arm positions (such as in warrior I, II, or III), cow arms, eagle arms, and inversions such as downward-facing dog, dolphin dive, headstand, and shoulderstand.

Early intervention is critical since chronic inflammation of the RTC tendons via microtrauma can lead to tendon degeneration at their humeral attachment

Case study

Initial examination: A 32-year-old female athlete and new mother presented with left shoulder pain and no previous medical history of shoulder injury or pain. She complained of night pain and an inability to lift her arm overhead without pain. Previous activity included prenatal yoga and walking. The mechanism of injury was nap nursing (breastfeeding). She awoke with her left arm in approximately 90 degrees of internal rotation and flexion with horizontal adduction. She knew this was an abnormal position for her arm, so she tried to carefully move it out of the position but experienced a tearing sensation (an audible pop) in her anterior arm, followed by immediate pain.

Objective measures: "+" Impingement (Hawkins-Kennedy, Neer tests), "+" full can; manual muscle test (MMT) 2+ to 3+/5 and painful, ROM not tested secondary to pain; mild scapular dyskinesis; global upper extremity weakness, superficial, deep front line, and arm line restriction.

Assessment/diagnosis: Stage III impingement with potential RTC tear/ impingement of left shoulder secondary to acute injury as a result of natural deconditioning occurring during pregnancy (postpartum × 2 weeks) limiting ADL completion. Postpartum routine was stroller walking and some yoga based on prenatal participation; required ADL include caregiving for her infant son, household management, and working part-time at a desk job.

Rotator cuff case study programs

Acute program

- A-D breath

- Spinal neutral (anterior/posterior (A/P), lateral)

- Transversus abdominis-assisted thoracodiaphragmatic (TATD) breath

- Shoulder lock for dynamic neuromuscular re-education

- Seated meditation for stress, neuroendocrine regulation, pain management, and centering

- Restorative postures for tissue extensibility (fascial, neural, and muscular) of the pectoralis and chest areas, fatigue, and stress management

- Additional restorative postures combined with manual therapy (joint mobilizations grade I–II for pain relief and gentle capsular mobility) to continue to address tissue extensibility, as above

- Arm floats moving from active assistive range of motion (AAROM) to active range of motion (AROM) with bamboo cane in a pain-free range while practicing spinal neutral, TATD breath, and activating periscapular and lumbopelvic stabilizers. Emphasis on TATD, serratus anterior and lower trapezius engagement and dampening of a dominant external abdominal oblique strategy. Started with 45–60 degrees flexion and progressed to 180 degrees flexion by end of 6 weeks

- Child's pose to upstretched mountain (AAROM) for subtle body (restorative, biofeedback, proprioception, neuromuscular re-education, and myofascial mobility) and gross body (lower trapezius work, upper trapezius downtraining, postural alignment, positioning for manual therapy as needed for scapular, supscapularis, and posterior capsule work)

- Child's pose progression *"reach, roll, and rise"*

- Upstretched mountain (AAROM – right hand assisted left)

- Standing postures without open kinetic chain arm movement or with AAROM.

Subacute program

- Moon salutation for closed kinetic chain activation of the rotator cuff from the functional movement assessment with continued focus on TATD breath, joint mechanoreceptors for rotator cuff and scapular dyskinesis (serratus anterior, upper trapezius and lower trapezius force couple), and lumbopelvic postural alignment via spinal neutral and TATD breath

- Arm spiral in closed kinetic chain for myofascial and neural (median nerve) integrity
- Shoulder opener in supine with yoga strap
- Upward-facing bow
- Scales
- Cow arms
- Fish pose over bolster
- Seated twist (for inferior joint mobilization glide)
- Downward-facing dog (strap-assisted and sometimes Theraband-assisted from forearms for glenohumeral external rotator strength)
- Strap-assisted plank
- Dolphin dive.

Advanced subacute progression

- Non-weight-bearing (NWB) inversion prep and inversions
- Strap-assisted dolphin as headstand and forearm balance preparation
- Wall-assisted NWB headstand.

Program impact

Pre-test

- Active range of motion (AROM) – abduction to 45 degrees without pain
- Pain analog scale (PAS) 7/10 with attempted activity
- Special tests:
  - Positive Hawkins–Kennedy impingement
  - Positive empty can
  - Manual muscle test (MMT) 2+/5 (flexion, abduction, external and internal rotation).

Post-test (16 weeks)

- Post-test active range of motion (AROM) – full, pain-free abduction
- Pain analog scale (PAS) – 0/10 with full activity
- Special tests – negative, pain-free
- Manual muscle test (MMT) – 5/5, pain-free
- Able to return to full ADL and activity without pain.

sites. Common pain patterns include radiating and diffuse pain to the deltoid tubercle due to the RTC's shared dermatomal innervation of the brachial plexus in C6–C8, as well as neck pain, headaches, upper back or trapezius pain.

Safe inversion progression prerequisites

These progressions include gender-sensitive sequences for headstand as well as a general sequence for headstand and an SRA (static restorative approximation) and dynamic-based postural sequence for shoulderstand. Shoulderstand follows headstand practice because it is traditionally considered "cooling" and comes at the end of a sequence after the heating practice of headstand. However, therapeutic intent may alter their order.

Gender-sensitive headstand preparation

This section provides brief sequence suggestions for gender-sensitive teaching and prescription. It also includes non-gender-based sequences for inversion preparation, and a preparatory sequence for both nonaxial loading headstands and shoulderstands.

Men

- Hip joint ROM
- Spinal extension — Locust (*salabasana*), upward-facing bow (*urdhva dhanurasana*)
- Twists + forward bends — Forward standing bend with twist (*uttanasana* with a twist), forward seated bend (*paschimottanasana*)

- Standing twists — Revolved triangle (*parivritta trkonasana*), triangle (*trkonasana*), tree (*vrkasana*)

- Seated twists — Half lord of the fishes (*ardha matsyendrasana*)

- Lumbopelvic strengthening — Boat (*navasana*), dolphin dive, half upward-facing bow and variations (*ardha urdhva dhanurasana*).

Women

- Upper quarter power (strength + endurance) — Caterpillar, dolphin dive (*astang pranam*), plank, side plank, downward-facing dog preparation, downward-facing dog (*adho mukha svanasana*)

- Inverted center of gravity balancing: dolphin preparation series, headstand at a wall, headstand with a chair and/or multiple spotters giving manual and verbal cuing

- Lumbopelvic strengthening: boat (*navasana*), dolphin dive (*astang pranam*), half upward-facing bow and variations (*ardha urdhva dhanurasana*)

- Pelvic floor strengthening (uptraining) or relaxation (downtraining) as well as giving consideration to neural mobilization, myofascial release, and other soft tissue or joint mobilization techniques. Women are at increased risk for incontinence, pelvic floor weakening, organ prolapse, pelvic pain, and conditions such as vaginismus, dyspareunia (painful intercourse), and vulvar vestibulitis (dysesthesia in the vulvar vestibule), or vulvodynia (pain in the vulvar area). Additional conditions such as age and gravity exerted forces, pregnancy, weight gain, birth (vaginal or cesarean section), menopause, hysterectomy, hormonal problems, poor hygiene, friction from recreational activities, sexual trauma or violence, abdominal surgery, or other psychophysiological issues can also negatively affect pelvic floor integrity and strength. Consideration must be given to menses and the psychophysiological, biochemical, and musculoskeletal effects it renders. Increased joint laxity, similar to that experienced during pregnancy, is common during menses. This alone warrants different prescription of yoga. In the week before and during menses consider avoiding the following:

- Full or extreme ranges of motion

- Full exertion or exhaustion

- Inversions.

Encourage:

- Downward flow of energy (*apana vayu*)

- Twists, squats, and other postures that encourage downward flow

- Restorative postures, breathing, and meditation for those with premenstrual syndrome (PMS) or premenstrual dysphoric disorder (PMDD).

Nonspecific gender preparations that should precede inversion practice can include:

- Lumbopelvic conditioning + healthy hip ROM (first screen femoral version): crane (*bakasana*), side crane (*parsva bakasana*), and legs-bound-by-shoulders (*bhujapidasana*)

- Lumbopelvic conditioning + back line fascia/neural/muscle extensibility — Staff (*dandasana*), forward seated bend (*paschimottanasana*) with "scales" lift off (modified *tolasana*), wide-angle forward seated bend (*upavista konasana*)

- Lumbopelvic conditioning + shoulder stabilization — Arm spiral in closed kinetic chain, downward-facing dog, followed by dolphin series

- Spinal pliability + fascial resilience — Prone, seated, and supine controlled twists (controlled flexibility) utilizing lumbopelvic stabilizers (TATD breath).

Nonaxial loading headstand preparation

1. Four-point

2. Four-point mini four-limbed staff dive

3. Downward-facing dog preparation in spinal neutral

4. Forearm downward-facing dog without strap

5. Forearm downward-facing dog with strap two finger-widths distal to elbow joint and over lateral extensor muscle mass, approximately

6. Three-legged downward-facing dog independent and with a partner to assist with alignment of the lower quarter and isolation of hip stabilizers

7. Full dolphin dive × 5, then rest in child's pose*

8. Child's pose triceps brachii extensibility

9. Headstand preparation from downward-facing dog (draw knee to chest)

10. Sofa or wall headstand

11. Corner headstand.

*Inability to perform a full, safe dolphin dive precludes student from progressing further. Dolphin dive must be mastered in order to safely perform a non-weight-bearing headstand.

Non-axial loading shoulderstand preparation

Static restorative approximation (SRA) series

1. Pre-plow* — Legs-up-the-wall (*viparita karani*) sequence

2. Supine over accordion-fold

3. Threading-the-needle (*parsva balasana*)

4. Bridge (*setu bandha*)

5. Two-foot posture (*dvipada pitham*)

6. Supported half upward-facing bow (*salamba ardha urdhva dhanurasana*)

7. Half upward-facing bow (*ardha urdhva dhanurasana*) — Practice finding pelvic neutral and lifting one or both legs from the floor using TATD breath to support the pose.

*Plow pose is rarely therapeutically indicated in any population and can be replaced by this series. Blankets will likely be needed under the shoulders to maintain a cervical lordosis and prevent lordotic reversal or other adverse neural tension. Chair-assisted shoulderstand (*sarvangasana*) can be utilized but is also an advanced pose contraindicated for most populations.

Review

Introducing partnership between yoga postures is known as sequencing, or a *vinyasa krama*, connecting postures together in a logical order for specific therapeutic benefit. The FMA in Chapter 5 is an example of an extended therapeutic sequence, an algorithm intended to streamline clinical decision-making and operationalize the use of yoga as both a simultaneous diagnostic and management tool. The sequences and case studies in this chapter, through consideration of the evidence base in rehabilitative sciences, effectively operationalize the FMA, including other postures and breathwork from this text. Keep in mind that the acute, subacute, and chronic progressions target postures and breath, and that the psychobiological substrates of BPS management happen in real time practice through customization of delivery method and instructional design, patient–provider relationship, therapeutic landscape, and language, all important facets of the common factors model (Miciak et al., 2012), which demonstrates that general effects overlap between psychotherapy and rehabilitation. The "king and queen" postures of yoga, the headstand and shoulderstand, respectively, are what most practitioners consider "5–10 year poses," which means 5–10 years of practice are usually necessary before a student is ready to conceptualize, respect, and safely perform them. It is from this perspective that prerequisite sequences are introduced for inversions, in order to ready the practitioner for eventual inclusion of some version of the "king and queen" postures.

This chapter provides practical tools for shifting the paradigm of dialogue in healthcare toward the inclusion of yoga in mainstream rehabilitation. Reducing barriers to the receipt of yoga in healthcare is critical to repair fractured healthcare systems that pit biomedical care against biopsychosocial (BPS) care. Guidelines for teaching and monitoring patients during yoga are presented, including considerations for differential diagnosis that identify red flags that may warrant outside referral. Options for outcome measures used in standardized assessment, especially as they affect patient adherence and empowerment, health promotion, and research, are presented. Finally, business practices and liability concerns are addressed in the context of healthcare practice.

How fractured healthcare affects you

The future of nations depends on the health of their individual citizens. The World Health Organization (WHO) reports epidemic proportions of chronic pain and chronic disease internationally (WHO, 2005), and provides clear evidence that our current approach to healthcare, disease prevention, and health promotion is flawed.

A successful intervention model requires four components:

1. An active patient theme that promotes self-care
2. Social support that provides help in meeting illness-related demands
3. Patient education to increase concern about disease consequences
4. Patient instruction.

In the biomedical model, the "patient" has historically been considered a passive recipient of "doctor's orders," and expected to adhere to a prescribed plan of care (Leventhal and Cameron, 1987; Horne and Weinman, 1998; WHO, 2003). Passive medicine disempowers the individual and can foster learned helplessness and even addictive behavior. A successful intervention model requires four components:

1. An active patient theme that promotes self-care
2. Social support that provides help in meeting illness-related demands
3. Patient education to increase concern about disease consequences
4. Patient instruction.

The first two of these are considered the most important (Garrity and Garrity, 1985; WHO, 2003). In developed countries, where adherence to long-term therapy averages only 50% (WHO, 2003), delivery of healthcare using a yogic model could improve adherence. As chronic disease is expected to exceed 65% of the global illness burden by 2020, action proposed in this text could impact health economics and quality of life through advocating for (1) coverage of yoga as medicine and (2) inclusion of yoga in medical education.

Chapter 12

An additional impetus for this text is consumer safety. If this text can improve adherence to long-term therapies for chronic disease, as well as disease prevention, then it provides an economically feasible methodology for improving patient safety, deemed vital by the World Health Organization (2003).

Addressing barriers to receipt of yoga in healthcare

A broken healthcare system can also shift blame to the patient. The WHO four-part intervention method outlined above supports the patient (WHO, 2003). Lack of individualized strategies, absence of multidisciplinary or interdisciplinary team approach, and training in cultural sensitivity and patient adherence are all modifiable barriers to successful outcomes (WHO, 2003).

Focusing on patient-centered care through a yogic lens can address the largest risk factors for chronic disease development through teaching stress management, facilitating healthy nutritional choices, and fostering commitment to an active lifestyle. The economic benefits are clearly embedded in improved adherence as well, with resulting reduced use of expensive health services needed for "disease exacerbation, crisis, or relapse" (WHO, 2003). Reduction in hospitalization, hospital stay, and outpatient visits are well documented when self-management programs are offered to patients with chronic disease (Holman et al., 1997; Ciechanowski et al., 2000; Massanari, 2000; Put et al., 2000; Rohland et al., 2000; Tuldra et al., 2000; Valenti, 2001; WHO, 2003). That makes yoga, when used through the scientific lens of healthcare, an ideal method for teaching self-management and lowering healthcare costs for the patient and the system.

Timing in medical intervention in yoga

The timing of an intervention also plays a critical role in overall patient outcomes. The difference between acute versus chronic treatment in medicine can mean the difference between life and death (Maiese, 2010).

The acute phase of injury or disease is defined in terms of a short-term time parameter. In an acute process symptoms can develop, change, or worsen rapidly (NIH, 2013), with the acute time frame varying from 1 to 2 days for dermatological issues, 1 week for cardiovascular issues, or up to 3 months for orthopaedic conditions.

Chronic pain is less succinctly defined and has several parameters for definition, making it more of an enigma. Chronic pain can be a period of time in which pain persists that is equal to or greater than 3–6 months (Turk and Okifuji, 2001; Debono et al., 2013). Other definitions shun the use of time as a defining parameter for chronic conditions and instead use the presence of low inflammation levels and persistent stress as a means for determining the presence of "chronic" high risk factors or disease processes (McEwen and Stellar, 1993; McEwen et al., 2012; McVicar et al., 2014). Despite the controversy of defining acute versus chronic parameters, there are some general guidelines to follow when prescribing intervention in each stage.

Acute phase intervention generally considers the following (Table 12.1):

1. Pain management — Reduction of patient distress is the chief intention of any first visit. Increasing comfort level and decreasing pain can allow for focus on long-range management instead of using passive administration of pain medication as a short-term means to an end.

2. Adequate rest and sleep hygiene — Sleep disorders are associated with neuroendocrine dysregulation, hypertension, depression, and obesity but can also contribute to adverse pregnancy outcomes such as preeclampsia, elevated serum glucose, depression, prolonged labor, and caesarean birth (Nodine and Matthews, 2013). Inadequate sleep in adolescence is related to shortened and disrupted sleep patterns, insomnia, daytime sleepiness, high-risk behaviors, psychosocial health, and overall somatic and physical health and functioning (Shochat et al., 2014). Sleep issues also affect healthcare providers, with sleep deprivation associated with anxiety, depression, and increased risk of medical errors (Mustahsan et al., 2013). The average

314

Table 12.1
Timing in intervention

Acute	Chronic
• Pain management	• Yoga for biopsychosocial benefit(s)
• Adequate rest and sleep hygiene	• Continued patient education to improve health literacy, self-efficacy, self-advocacy, motivation, and coping skills
• Patient education and interviewing to improve health literacy and self-efficacy	
• Patient counseling on anti-inflammatory-based nutritional changes	• Advocacy or referral for managing long-term lifestyle change
• Yoga breathwork, postures, and meditation in restoratives for immediate pain and stress management	• Provision of support via community resources
• Manual therapies	• Primary emphasis on active therapies for patient empowerment
• Meditation	
• Prescription of holistic or pharmaceutical medications as necessary	

adult gets approximately 6.9 hours of sleep per night (about 90 minutes less than 100 years ago); however, 7–9 hours of sleep per night is recommended (Ramar and Olson, 2013; Schochat et al., 2013).

3. Patient education and interviewing to discern change readiness and associate lifestyle choices with current health status.

4. Patient counseling on anti-inflammatory-based nutritional changes to affect C-reactive protein (CRP) levels and lower all-health outcome risks for chronic non-communicable diseases including cardiovascular disease (Pearson et al., 2003), metabolic syndrome, obesity, osteoarthritis, and cancer (Liu et al., 2013; Mahalle et al., 2013). Nutritional impairment, and its correlation

with systemic inflammation, is also associated with poor performance status, shorter survival, and increased mortality in patients with cancer (Pinato et al., 2012). A diet high in polyunsaturated fats plays a role in modulating pro-inflammatory cytokines (Liu et al., 2013). Low levels of vitamin B12 could be a causative factor in increasing homocysteine (Hcy) levels, which are associated with insulin resistance and inflammatory markers (Mahalle et al., 2013). A diet high in flavonoids, polyphenolic compounds found in fruits and vegetables, is correlated with anti-diabetic effects and reduction of oxidative stress in muscle and fat (Babu et al., 2013). Overall, high plant intake, giving consideration to both fiber and micronutrients with a "recognized antioxidant capacity," positively affects pro-inflammatory activity and has a role in the reduction of risk factors and the incidence of the above-mentioned chronic diseases (Hermsdorff et al., 2010; Yang et al., 2013).

5. Yoga breathwork and postures with an emphasis on meditative restorative postures — Restorative postures in this phase generally include open-packed joint position in a pain-free range of motion (ROM). Introduce one degree of freedom at a time in postures to identify and address biomechanical variables that contribute to functional impairment. Use yoga props (aka "toys") that facilitate postural modification for safety and efficacy during growth and remodeling phases. These include blocks, straps, blankets, fascial tools, or a wall, chair, ball, or aquatic therapy.

6. Manual therapies — These are outlined in the Touch therapy guidelines section in this chapter and should be provided under the appropriate medical scope of practice in osteopathic, physical therapy, chiropractic, orthopaedic, massage therapy, occupational therapy, or related practitioner practice, for example.

7. Meditation — Use of guided progressive relaxation, transcendental meditation, mindfulness-based stress reduction, therapeutic yoga scan, and

Chapter 12

guided imagery can be considered for meditation's systemic impact on health.

> **Code 12.1** (free code)
> Resources on meditation practice
>
>

8. Prescription of holistic or pharmaceutical medications as necessary.

Subacute and chronic phase intervention (see Table 12.1) should progress toward inclusion of the following:

1. Yoga for BPS benefit plus strength, tissue resilience, functional mobility and sport- or activity-specific training, and neuromuscular re-education

2. Continued patient education and work toward improving health literacy, self-efficacy, self-advocacy, motivation, and coping skills

3. Advocacy or referral for managing long-term lifestyle change and acceptance of any remaining disability

4. Provision of support through individual or group/community resources

5. Passive therapies such as manual therapy can be used less as a primary intervention unless there are unresolved manual therapy needs. Primary emphasis is on active therapies in order to shift responsibility of long-term care to, and empower, the patient.

Biopsychosocial outcome measures

Yoga's systemic benefits should be objectively measured and tested to increase its acceptance and use as a valid intervention in medicine. Standardized outcome measures and the provision of study fidelity through standardization of application provided in this text are reliable ways to capture efficacy. There are as many outcome measures as there are yoga postures, given the vast number standardized tests available across multiple rehabilitation professions, and therefore the list in Table 12.2 is not exhaustive, but provides options for BPS measurement using validated

Table 12.2
Biopsychosocial outcome measures

General musculoskeletal	Neuromuscular and vestibular
• Oswestry Disability Index	• Dynamic Gait Index
• Roland–Morris Disability Questionnaire	• Five Times Sit-to-Stand test
• McGill Pain Questionnaire	• Activities-Specific Scale
• Lower Extremity Functional Scale	• Dizziness Handicap Inventory
• Pelvic Girdle Pain Questionnaire	• Balance Error Scoring System
• Pelvic Floor Distress Inventory-20	• Sensory Organization Test
• Pelvic Floor Impact-7 Questionnaire	• Berg Balance Scale
	• The ImPact Tool
Neuroendocrine and cardiorespiratory	**Psychoemotional and all-health**
• Heart rate variability	• Fear-Avoidance Beliefs Questionnaire
• Resonant frequency analysis	• Pain Catastrophizing Scale
Sensory Profile	• SF-36
• Sensory Profile™ test	• Sleep quality (VAS)
	• Social Occupational Functioning Scale
	• World Health Organization Quality of Life Abbreviated Form

outcome measures in order to facilitate the creation of clinical guidelines for the use of yoga in healthcare.

General musculoskeletal measures

• The Oswestry Disability Index (ODI) is a validated (Fairbank and Pynsent, 2000) 10-question tool that quantifies low back pain disability by relating pain to activity.

- The Roland–Morris Disability Questionnaire (RMD) is a validated (Bombardier, 2000) 24-question tool that measures activities affected by back pain.

- The McGill Pain Questionnaire (MGP) is "designed to measure the qualities of both neuropathic and non-neuropathic pain in research and clinical settings" (Melzack and Katz, 2013, p. 3).

- The Lower Extremity Functional Scale (LEFS) is a validated 20-item test applicable for a broad population of patients with lower extremity problems (Binkley et al., 1999).

- The Pelvic Girdle Pain Questionnaire (PGP) is a reliable and valid 20-item test for use in women with pelvic girdle pain (Grotle et al., 2012).

- The Pelvic Floor Distress Inventory-20 (PFD) and the Pelvic Floor Impact-7 Questionnaire (PFI) are both valid and reliable forms used together to assess women with pelvic floor disorders (Barber et al., 2005).

Neuromuscular and vestibular measures

- The Dynamic Gait Index (DGI) uses eight items to assess gait stability during head motions with speed changes with and without obstacles (Alsalaheen et al., 2010; Lei-Rivera et al., 2013).

- The Five Times Sit-to-Stand (FTSTS) test is a valid outcome measure for gait and postural stability (Alsalaheen et al., 2010).

- The Activities-Specific Balance Confidence (ABC) Scale confidently measures a person's ability to complete functional tasks without loss of balance (Alsalaheen et al., 2010).

- The Dizziness Handicap Inventory (DHI) includes 25 items that quantitatively assess dizziness on physical, emotional, and functional health (Alsalaheen et al., 2010).

- Balance assessment outcome measures include the Balance Error Scoring System (BESS), the Sensory Organization Test (SOT) (Aligene and Lin, 2013; Lei-Rivera et al., 2013), and/or the Berg Balance Scale (BBS).

- The ImPact Tool (Post-Concussion Impact Assessment and Cognitive Testing) identifies cognitive versus neurophysiological functioning, and is suggested as a screening tool measuring subtle functional changes (Aligene and Lin, 2013).

Note: Differential diagnosis for cervicogenic-induced vertigo should also be completed, via ruling out impairment of neck mobility and presence or absence of neck pain (Aligene and Lin, 2013). The Canalith Repositioning (Hall-Pike) Maneuver (Alsalaheen et al., 2010; Aligene and Lin 2013) is a first-line test to rule out benign paroxysmal positional vertigo (BPPV).

Neuroendocrine and cardiorespiratory measures

Heart rate variability (HRV) – the difference in intervals between heartbeats (McCraty and Shaffer, 2015) – is considered a gold standard for predicting all health outcomes in both healthy and affected populations. HRV is reflective of systematic autonomic status, and low variability of resonant frequency is associated with many adverse health outcomes, including increased CRP (systemic inflammation), depressed immune function, and cardiovascular disease, including decreased longevity (Kemp and Quintana, 2013); diabetes, cardiovascular disease, fibromyalgia, and chronic pain (Staud, 2008; Meeus et al., 2013); depression, anxiety, and female sexual dysfunction (Stanton et al., 2015), bipolar disorder (Levy, 2014), and post-traumatic stress disorder (Sammito et al., 2015). It is also associated with predicting the development and prognosis of some disease processes (Mazzeo et al., 2011; Chandra et al., 2012; Melillo et al., 2012; Xhyheri et al., 2012; Wang et al., 2013). Increasing respiratory sinus arrhythmia (RSA) amplitude through biofeedback is the most accurate way to individualize improving HRV (Lehrer et al., 2000; Vaschillo et al., 2006), since the breaths per minute (BPM) at which HRV is maximized can vary from 4 to 7 BPM (Lehrer et al., 2000). Paced breathing practice without biofeedback can still be effective, however, as evidenced by the excellent HRV of experienced yogic breathers. The speed, or BPM, where the RSA is highest, is known as "resonant frequency" (Lehrer et al., 2000), and is the target of resonant frequency analysis in measuring HRV.

An application available for patient education and outcome measurement is Breathpacer (available on Android and iPhone); HRV Software – HeartMath (Power Spectrum portion).

Note: Vital signs, including blood pressure, respiratory rate, and pulse, are influenced by baroreflex sensitivity, and can be accurately represented and influenced through HRV measurement and intervention. Pulmonary function testing, salivary diurnal cortisol levels as a measure of hypothalamic–pituitary–adrenal (HPA) axis regulation and allostatic load, CRP levels as a measure of systemic inflammation, and blood lipids can also be considered for use.

Psychoemotional and all-health measures

- Fear-Avoidance Beliefs Questionnaire (FABQ) — This provides a measure of a patient's fear related to low back pain and how these beliefs may affect physical activity and work.

- Pain Catastrophizing Scale (PCS) — This quantifies the negative belief that experienced pain will ultimately result in the worst possible outcome. Pain catastrophizing is linked to the development of chronic low back pain, low diurnal cortisol variability, HPA axis dysregulation, and a wide range of other conditions, including narcotic dependency, depression, and repeat healthcare provider visits (Quartana et al., 2009).

- SF-36 — The SF-36 is a standardized and well-validated (McHorney et al., 1994) health survey helpful in measuring functional health and well-being from the patient's perspective. (Quality Metric; SF Health Surveys, 2013). The SF-36 is a BPS measure that quantifies health beliefs, patient satisfaction, self-efficacy, pain, disability, functional physical and emotional impairment, and limitations in social or physical activities due to health problems. However, it fails to screen for nutritional habits and sleep hygiene. Those two areas are vital in influencing health, and should be included in future SF-36 validation studies.

- Other measures which could be utilized include reporting of sleep (VAS) quality, or use of the Social Occupational Functioning Scale (SOFS) or World Health Organization Quality of Life Abbreviated Form (WHOQOL-BREF).

Sensory profile measures

The Sensory ProfileTM test, in its various forms, screens for sensory integration patterns in infants, children, adolescents, and adults (Brown and Dunn, 2002; Dunn, 2006, 2009). Dunn's model of sensory processing (Dunn, 1997) recognizes that each person has a neurological threshold and different inherent strategies for self-regulating the way they interact with themselves and the world around them.

Guidelines to practice and intervention

Guidelines overview:
- Breath practice
- Hand posture
- Posture
- Safety
- Touch therapy
- Myofascial release
- Manual positioning
- Neural mobilization
- Teaching
- Sequencing
- Meditation.

Teaching yoga requires yoga practice. According to Yoga Sutras 1.13 and 1.14 (see box opposite), practice must be consistent in order to attain a steady mind. Any posture should be evaluated not only physically, but utilizing the entire BPS model. Beyond monitoring the individual's face, eyes, secondary muscles of respiration, including the sternocleidomastoid, the scalenes, platysma, upper trapezius, muscles of facial expression, and stance, ask the following questions:

> **Yoga Sutra 1.13**
>
> Of these two (practice and nonattachment), effort toward steadiness of mind is practice.
>
> **Yoga Sutra 1.14**
>
> Practice becomes firmly grounded when well attended to for a long time, without break and in all earnestness.

- Is there a maturity and health to the pose that reflects psychoemotional health?

- Does the posture reflect intellectual health, or an attitude of openness for learning what a pose can teach?

- Does the practice inspire spiritual readiness and openness?

- What does the energetic health of the pose look like?

Not all individuals will learn by, or be comfortable with, the same cue. Some of the types of cues that exist in learning style inventories, such as the VARK® Questionnaire, can be extrapolated for the "classroom" of patient–provider interaction/education, including use of:

- Aural or auditory cues

- Kinesthetic or tactile cues, including biomechanical cues for safety, alignment, and efficacy

- Written or verbal cuing or resources, such as guided imagery or metaphorical cuing, and/or

- Visual cues.

Guidelines for breath, posture, safety, touch and myofascial therapy, manual positioning, neural mobilization, teaching, sequencing, and meditation are provided for clinical practice with individuals or groups.

Breath practice (*pranayama*)

The breath is the fourth limb in the eight-limbed practice of Ashtanga yoga. Because yoga posture (*asana*) practice (third limb) depends on the breath, the breath (fourth limb) should precede posture practice. Without the breath, the pose cannot exist. The following guidelines are suggestions for optimizing breath practice:

- Frequency — Adopt a daily breath practice.

- Duration — Novice practitioners may require 5–10 minutes of practice to achieve resonant frequency and relaxation response; however, experienced practitioners may achieve it in as little as 1–2 breaths.

- Time of day — If morning practice (recommended) is adopted, attend to hygiene practices first, such as teeth brushing, tongue scraping, elimination of bowel and bladder. Traditional recommendation was morning practice (Iyengar, 1976), hence the advice to practice on an empty stomach; however, a breath practice should facilitate a relaxation response, focus, or sleep as needed, which means breath practice can be done at any time throughout the day and/or night.

- Position — Find a comfortable position to practice, such as seated against a wall on graded quarter-folded blankets with blocks at the lumbosacral junction and under the legs. Free-sitting (unsupported) may be uncomfortable or physically impossible. If so, consider the yoga couch, sidelying, or supine corpse.

- Pose type — There is no specific pose that should attend a breath practice. Corpse was traditionally recommended; however, a practice should be calibrated to the practitioner in order to meet her/his functional and activities of daily living needs.

- Location — A quiet place to practice, free of distraction, may be optimal for novice practitioners; however, mature practitioners can practice in distracting or challenging environments.

- Progress — Monitor the orofacial area, including mask of the face, width of the airway, root of the tongue, and perceived pressure in the ears and cranium:

  - Begin practice with exhalation (parasympathetic input) and end on inhalation (sympathetic input)

- Breathe through the nose unless otherwise specified. Open-mouth breathing can restrict upper airway flow via reduction of the retropalatal and retroglossal areas (Lee et al., 2007), which can exacerbate sleep apnea and disordered sleeping (Kim et al., 2011) and orofacial dysfunction, as discussed in Chapter 4

- Inhalation can be grossly equal to exhalation unless otherwise specified

- Do not valsalva.

- Visual input — The choice of practice with the eyes open or closed is determined by the position that optimizes relaxation and concentration response. For example, those using Ayurveda to prescribe yoga may find that air/ether (*vata*) and fire/water (*pitta*) types need to meditate with the eyes open, while earth/water (*kapha*) types can practice with the eyes closed.

- Finishing — Always end with corpse or a similarly calibrated posture to allow time for introspection, active rest, and relaxation response.

Hand posture (*mudra*)

If hand postures (*mudras*) are used during practice, consider the following guidelines:

- The fingers should lightly touch without rigidity.

- Practice in a comfortable pose. Performed in any posture, most often hand postures are conjoined with meditation.

- Maintain a steady, slow breath.

- Hold the posture from three breaths to upwards of 45 minutes as needed. It may take a 5-minute practice to initially feel an effect, whereas with practice it may only take three breaths to feel change.

Posture (*asana*)

The third of the eight limbs of Ashtanga yoga, postures can be flowing or held for several breaths and should be introduced after mastering breath control:

- The breath takes priority over the posture. If the breath is lost in a pose, stop and begin again or adapt the pose to accommodate successful breathing.

- Practice of *asana* without ethics, goodwill and discipline (*yama*), and social conduct (*niyama*) is not yoga.

- Frequency — Practice can be daily, but is determined by therapeutic intention.

- Duration — The conditions for each pose, whether holding for a determined number of breaths or flowing from posture to posture, is determined by therapeutic intention.

- Time of day — The ideal time for practice depends on therapeutic intention. A morning practice is safely self-limiting due to joint stiffness and the mind will be most alert and fresh, whereas an evening practice may remove fatigue and stress. However, an evening practice can carry a higher risk for injury if physical limits and fatigue are not identified and respected. If practice occurs around mealtime, the meal should be light.

- Empty bladder and bowel before practice.

- Use of a yoga mat is optional but can improve safety and efficacy by reducing risk of falls or slippage on the floor. For air/ether (*vata*) types who tend to be thinner and have more bony "hotspots" or angles, a yoga mat covered with a yoga rug is helpful.

- Progress — Monitor orofacial and respiratory status (Chapter 4).

- Visual input — Beginners practice with eyes open for biofeedback to carefully observe movements, monitor biomechanical stability and safety, and cultivate proprioceptive awareness. Experienced practitioners with excellent proprioceptive awareness can close the eyes.

- The mind observes, rather than judges, during practice.

- Nostril breathing is used unless otherwise specified.

- Do not valsalva in any pose.

- Finishing — See breathing guidelines.

- Practice during menstrual cycle — Women just prior to or during their menstrual cycle or lochia flow (postpartum) may prefer to exclude inversions due to urogynecological and orthopaedic comfort. Ligamentous or joint laxity can increase during ovulation and/or 1 week prior to menstruation, and also persists during pregnancy and immediate post-partum (which is prolonged in breastfeeding mothers), which could increase risk for injury. Limit ROM excursion in postures during these times.

- Experienced practitioners — Beware of complacency in a pose. The pose should be new with each practice.

- Postpartum — After giving birth, practice may be resumed with the collaboration of the midwife, physician, and/or pelvic practitioner. Breathwork can begin immediately, along with appropriate yogic lock work. Postures can begin as early as 0–7 days (to include breathing and light yoga lock and/or restorative practice). Heavier postural practice can typically resume, with medical provider clearance, approximately 4 weeks after a vaginal delivery, and 6 weeks after a caesarean section.

- Coordinate your plan of care with the treating physician and/or therapist prior to initiation of a yoga program where necessary.

Safety

- Have patients or participants read and sign liability waiver(s), informed consent, and medical intake forms.

- Therapists have a legal liability and authority to limit class size. Never have more students in a class or session than you have adequate props for and can safely monitor.

- If you question someone's ability to follow instruction(s), suggest a private follow-up to determine cognitive status and instructional adherence. It may be necessary to recommend a more appropriate class or a one-on-one appointment.

- Follow the 10 precepts of Medical Therapeutic Yoga (see Table 1.1).

- Work slowly from simple to complex postures. Introduce one degree of freedom or plane of motion at a time in order to safely progress a posture but

also to determine which movement variable is influencing safe kinematics, biomechanics, and load transfer.

- Only introduce postures that can be appropriately monitored in a group setting, and that you have personally experienced and can safely instruct.

- Watch for signs of exhaustion, confusion, or lack of understanding, which may include breath-holding, wincing, or skin changes, etc. Pay attention, and respond to participant needs.

- Only use partner poses if they are the best method for proving a teaching point or concept.

Touch therapy

Therapeutic touch is within the legal scope of practice of many licensed healthcare professionals and includes such techniques as indirect or direct positional release, acupressure, acupuncture, Marma point massage, dry needling, trigger point therapy, muscle energy, myofascial release, visceral mobilizaiton, Thai yoga massage, joint mobilization and manipulation, craniosacral therapy, Feldenkrais, Reiki, polarity, and other soft tissue mobilization. Consult your practice act to determine what is allowed under your legal scope of practice. Consider the following general guidelines prior to giving therapeutic touch:

- Respect personal space and vulnerable regions of the body, especially the chest and pelvis.

- Ask permission from the student to give manual positioning to him/her before touching them or making any adjustment.

- Use the breath as the first therapeutic tool for myofascial release. Observe first, touch second. Secondary to breathing as a manual therapy tool is use of the hands, whether by the patient or practitioner.

- Through observation of the breath and movement, identify:
  - affected short or restricted tissues and assess them (within the breath first, and posture second)
  - the agonist and the antagonists of the affected joint(s) and if they are implicated

- improper movement strategies, such as an inability to isolate a muscle contraction on demand or improper initiation or recruitment of a muscle within a yoga pose.

- Have the individual progress slowly through the posture by breaking down the posture into components. For example, tree pose is broken down into five distinct movement patterns in Chapter 5, in order to isolate and identify movement impairment(s) and improper load transfer that could be related to fascial restriction. Breaking down postures and breath techniques into multiple complex components for myofascial release can greatly increase clinical efficacy.

Myofascial release

- Always attend to orofacial tone and presentation (see breathing guidelines).

- Use skin-on-skin palpation and treatment when possible.

- Provide gradual increase of pressure to the tissues. Imagine the fascia is akin to a large boat in the water. If you went up to this boat and gave it a swift kick, it would not create movement (though it might injure your foot). However, if you approached movement of the boat with a slow and steady prolonged "lean" against the boat's surface, it would eventually respond with movement. Providing myofascial release happens in a similar fashion, whether by direct or indirect approaches.

To progress:

- Determine and refine the level of pressure given by constantly listening and looking for patient response. The terms "micromovement," fascial "unwinding," and "release," have been used to describe the neurobiologic response to therapist touch (Minasny, 2009).

- Monitor skin temperature and any histamine response (which is active in the inflammatory response), as well as vitals (BPM, heart rate, and blood pressure), in response to the pressure or mobilization.

- Hold or apply treatment 2–5 minutes (Chapter 3).

- Ask and allow for deepening of feeling or proprioception during treatment.

- Slower yoga practice reflects an increased sensitivity to assessment of both myofascial health and movement strategy quality, especially when myofascial release is being delivered in a yoga posture.

- Facilitate release, do not manipulate it.

Myofascial release can be actively or passively administered but may be most effective if following guidelines for affecting mechanoreceptors (adapted in part from Schleip, 2003):

- *Type I mechanoreceptors* include tissues with higher density mechanoreceptors, such as myotendinous junctions (i.e. suboccipital area), ligaments of peripheral joints, and attachment areas of aponeuroses, for example areas such as the palmar and plantar fascia and transversalis fascia. Assess for contributions to fascial restriction. These areas respond to muscular contraction and strong stretch via Golgi tendon receptors with "tonus decrease in related striated motor fibers" (Schleip, 2003, p. 1).

- *Type II mechanoreceptors* include Pacini receptors, which are found in myotendinous junctions, deep capsular layers, spinal ligaments, and investing muscular tissues, and respond to rapid pressure changes and vibrations. When stimulated they provide proprioceptive feedback for affecting movement strategies. Ruffini receptors are also type II receptors and, through lateral stretch and sustained pressure, can potentially inhibit sympathetic activity. They are found in the dura mater, dorsal hand fascia, and superficial joint capsules.

- *Type III and IV mechanorecptors* are interstitial and are constitute the majority of receptors, especially in periosteum. They may be most closely connected to autonomic regulation. They respond to rapid and sustained pressure by affecting vasodilation and plasma extravasation. It is thought that the majority of these receptors are unmyelinated (90% of type IV). The receptors' primary role is thought to include not only mechanoreception but also thermoception, nociception, and/or chemoception.

Manual positioning

When making adjustments in a group setting, use the following guidelines:

1. First, ask permission to touch the person.

2. Assure the adjustment is comfortable and pain free.

3. Stay with the student until they have self-corrected and are safe with the adjustment given.

4. Avoid using the fingers to make an adjustment. Use heels of the hands, forearms, elbows, shoulders, foot, or the side of the hip instead.

5. In all standing postures, for example during right warrior I, II, or III, position yourself on the ipsilateral stance leg of the patient and provide manual cuing with your hip so that the pelvis is not directly facing a student's body.

6. When appropriate, follow up with the student after the session.

Neural mobilization

Neurodynamic testing assesses neural tissue mechanosensitivity and its ability to withstand reasonable tensile and/or gliding force. These guidelines serve as a neurological safety net for identification of neural tension and may represent, for many patients, a new experience in yoga. Most importantly, the guidelines allow for recognition of warning signs to know when to refer a patient for, or perform, a more extensive neurological work-up. Even the most benign of postures can reveal neural tension if aligned carefully and mindfully:

1. Do not assume anything about a patient's experience or expertise in a yoga posture. For example, someone in a full manifestation of rarely therapeutically taught postures such as lotus, plow, or shoulderstand may not be sensitized to the subtle circulatory and neuromuscular input the pose should provide when carefully aligned. Almost always in yoga prescription, the mantra "less (movement) is more" is most effective.

2. Watch nonverbal communication and body language for clues about fatigue, pain, discomfort, and safety.

3. Ask direct questions of the patient while in the posture, acting immediately to give modifications based on the subjective or objective identification of pain associated with neural tension.

4. Discerning if a sensory experience in a pose (related to neural tension) should be encouraged or discouraged depends on knowing the frame or reference. Delineate the "when, how, and what" of the sensation to determine the proper course of action, either continuing to progress in the pose or limiting the degrees of freedom in a pose to diminish mechanical neural tension. For example:

   • Does it recreate injury or functional impairment?

   • Does it provoke radicular pain? Ask questions such as "In what pose, when during the pose, and when does your pain occur during the day or your practice?"

5. A single neural tension test is not as reliable as the diagnostic accuracy of finding two or more tests that are positive, particularly in lower limb tension testing (Walsh and Hall, 2009).

6. Neural mobilization can be self-guided and/or administered by the clinician and can occur with or without gross movement. Static mobilization uses joint traction or gliding of tissue that direct tensile or compressive force to the joint capsule. Mobilization with movement refers to the concurrent application of a sustained accessory mobilization applied by a clinician and/or an active physiologic movement applied by the patient within a functional movement such as a yoga posture.

Precautions and contraindications   (Butler, 1991)

• An increase in neurological signs and symptoms that range from: numbness, tingling, sensation of hot or cold, general impaired or loss of sensation, weakness, loss of motor coordination, or paralysis.

- General health problems. Other medical conditions such as cancers, diabetes, multiple sclerosis and other neurological disorders can create neurological signs.

- Dizziness (vertebrobasilar insufficiency or cord tethering) during neck movements or full spinal flexion.

- Circulatory interruptions related to the close connections of the nervous and circulatory systems. Butler describes these as "neurovascular bundles which are tortuous in the course." Butler writes that blood is "far more compressible than nervous tissue."

- Loss of bowel or bladder control or paralysis is a medical emergency.

- Cauda equina (bowel and bladder function) lesions.

- Spinal cord injury.

- Any existing disc injuries, bulges, or previous medical history of herniated discs in the vertebral column require a neurological referral.

- Frank cord injury. This describes those students who may already present with a minor cord injury and end up with a major cord injury resulting in partial or full paralysis secondary to a vigorous practice.

Lower limb neural tension screen

Lower limb tension testing can be completed from a range of functional yoga positions. The types of neural mobilization that may elicit sensitivity in the lower extremities include the following movements:

- Sciatic nerve — Hip flexion or straight leg raise to 90 degrees. Asymptomatic persons may feel a stretch of the hamstrings, while symptomatic persons will feel pain, paresthesia, or other neurological signs past the knee due to adverse tensile force of the sciatic nerve. Hip adduction and/or hip internal rotation could also identify sciatic tract tension secondary to the lateral location of the nerve relative to the ischial tuberosity.

- Intensification of sciatic nerve tension can be tested via:

- tibial tract tension – add ankle dorsiflexion

- common peroneal tract tension – add ankle plantarflexion/inversion.

- Obturator nerve — Supine or seated hip flexion and knee flexion (up to 90 degrees) followed by patient-led passive hip abduction. To intensify, add active cervical flexion with hip abduction. Asymptomatic persons will feel no change with either movement in the adductor area other than a stretch or elongation, while symptomatic persons may feel pain, dull aching, or other neurological signs which run to the knee and could implicate hip joint or pelvic floor.

- Pudendal nerve — Any neural tension or compression of this nerve would result in saddle-type (external genitals, urethra, anus, and perineum) pain, paresthesia, increased sensitivity or sensations such as stinging, burning, stabbing, aching, cramping or spasming, and/or an inability to sit or wear tight clothing.

Upper limb neural tension screen

The types of neural mobilization that may elicit sensitivity in the upper extremities, neck, and head include the following movements:

- Median nerve — Arm spiral screen (Chapter 5). Asymptomatic persons may feel a stretch of the bicep or pectoralis, while symptomatic persons may feel pain, paresthesia, or other neurological signs or symptoms in the median nerve distribution, especially with added wrist extension in arm spiral at 90 degrees glenohumeral joint abduction.

- Ulnar nerve — Arm spiral screen (Chapter 5). Asymptomatic persons may feel a stretch of the triceps of pectoralis, while symptomatic persons may feel pain, paresthesia, or experience other neurological signs or symptoms in the ulnar nerve distribution.

- Radial nerve — Reverse arm spiral screen. Position the arm(s) in glenohumeral joint abduction (45 degrees), full internal rotation, and mild horizontal abduction and extension. Add wrist and finger flexion at the end. Asymptomatic persons may feel a stretch of the wrist extensors, pectoralis, or biceps, while symptomatic persons may feel pain, paresthesia, or experience other neurological signs or symptoms in the radial nerve distribution.

During upper limb screening, the following variables should be considered:

- Differential diagnosis for neurogenic or vascular thoracic outlet syndrome (TOS). Neurogenic is the most common type of TOS, comprising 90–95% of TOS cases; while venous and arterial TOS is much rarer, making up only 5% and 1% of cases, respectively (Moore and Wei Lum, 2015). Referral out for TOS testing is appropriate if any motor, sensory, or circulatory impairments are noted during subjective or objective intake. However, arm spiral may serve as a preliminary and/or adjunct screen.

   TOS screen:

- Perform passive arm spiral without forearm pronation above and below 90 degrees glenohumeral abduction while constantly monitoring the pulse at the wrist. The pulse should remain steady and full at any arm position. Any variation requires further screening.

- Repeat the test with active arm spiral. This action may identify additional proximal impairment driven by improper motor strategies or load transfer that could exacerbate or cause TOS via compressive or tensile force on the brachial plexus compression or vascular structures. Neural tension with active scapular depression which reproduces symptoms could be indicative of neurogenic or vascular TOS.

General spinal neural tension

- General dura mater tension — Combination of neck flexion, trunk flexion, hip flexion, knee extension, and ankle dorsiflexion would equate to the slump test. Neck flexion and upper thoracic flexion in asymptomatic persons would elicit only a stretch sensation at the cervicothoracic junction. Symptomatic persons may feel pain, paresthesia, or other neurological signs due to adverse tension during lengthening of the spinal meninges.

Asymptomatic individuals would feel a stretch but without neurological signs.

Modifications

Modifications in neural tension testing are not typically required for the upper extremity or slump test, since all neural tension testing can be done in seated, supine, or sidelying. The slump test can be done in seated from a chair or supine in bed by performing bilateral hand-to-big toe using a strap with combined cervical flexion. The forward seated bend in long-sitting, partial and full plow are only used in higher level athletes who may be experiencing neural symptoms in sport or activity that require full spinal flexion under loaded conditions.

Neural screening overview

Neural tension screening can reveal potential minor nerve impairments influenced not by conduction deficits but rather nerve mechanosensitivity (Lai et al., 2013). Radicular symptoms that are unrelated to functional impairment or complaints do not necessarily indicate a positive neurodynamic text. Both symptom recreation and structural indication of neural tension must be present in order to implicate neural tension as a clinical problem or diagnosis.

Teaching

1. Prepare yourself. Work with pure intention and protect your own energy by meditating prior to patient care or teaching a group.

2. Practice moderation. Avoid the pendulum swing of extreme language use. As biomedically trained professionals, using yoga in healthcare requires a new language steeped in both biomedicine and yoga. Biomedical training offers distinct advantages for patient care, but strict use of only East or West language diminishes the impact of our work. Yoga without philosophy and the practice of all limbs looks and sounds like traditional biomedical rehabilitation. We must respect the medicine of both cultures and instead emerge with a new language from the fusion of the two, which is no small task. This is the language of MTY.

3. Never stop learning. Vocalizing this new language through patient care preparation and being a perpetual student demands a sort of prose-driven language, but one of beauty and depth of meaning. Reading inspirational texts, spiritual texts, and other poetry and readings helps to develop this language. The following checklist has been in development for almost two decades, and serves as a guide to fully develop your MTY voice and skillset.

Teaching checklist

Teaching will feel difficult in the beginning, but with time and practice, verbalizing the nuances of yoga becomes like breathing. To get you started, follow the teaching checklist below. Whether teaching a group or an individual, or a general or population-specific session, the list is instrumental in fostering creativity in instructional design and execution.

- *Instructor mechanics*:

  - calm breath – the student will mimic your quality of breath

  - use of safe body mechanics during cuing

  - give rationale for use of sequence.

- *Qualitative cuing* — Vary cues in a group setting. It is challenging to develop a yoga language not steeped in clinical, antiseptic jargon. As healthcare professionals, we have an expansive and intricate knowledge of medical terminology vocabulary. Consider this not as a liability, but as an asset. Use knowledge of medical terminology and kinesiology to facilitate the development of yoga "poetry" or language, considering:

  - proprioceptive cuing – identify joints used in poses and formulate cues based on this to help students identify where they are in space

  - discriminative touch cuing – gripping and overworking is common in postures and can create incorrect psychobiological emphasis or physiological pressure(s). Use knowledge of where light touch should be felt in a pose to cultivate awareness of a feeling they should have in a pose

  - deep pressure cuing – deep pressure is part of every pose, depending on what body part contacts the earth. Use knowledge of deep pressure feedback to bring awareness to where they should and should not feel deep pressure in a pose

  - internal imagery cuing – what is going on internally as a result of the student's outside "shape" in a pose?

  - modifications – offer suggestions for safety during the entire pose, especially during transitions. If someone struggles, help them. Err on the side of caution.

- *Quantitative cuing* — This cuing is as important as qualitative cuing. However, excessive use of quantitative cuing (for example, put the hand here or repeat 5 times) typically prefers clinical language and begins to resemble biomedical rehabilitation instead of yoga rehabilitation:

  - speaking pace and cue pauses – give students time to *"rest and digest"* what you are asking of them

  - cue frequency – excessive cues results in overload and frustration in the student, but too few can leave the student confused and uncertain of what to do

  - modification type – be prepared to give more than one type of modification, as not all bodies respond to the same cue.

- *Unspoken language* — Where can you see or feel tension in a person's unspoken language? Practice interpreting class "energy" as each student comes into the room. What do you notice? Offer tips for alignment or adjustment in poses that allow for release of those stressors you feel intuitively or via direct observation. Consider:

  - using psychoemotional text

  - balance of clinical versus poetic language (metaphors, analogies, having intention versus goals)

  - using humor to disarm or relax students – humor is good medicine

- character *"Golden Rule"* (*yama* or *niyama*) lesson – study and practice the yogic texts of other philosophies and of your own spiritual foundation(s) to guide students toward enriching interpersonal and intrapersonal relationships with all living things. To embody yoga, we must embrace one other with the *"Golden Rule"* of treating others as we would like to be treated

- inspirational readings – use poetry or other readings to inspire motivation or renewal.

- *Observational skills* — Recognize danger signs such as:

  - bulging or strained eyes

  - tight toes or gripping fingers

  - crinkled forehead, pinched mouth, clinched jaw

  - nonoptimal motor strategies that influence safe alignment.

- *Objective cues versus subjective cues* — As healthcare professionals we are trained to speak in the objective sense, asking few subjective questions and limiting subjective explanations or cues. To embody yoga in healthcare, we must transcend the objective and subjective and embrace the yogic language. For example, an indication of an effective song is that it shows you a concept or a feeling rather than telling you. The difference between good and bad instruction and song lyrics is the same. A good song lyric is open to interpretation, much like asking a closed versus an open-ended question. Hold space for individual growth while still maintaining safety by preferring figurative language over literal.

- *Biomechanical alignment* — Biomedical knowledge is critical to safe alignment. This skill is developed over time, but it is one of the forefront skills in successfully managing disorders, dysfunctions, and diseases through Medical Therapeutic Yoga. Always scaffold instruction via introduction of one degree of freedom at a time, when possible. Use of manual, verbal, and/or visual cuing while also considering partner-assist in poses can increase safety and efficacy.

Vocal characteristics:
- Anticipatory
- Authoritative
- Authentic
- Boisterous or demanding
- Calming
- Clinical
- Concerned
- Compassionate
- Crisp and clear
- Dictatorial
- Decongesting (good for kapha types)
- Encouraging
- Empathetic
- Empowering
- Energetic
- Engaging
- Excessive vata, pitta, or kapha
- Forgiving
- Fun
- Gentle around the edges (good for savasana, for example)
- Grounding
- Immersing
- Invitation to move past five senses
- Love of craft
- Motivated
- Natural vs. contrived
- Perky/sunny
- Personal
- Relaxed

- Sedating
- Self-searching
- Sisterly/brotherly (protective of student)
- Slowing or thoughtful (good for vata types)
- Thoughtful or academic
- Understanding
- Without ego or judgment (ahamkara).

- *Vocal quality* — The "whats and hows" of teaching are important, but the sound quality of knowledge delivery is perhaps most important. The quality of the voice dictates your clinical success and includes:

  - projection – the voice should project to the entire room without being too loud for the front row

  - cadence – pace of speaking should allow for mental digestion of knowledge shared, and should be easy to understand

  - pitch – vocal range should be determined for vocal protection and freeing the voice. Pitch should modulate during sentence production without pitching up so the end of every phrase sounds like a question

  - resonation – pitch is dependent on resonation, and all resonant cavities in the body (gut, chest, sinuses, skull) should be utilized not only for effective teaching, but for preserving the vocal folds. Clinicians and educators who speak for long stretches at a time can end up suffering from repeat laryngitis, hoarseness, or vocal nodules.

  - see Code 12.2 for resources on vocal training

Code 12.2 (free code)
Resources on vocal training

- vitality (*prana*) – the voice should reflect the patient demographic. Energy of the voice should be steady and sure, as well as:

- welcoming (as opposed to alienating)

- grounding (as opposed to distancing)

- empowering (as opposed to critical)

- compassionate (as opposed to condescending or apathetic).

Sequencing

Sequencing can define success in prescription. Not sequenced properly, prescription can hurt rather than help. This is a skill developed with time and training, but give careful thought to posture choice by considering the following:

1. Breath work coincides with movement and can facilitate or prevent movement. Beginners may impede movement with the breath, whereas someone advanced may facilitate movement with the breath. Breath work can also be used to expend or conserve energy.

2. Primary, secondary, tertiary purpose — Teach with a purpose, not necessarily a goal. If you decide what the primary purpose of a pose is, consider the secondary purpose or even the tertiary purpose too. This can help determine what pose(s) should follow.

3. Oppositional cuing — *Hatha yoga* means a union of a pair of opposites. The beauty of yoga is that it is balancing for the body and mind. Providing oppositional cuing (such as "Let the pose contract but mind the expand" or "Lengthen the bicep but strengthen the tricep") can allow for embodiment of Hatha yoga's meaning.

4. Pose and counterpose theory (moving from one extreme ROM to the opposite ROM) is often used traditionally but may not always be favorable for functional sequencing, especially in those populations with contraindications to the pose or its counterpart) (for example, acute spinal posterior disc lesions may need to avoid spinal flexion and focus only on spinal extension during the acute phase). Sequencing should be determined by functional person-centered goals and the rehabilitative evidence base.

5. Develop the agonist, antagonist, and synergists for healthy form and force closure and neuromuscular patterning.

6. Develop internal and external balance in joints, remembering the spin and roll arthrokinematics of each joint, not just the gross osteokinematics of the bones (ROM).

7. If you are aligning postures slowly and carefully according to the 10 precepts, functional impairments are easily identified.

8. Sequencing a class or session can consider the following options: (1) postural chronology (for example, progress *asana* from standing to sitting to prone to supine); (2) therapeutic prescription or pathophysiology; (3) Ayurvedic constitution or *dosha* of the person, disease or condition, the environment, or the climate or the *dosha* of the *asana*, *mudra*, or *pranayama**; (4) time of day, season of year, or season of life or age; or (5) *chakra* therapy*.

*Note: The concepts of Ayurvedic *doshas* and *chakras* are outside the scope of this text; however, there is some early evidence to support phenotype with the constitutional analysis of the *doshas*; and, in the case of *chakras*, there is some functional, scientific overlap in sound, color, and endocrine system function.

Meditation

(see Code 12.1)

Meditation is the cornerstone of yoga and is supported by a plethora of scientific evidence. It is a complex practice with simple foundations. Despite the many types of meditation that exist, all that is needed to begin is time, space, and intention. Think of meditation less as a lengthy investment of time requiring equipment and an experienced teacher, more as an invitation to equanimity and calm, no matter what your background or training.

Accountability measures may be helpful to begin or sustain a meditation practice. Those measures could include gratitude journaling, scheduling a set time each day, sharing your plans with a friend, using tangible reminders such as a gentle alarm or colored stickers ("green dot therapy") placed in unexpected places that will remind you to stop, breathe, and then do. Consider the following:

- Meditation should be suitably conjoined with your belief system. Yoga does not ask you to follow a spiritual path that is not your own.

> *Out beyond ideas of wrongdoing and right doing, there is a field. Meet me there.*
> Rumi

- Meditation is not an escape or journey into negativity.

> *Each one of us is merely a small instrument. When you look at the inner workings of electrical things, often you see small and big wires, new and old, cheap and expensive, lined up. Until the current passes through them, there will be no light. That wire is you and me. The current is God. We have the power to let the current pass through us, use us, produce the light of the world. Or, we can refuse to be used and allow darkness to spread.*
> Mother Teresa

- Choose your object of meditation carefully, for this will permeate all of your thoughts and actions.

> *As a result of contentment, one gains supreme happiness.*
> Yoga Sutras

- Choose a practice you can sustain, a posture you can sustain for an extended period of time, without distraction.

> *Lack of true knowledge is the source of all pains and sorrows.*
> Yoga Sutras

> *You must learn to be still in the midst of activity and to be vibrantly alive in repose.*
>
> Indira Gandhi

- Meditation is an individual path. Your teacher's path may not necessarily coincide with your own. You must constantly reassess if your meditation practice is beneficial.

> *Hell is the place where nothing connects.*
>
> T.S. Eliot

> *For as he thinketh in his heart, so is he.*
>
> Proverbs 23:7

> *Very often, understanding and practice do not go together. One student may be better able to understand, while another may have better skill in practice. In each case, he has to develop uniformity in skill and intelligence and use them harmoniously.*
>
> B.K.S. Iyengar

Business practice and liability concerns

Medical documentation

Medical documentation has historically followed a general pattern known by the acronym SOAP – subjective, objective, assessment, and plan. MTY uses the same documentation format where the clinician, after collecting subjective and objective information, makes a conclusion about the findings in the assessment section and then generates a list of problems to justify the diagnosis. In the plan section, a list of therapies to be administered is documented and encased in a specific time frame, including short range and long range plans. On the first visit, the note should also include any treatment given on the first day, as well as a note to the referring practitioner, if applicable, thanking them for the referral and informing him/her of the findings.

Documentation for inclusion of yoga postures and breathwork should include the clinical rationale for the postural/movement sequence, rather than simply being a list of the yoga postures included. The list is an adjunct, if included, to the scientific rationale for treatment.

Documentation tips

- Document the English rationale for use of yoga breath and/or postures, not necessarily the actual postures and breath used. However, as a clinician, documenting both is very valuable for accurate record keeping and progression of a patient's program.

- Functional carry over — Document the movement impairments that affect everyday activities. Also document their associated BPS impact, so that patterns can be established between functional movement and discomfort.

- Test–retest — Test the impaired or painful movement prior to treating the area. Then retest it again after treatment. This strategy includes performing myofascial release in the context of daily functional activities such as squatting, standing, or sitting and allows the patient to make a connection between their actions and their progress or pain.

- Include a note to the referring practitioner to facilitate and maintain partnership theory relationship.

Coding

Coding that is used to obtain insurance reimbursement for use of skilled rehabilitative services performed by licensed therapists can also be used for skilled MTY service reimbursement, when delivered by a licensed medical provider. The following CPT codes can include skilled yoga prescription delivered by a licensed therapist or physician:

- 97110 – Therapeutic exercise
- 97112 – Neuromuscular re-education, balance, coordination
- 97140 – Manual therapy
- 97530 – Therapeutic activity

- 97532 – Cognitive training
- 97533 – Sensory integration
- 97535 – Self-care management training.

Patient education (98960) should be a reimbursable service, since the majority of our time in healthcare is spent educating our patients. Unfortunately, this code is rarely, if at all, reimbursed. Aquatic therapy (97113), biofeedback (90901 and 90911), and oftentimes group therapy (97150) are also not covered or poorly reimbursed services (respectively) under Medicare and many major insurance policies, at least in the United States. Please check with service provider contracts to determine what codes are eligible for reimbursement under your scope of practice.

Referral to an appropriate medical practitioner should happen when (Delitto et al., 2012):

- The patient's clinical findings are suggestive of serious medical or psychological pathology
- The reported activity limitations or impairments of body function and structure are not consistent with those presented with diagnosis or classification
- The patient's symptoms are not resolving with interventions aimed at normalization of the patient's impairments of body function.

Liability concerns

A practitioner's scope of practice that includes touch or movement therapy is an umbrella that includes yoga when it is used as in the section on Coding. Yoga as a contemplative science is a skilled therapy requiring additional training or schooling in order to prescribe, particularly under the auspices of a licensed healthcare professional. In some cases, practitioners may feel the need to purchase additional liability insurance to cover their inclusion of yoga as a therapeutic modality. However, using the example of internal pelvic physical therapy, no additional insurance or release of liability is needed in order to practice or perform internal physical exams. A practitioner, once licensed in a medical field, is always held to the highest tiered licensure. In other words, a therapist is always a therapist and will be legally held to the scope

of practice in his or her practice act. Healthcare professionals, then, with adequate training in using rehabilitative yoga, can be ideally suited to use yoga on the frontlines of medicine.

Review

This chapter introduces methods and outcome measures for self-management programs to both improve our collective healthcare and well-being while also reducing the burden of healthcare costs. In this way, Medical Therapeutic Yoga is a low-cost, inexpensive method that can improve health outcomes, empower patients in this age of illness, and decrease healthcare costs.

Conclusion

Yoga has been evolving since the moment it was born. The methodology presented in this text is not yoga's first evolution, as evidenced by many yoga historians (De Michelis, 2005; Singleton, 2010; Horton, 2013), which places us in a postmodern era of contemplation about yoga. Still yet, the application of the evidence base to yoga has occurred only in very recent history. Current practice has been termed "modern postural yoga" (De Michelis, 2005), while early yoga shunned the physical practice of yoga as hedonistic and derogatory toward Hindu spirituality and overall spiritual growth and refused to include it as part of yoga (Singleton, 2010).

Clearly, the yoga of India has evolved over the centuries and should continue to evolve globally in order to meet the needs of its citizens. Healthcare concerns in the 21st century worldwide include increasing amounts of chronic disease and chronic pain (WHO, 2005). Safety, as well as relevancy, based on what we know about the human body, especially in the biomedical fields of orthopaedics, biomechanics, microbiology, neuroendocrinology, and even quantum physics, should be the chief concerns in the utilization of yoga postures and breath practice in medicine.

Additionally, the persistence of any gender bias or lack of specific application of yoga for women's needs due to patriarchal domination of modern yoga is damaging to the fabric of yoga. Cultural conditioning that would hinder the evolution of medicine and yoga can be addressed by a nurturing partnership to join the hands of yogic and biomedical medicine.

Mainstreaming the use of yoga in healthcare can reduce barriers to the receipt of conservative rehabilitative care and reduce the need for invasive medical procedures and pharmacology that may carry significant risks and/or side effects, while also broadening the spectrum of how we can address psychobiological pathophysiologies, which can directly address the stigma that often prevents our patients from seeking out mental healthcare. The use of yoga in healthcare can also reconcile the impact of neuroendocrine dysregulation on orthopaedic pain and trauma management, which can have massive implications for shifting the paradigm of practice in rehabilitative care. We are on the boundary of a new frontier in rehabilitation and medicine. All we need to do to cross it is to work together, through interdisciplinary education and research, to embrace the full potential of yoga's transformative and healing power.

GLOSSARY

The purpose of this section is to define the therapeutic template abbreviations, terms, and blanket-fold types found in Chapters 4–10. The terms are defined in a therapeutic manner for medical professionals to use in patient evaluation and management within their scope of practice. Some terms are mentioned for the first time in therapeutic yoga and yoga literature.

Abbreviations

DMs (dynamic modifications) – A phrase to describe modification of posture or breath. DMs are modifications made, with or without internal musculoskeletal or external props, in order to assist in pose entry, maintenance, or exit. Most often these postures are performed in a gravity-dependent position.

SP (starting position) – Where a person starts in order to enter a pose.

SRAs (static restorative approximations) – A phrase to describe alternative postures used with or without external props that serve to approximate the therapeutic intent of the original posture when a person is unable to perform the dynamic version. Most often these postures are performed in a gravity-minimized position.

TI (therapeutic intention) – A preferred term to "goal," which suggests a means to an end only, "TI" is used as a clinical prediction guideline to aid decision-making. Yoga is, rather than a means to an end, about "being" as well as about the power of transformation through observation and action with detachment (*pratyahara*). For medical care, goals will need to be set in order to receive third party reimbursement, as well as to chart objective progress for a patient. Goal-setting for objective management is acceptable, but should be functional and meaningful to the patient. Of utmost importance is the invitation of yoga to enjoy an open-minded and open-ended "intention," enjoying the process and the journey and being open to what it brings, instead of only seeking the end.

TTCP (teaching and tactical cuing primer) – This primer includes practical recommendations for instructing and modifying movement.

Terms

Arm spiral – A postural practice specific that facilitates shoulder complex stability and controlled flexibility.

Contraindications – Precautions, including relative and absolute contraindications that would require either (1) modification or (2) elimination and substitution of another pose, perhaps from SRAs (static restorative approximations).

Gateway posture – A gateway posture is a pose that helps prepare and transition you toward more biomechanically complex yoga postures.

Hip lock – Utilization of the hip rotator cuff, the gluteals, and occasionally the hamstrings to synergistically support TATD (transversus abdominis-assisted thoracodiaphragmatic) breath.

Hip telescoping – A phrase that describes supine, gravity-minimized multiplanar hip range of motion.

Partial chin lock, abdominal lock, root lock, anterior and posterior – mild *jalandhara bandha*, mild *uddiyanda bandha*, mild *mula bandha* and *ashwini mudra* – These are locks or *bandha* techniques recalibrated by the evidence base in rehabilitation and used to improve safety or energetic retention of a pose.

Shoulder lock – A combination of scapulohumeral stabilization and neuromuscular re-education for plumb line posture during prayer hands posture (*anjali mudra*). Shoulder lock can also be performed in various closed kinetic chain or simulated closed kinetic chain postures, and in open kinetic chain postures when combined with arm spiral.

Shoulder opener, arm floats (supine and standing) – A foundational pre-posture focusing on scapular stabilization and simultaneous safe glenohumeral osteokinematic joint range of motion in addition to the osteokinematic and arthrokinematic motion of the acromioclavicular, scapulothoracic, and sternoclavicular joints and lumbopelvic stability and awareness.

TATD (transversus abdominis-assisted thoraco-diaphragmatic breath) – A breath technique used during active practice unless otherwise noted in posture description and instruction.

Blanket-fold techniques

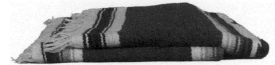

Figure G.1 Two-tier approach blanket-fold

Two-tier approach (Fig. G.1) – A blanket-folding technique primarily used for posterior tissue preservation in seated postures (*asana*). Two blankets are folded in quarters and then halved and stacked in an offset or scaffolded fashion. Use two separate yoga blankets to create a "tier" in which the ischial tuberosities rest on the second or highest "tier" and the hamstrings can rest on the loft of the first or lowest tier, allowing for gentle graded decline for supported sitting rather than the abrupt drop typically offered, which allows large gaps from which the hamstrings or fascia could be potentially strained from excessive biomechanical length/tension.

Code G.1 (free code)
Two-tier approach
to yoga couch

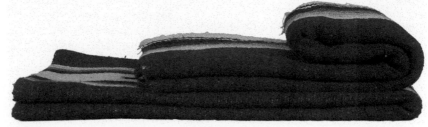

Figure G.2 Three-tier approach "yoga couch" blanket-fold

Three-tier approach (yoga couch) (Fig. G.2) – A blanket-folding technique utilizable in a wide range of postures. Two blankets are folded in a tri-fold and then halved and stacked in a vertically offset fashion to create a "three-tier" look.

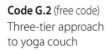

Code G.2 (free code)
Three-tier approach
to yoga couch

Figure G.3 Ganesha-fold blanket-fold

Ganesha-fold (Fig. G.3) – A blanket-folding technique which allows for asymmetrical support of postures, usually in SRAs (static restorative approximations). Two yoga couch-folded (tri-fold) blankets are used and placed end to end to create the shape of two airborne elephants' trunks "kissing."

Code G.3 (free
code)
Ganesha-fold

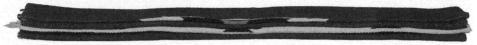

Figure G.4 Accordion-fold blanket-fold

Accordion-fold (Fig. G.4) – A blanket-folding technique which spans the width of the palm when the blanket is turned back and forth on each other, resulting in a narrow lengthwise stack about 6 inches tall.

Code G.4 (free code)
Accordion-fold

REFERENCES

Chapter 1

American Occupational Therapy Association (2011), Complementary and Alternative Medicine Supplement. American Journal of Occupational Therapy 65(6): S26–S31.

Anderzen-Carlsson A, Persson Lundholm U, Kohn M et al. (2014), Medical yoga: another way of being in the world. A phenomenological study from the perspective of persons suffering from stress-related symptoms. International Journal of Qualitative Studies on Health and Well-being 9: 23033.

Beckie TM (2012), A systematic review of allostatic load, health, and health disparities. Biological Research for Nursing 14(4): 311–346.

Bella SD, Kraus N, Overy K et al. (2009), The neurosciences and music III: disorders and plasticity. Annals of the New York Academy of Sciences 1169: 225–233.

Bengtsson SL, Ullen F, Ehrsson HH et al. (2009), Listening to rhythms activates motor and premotor cortices. Cortex 45(1): 62–71.

Bernard P (2004), Music as Yoga: Discover the Healing Power of Sound. Mandala, San Rafael, CA.

Bharati SJ (2013), Is Yoga a religion? wwwswamijcom (last accessed September 6, 2013).

Bhushan P, Kalpana J, Arvind C (2005), Classification of human population based on HLA gene polymorphism and the concept of Prakriti in Ayurveda. Journal of Alternative and Complementary Medicine 11(2): 349–353.

Bordoni B, Zanier E (2013), Anatomic connections of the diaphragm: influence of respiration on the body system. Journal of Multidisciplinary Healthcare 6: 281–291.

Brandes VM et al. (2008), Special receptive music therapy in the ambulatory treatment of depressive states. First results of a longitudinal study. Poster presentation, Paracelsus Science Get Together – Life Science, Salzburg, Austria, June 13, 2005.

Brandes V, Terris DD, Fischer C et al. (2009), Music programs designed to remedy burnout symptoms show significant effects after five weeks. Annals of the New York Academy of Sciences 1169: 422–425.

Brown RP, Gerbarg PL (2009), Yoga breathing, meditation, and longevity. Annals of the New York Academy of Sciences 1172: 54–62.

CAMDOC Alliance (2010), The regulatory status of complementary and alternative medicine for medical doctors in Europe. http://wwwcamdoceu/Pdf/CAMDOCRegulatoryStatus8_10pdf (last accessed February 11, 2014).

Chvatal SA, Ting LH (2013), Common muscle synergies for balance and walking. Frontiers in Computational Neuroscience 7: 48.

Cohen S, Janicki-Deverts D, Doyle WJ et al. (2012), Chronic stress, glucocorticoid receptor resistance, inflammation, and disease risk. Proceedings of the National Academy of Sciences of the United States of America 109(16): 5995–5999.

Conway CM, Pisoni DB, Kronenberger WG (2009), The importance of sound for cognitive sequencing abilities: the auditory scaffolding hypothesis. Current Directions in Psychological Science 18: 275–279.

Creer T, Renne C, Christian W (1976), Behavioral contributions to rehabilitation and childhood asthma. Rehabilitation Literature 37: 226–232, 247.

Danese A, McEwen BS (2012), Adverse childhood experiences, allostasis, allostatic load, and age-related disease. Physiology and Behavior 106(1): 29–39.

De Michelis E (2005), A History of Modern Yoga. Continuum, London.

Devi S (2011), Doctors in distress. Lancet, 377(9764): 454–455.

Eisler RT (2007), The Real Wealth of Nations: Creating a Caring Economics. Berrett-Koehler, San Francisco, CA.

Eisler RT, Potter TM (2014), Transforming Interprofessional Partnerships: A New Framework for Nursing and Partnership-based Health Care. Sigma Theta Tau International, Indianapolis, IN.

Elliott AM, Smith BH, Hannaford PC et al. (2002), The course of chronic pain in the community: results of a 4-year follow-up study. Pain 99(1–2): 299–307.

Engel GL (1977), The need for a new medical model: a challenge for biomedicine. Science 196: 129–136.

Fiabane E, Giorgi I, Musian D et al. (2012), Occupational stress and job satisfaction of healthcare staff in rehabilitation units. La Medicina del Lavoro 103(6): 482–492.

REFERENCES

Fitzgerald CM, Mallinson T (2012), The association between pelvic girdle pain and pelvic floor muscle function in pregnancy. International Urogynecology Journal 23(7): 893–898.

Friedman EM, Karlamangla AS, Almeida DM et al. (2012), Social strain and cortisol regulation in midlife in the US. Social Science and Medicine 74(4): 607–615.

Garner G (2001), Professional Yoga Therapy Studies Professional Yoga Therapy Course Manuals. Living Well, Emerald Isle, NC.

Garner G (2014), The role of relationship and creativity. In: M Taylor (ed.), Fostering Creativity in Rehabilitation. Nova Science Publishers, New York City, ch 6.

Ghodke Y, Joshi K, Patwardhan B (2011), Traditional medicine to modern pharmacogenomics: Ayurveda Prakriti type and CYP2C19 gene polymorphism associated with the metabolic variability. Evidence-Based Complementary and Alternative Medicine, eCAM, 2011: 249528.

Goldberg DS, Mcgee SJ (2011), Pain as a global public health priority. BMC Public Health 11: 770.

Gray C (1997), Growing popularity of complementary medicine leads to national organization for MDs. Canadian Medical Association Journal (Journal de l'Association Médicale Canadienne) 157(2): 186–188.

Hall P, Weaver L (2001), Interdisciplinary education and teamwork: a long and winding road. Medical Education 35(9): 867–875.

Hankey A (2005), A test of the systems analysis underlying the scientific theory of Ayurveda's Tridosha. Journal of Alternative and Complementary Medicine 11(3): 385–390.

Hellwig JP (2013), State of the world's mothers: new report from Save the Children. Nursing for Women's Health 17(4): 347–349.

Hodges PW, Richardson CA (1997), Feedforward contraction of transversus abdominis is not influenced by the direction of arm movement. Experimental Brain Research 114(2): 362–370.

Hodges P, Richardson C, Jull G (1996), Evaluation of the relationship between laboratory and clinical tests of transversus abdominis function. Physiotherapy Research International 1(1): 30–40.

Iliceto P, Pompili M, Spencer-Thomas S et al. (2013), Occupational stress and psychopathology in health professionals: an explorative study with the multiple indicators multiple causes (MIMIC) model approach. Stress 16(2): 143–152.

Institute of Medicine (US), Committee on Building Bridges in the Brain, Behavioral, and Clinical Sciences, Division of Neuroscience and Behavioral Health (2000), Bridging Disciplines in the Brain, Behavioral, and Clinical Sciences. National Academy Press, Washington DC.

Institute of Medicine, Committee on Advancing Pain Research, Care, and Education (2011), Relieving Pain in America: A Blueprint for Transforming Prevention, Care, Education, and Research. National Academies Press, Washington DC.

Institute of Medicine (2013), Establishing Transdisciplinary Professionalism for Improving Health Outcomes: Workshop Summary. National Academy of Sciences, National Academies Press, Washington DC, prepublication copy, uncorrected proof.

International Digest of Health Legislation (1993), Regulations respecting the practice of acupuncture by persons other than physicians. International Digest of Health Legislation 44: 208.

Irving JA, Dobkin PL, Park J (2009), Cultivating mindfulness in health care professionals: a review of empirical studies of mindfulness-based stress reduction (MBSR). Complementary Therapies in Clinical Practice 15(2): 61–66.

Iyengar BKS (1966, 1968, 1976), Light on Yoga: Yoga Dīpikā. Schocken, New York.

Iyengar BKS (1993), Light on the Yoga Sūtras of Patañjala: Patañjala Yoga Pradīpikā. Aquarian Press, London.

Janssens L, Brumagne S, McConnell AK et al. (2013), Greater diaphragm fatigability in individuals with recurrent low back pain. Respiratory Physiology and Neurobiology 188(2): 119–123.

Jull GA, Richardson CA (2000), Motor control problems in patients with spinal pain: a new direction for therapeutic exercise. Journal of Manipulative and Physiological Therapeutics 23(2): 115–117.

Kjaer M, Hansen M (2008), The mystery of female connective tissue. Journal of Applied Physiology 105(4): 1026–1027.

Kolar P, Sulc J, Kyncl M et al. (2010), Stabilizing function of the diaphragm: dynamic MRI and synchronized spirometric assessment. Journal of Applied Physiology 109(4): 1064–1071.

Kolar P, Sulc J, Kyncl M et al. (2012), Postural function of the diaphragm in persons with and without chronic low back pain. Journal of Orthopaedic and Sports Physical Therapy 42(4): 352–362.

Lee D (2011), The Pelvic Girdle: An Integration of Clinical Expertise and Research, 4th edition. Churchill Livingstone/Elsevier, Edinburgh, UK.

Levitan D (2007), This is your Brain on Music: The Science of a Human Obsession. Penguin, USA.

Logan JG, Barksdale DJ (2008), Allostasis and allostatic load: expanding the discourse on stress and cardiovascular disease. Journal of Clinical Nursing 17(7B): 201–208.

McEwen BS (1998), Protective and damaging effects of stress mediators. New England Journal of Medicine 338(3): 171–179.

McEwen BS, Seeman T (1999), Protective and damaging effects of mediators of stress: elaborating and testing the concepts of allostasis and allostatic load. Annals of the New York Academy of Sciences 896(1): 30–47.

McEwen BS, Stellar E (1993), Stress and the individual mechanisms leading to disease. Archives of Internal Medicine 153(18): 2093–2101.

McEwen BS, Eiland L, Hunter RG et al. (2012), Stress and anxiety: structural plasticity and epigenetic regulation as a consequence of stress. Neuropharmacology 62(1): 3–12.

McVicar A, Ravalier JM, Greenwood C (2014), Biology of stress revisited: intracellular mechanisms and the conceptualization of stress. Stress and Health 30(4): 272–279.

Maddalena S (1999), The Legal Status of Complementary Medicines in Europe — A Comparative Analysis. Stämpfli Verlag, Bern, Switzerland.

Mohan AG, Miller K (2002), Yoga for Body, Breath, and Mind: A Guide for Personal Reintegration. Boston, Shambhala.

Mohan AG, Mohan G (2010), Krishnamacharya: His Life and Teachings. Boston, Shambhala.

Morandi A, Tosto C, Sartori G et al. (2011), Advent of a link between Ayurveda and modern health science. Proceedings of the First International Congress on Ayurveda, Ayurveda: The Meaning of Life-Awareness, Environment, and Health, March 21–22, 2009, Milan, Italy. Evidence-Based Complementary and Alternative Medicine, eCAM, 2011: 929083.

Morgan N, Irwin MR, Chung M et al. (2014), The effects of mind–body therapies on the immune system: meta-analysis. PloS one 9(7): e100903.

Murrock CJ, Higgins PA (2009), The theory of music, mood and movement to improve health outcomes. Journal of Advanced Nursing 65(10): 2249–2257.

Nahin RL, Barnes PM, Stussman BJ et al. (2009), Costs of complementary and alternative medicine (CAM) and frequency of visits to CAM practitioners: United States (2007). National Health Statistics Reports (18): 1–14.

National Center for Complementary and Alternative Medicine (2013), Complementary, Alternative, or Integrative Medicine What's in a Name? October (2008). Last updated May (2013). D347 wwwnccamnihgov.

National Center for Complementary and Integrative Medicine (2015), Complementary, Alternative, or Integrative Medicine: What's in a name? https://nccihnihgov/health/integrative-health (last accessed August 5, 2015).

National Institutes of Health Revitalization Act (1993), Public Law 103–143, 10 June 1993, United States of America.

Nilsson U (2008), The anxiety- and pain-reducing effects of music interventions: a systematic review. AORN Journal 87(4): 780–807.

Novak M, Costantini L, Schneider S et al. (2013), Approaches to self-management in chronic illness. Seminars in Dialysis 26(2): 188–194.

Palkhivala A (2006), Fire of Love: Teaching the Essence of Yoga. Innerworks Company, Bellevue, WA.

Paine NJ, Bosch JA, Van Zanten JJ (2012), Inflammation and vascular responses to acute mental stress: implications for the triggering of myocardial infarction. Current Pharmaceutical Design 18(11): 1494–1501.

Parliamentary Paper No 102/1977 (1977), Chiropractic, osteopathy, homeopathy and naturopathy: report of committee of inquiry. Acting Commonwealth Government Printer, Canberra, Australia.

Penman S, Cohen M, Stevens P et al. (2012), Yoga in Australia: results of a national survey. International Journal of Yoga 5(2): 92–101.

Pergolizzi J, Ahlbeck K, Aldington D et al. (2013), The development of chronic pain: physiological change necessitates a multidisciplinary approach to treatment. Current Medical Research and Opinion 29(9): 1127–1135.

Porges S (2011), Polyvagal Theory, Neurophysiological Foundations of Emotions, Attachment, Communication, and Self-Regulation. Norton Series on Interpersonal Neurobiology. WW Norton and Company, New York.

Pomeroy C (2012), Health disparities and social justice: a call to action for academic health centers: prioritizing health disparities in medical education to improve care. Lecture, New York Academy of Sciences, October 2.

Prasher B, Negi S, Aggarwal S et al. (2008), Whole genome expression and biochemical correlates of extreme constitutional types defined in Ayurveda. Journal of Translational Medicine 6: 48.

Rastogi S (2010), Building bridges between Ayurveda and modern science. International Journal of Ayurveda Research 1(1): 41–46.

Rohleder N, Aringer M, Boentert M (2012), Role of interleukin-6 in stress, sleep, and fatigue. Annals of the New York Academy of Sciences 1261: 88–96.

REFERENCES

Ross A, Thomas S (2010), The health benefits of yoga and exercise: a review of comparison studies. Journal of Alternative and Complementary Medicine 16(1): 3–12.

Satchidananda, Patañjali (1990), The Yoga Sutras of Patanjali. Integral Yoga Publications, Yogaville, VA.

Save the Children (2013), State of the World's Mothers. Save the Children, London, UK, and Fairfield, CT.

Sharma H, Chandola HM, Singh G et al. (2007), Utilization of Ayurveda in health care: an approach for prevention, health promotion, and treatment of disease. Part 1 – Ayurveda, the science of life. Journal of Alternative and Complementary Medicine 13(9): 1011–1019.

Singleton M (2005), Salvation through relaxation: proprioceptive therapy and its relationship to yoga. Journal of Contemporary Religion 20(3): 289–304.

Singleton M (2010), Yoga Body: The Origins of Modern Posture Practice. Oxford University Press, Oxford and New York.

Singleton M, Byrne J (2008), Yoga in the Modern World: Contemporary Perspectives. Routledge, London and New York.

Smith DW (2013), 'Phenomenology', in the Stanford Encyclopedia of Philosophy. http://platostanfordedu/archives/win2013/entries/phenomenology/ (last accessed June 13, 2014).

Stokes IAF (2010), Intra-abdominal pressure and abdominal wall muscular function: spinal unloading mechanism. Clinical Biomechanics 25(9): 859–866.

Streeter CC, Whitfield TH, Owen L et al. (2010), Effects of yoga versus walking on mood, anxiety, and brain GABA levels: a randomized controlled MRS study. Journal of Alternative and Complementary Medicine 16(11): 1145–1152.

Streeter CC, Gerbarg PL, Saper RB et al. (2012), Effects of yoga on the autonomic nervous system, gamma-aminobutyric-acid, and allostasis in epilepsy, depression, and post-traumatic stress disorder. Medical Hypotheses 78(5): 571–579.

Taylor M (2007), What is Yoga Therapy: An IAYT Definition. Yoga Therapy in Practice, December.

Taylor SE, Way BM, Seeman TE (2011), Early adversity and adult health outcomes. Development and Psychopathology 23(3): 939–954.

Thaut MH, McIntosh GC (2010), How music helps to heal the injured brain: therapeutic use crescendos thanks to advances in brain science. Cerebrum, March 24. http://dana.org/Cerebrum/2010/How_Music_Helps_to_Heal_the_Injured_Brain__Therapeutic_Use_Crescendos_Thanks_to_Advances_in_Brain_Science/ (last accessed May 23, 2016).

Thaut MH, Gardiner JC, Holmberg D et al. (2009), Neurologic music therapy improves executive function and emotional adjustment in traumatic brain injury rehabilitation. Annals of the New York Academy of Sciences 1169: 406–416.

Ting LH, Chvatal SA, Safavynia SA et al. (2012), Review and perspective: neuromechanical considerations for predicting muscle activation patterns for movement. International Journal for Numerical Methods in Biomedical Engineering 28(10): 1003–1014.

Torres-Oviedo G, Ting, LH (2010), Subject-specific muscle synergies in human balance control are consistent across different biomechanical contexts. Journal of Neurophysiology 103(6): 3084–3098.

US Department of Health and Human Services, Health Resources and Services Administration, Maternal and Child Health Bureau (2007), Women's Health USA. US Department of Health and Human Services (2006), Rockville, MD.

Van Hecke O, Torrance N, Smith BH (2013), Chronic pain epidemiology and its clinical relevance. British Journal of Anaesthesia 111(1): 13–18.

Wallace JE, Lemaire JB, Ghali WA (2009), Physician wellness: a missing quality indicator. Lancet 374(9702): 1714–1721.

World Health Organization (2001), Legal Status of Traditional Medicine and Complementary/Alternative Medicine: A Worldwide Review. World Health Organization, Geneva.

World Health Organization (2002), Towards a Common Language for Functioning, Disability and Health: ICF. World Health Organization, Geneva.

World Health Organization (2005), Preventing Chronic Diseases – A Vital Investment: WHO Global Report. World Health Organization, Geneva.

World Health Organization (2010), Framework for Action on Interprofessional Education and Collaborative Practice. WHO Department of Human Resources for Health, Geneva.

Yee R, Zolotow N (2002), Yoga: The Poetry of the Body. Thomas Dunne Books/St Martin's Griffin, New York.

Chapter 2

Abramowitz SA, Flattery D, Franses K et al. (2010), Linking a motivational interviewing curriculum to the chronic care model. Journal of General Internal Medicine 25(Suppl. 4): S620–S626.

Anderson JG, Taylor AG (2011), The metabolic syndrome and mind–body therapies: a systematic review. Journal of Nutrition and Metabolism 2011: 276419.

REFERENCES

Andrade PM, Haase VG, Oliveira-Ferreira F (2012), An ICF-based approach for cerebral palsy from a biopsychosocial perspective. Developmental Neurorehabilitation 15(6): 391–400.

Arnow BA, Hunkeler EM, Blasey CM et al. (2006), Comorbid depression, chronic pain, and disability in primary care. Psychosomatic Medicine 68(2): 262–268.

Awad H, Alghadir A (2013), Validation of the comprehensive International Classification of Functioning, Disability and Health core set for diabetes mellitus: physical therapists' perspectives. American Journal of Physical Medicine and Rehabilitation 92(11): 968–979.

Ayuso-Mateos JL, Avila CC, Anaya C et al., Bipolar Disorders Core Sets Expert Group (2013), Development of the International Classification of Functioning, Disability and Health core sets for bipolar disorders: results of an international consensus process. Disability and Rehabilitation 35(25): 2138–2146.

Bair MJ, Robinson RL, Katon W et al. (2003), Depression and pain comorbidity: a literature review. Archives of Internal Medicine 163(20): 2433–2445.

Baker DW, Wolf MS, Feinglass J et al. (2007), Health literacy and mortality among elderly persons. Archives of Internal Medicine 167(14): 1503–1509.

Baker DW, Wolf MS, Feinglass J et al. (2008), Health literacy, cognitive abilities, and mortality among elderly persons. Journal of General Internal Medicine 23(6): 723–726.

Bartlett DJ, Lucy SD (2004), A comprehensive approach to outcomes research in rehabilitation. Physiotherapy Canada 56: 237–247.

Benarous X, Legrand C, Consoli SM (2014), Motivational interviewing use for promoting health behavior: an approach of doctor/patient relationship. La Revue de Médecine Interne 35(5): 317–321.

Bennett IM, Chen J, Soroui JS et al. (2009), The contribution of health literacy to disparities in self-rated health status and preventive health behaviors in older adults. Annals of Family Medicine 7(3): 204–211.

Bijlani RL, Vempati RP, Yadav RK et al. (2005), A brief but comprehensive lifestyle education program based on yoga reduces risk factors for cardiovascular disease and diabetes mellitus. Journal of Alternative and Complementary Medicine 11(2): 267–274.

Bonaz BL, Bernstein CN (2013), Brain–gut interactions in inflammatory bowel disease. Gastroenterology 144(1): 36–49.

Brandt C, Pedersen BK (2010), The role of exercise-induced myokines in muscle homeostasis and the defense against chronic diseases. Journal of Biomedicine and Biotechnology 2010: 520258.

Cirelli C (2013), Sleep and synaptic changes. Current Opinion in Neurobiology 23(5): 841–846.

Conrad A, Coenen M, Schmalz H et al. (2012), Validation of the comprehensive ICF core set for multiple sclerosis from the perspective of physical therapists. Physical Therapy 92(6): 799–820.

Cramer H, Lauche R, Langhorst J et al. (2013), Predictors of yoga use among internal medicine patients. BMC Complementary and Alternative Medicine 13: 172.

De Couck M, Mravec B, Gidron Y (2012), You may need the vagus nerve to understand pathophysiology and to treat diseases. Clinical Science 122(7): 323–328.

Dean E (2009), Physical therapy in the 21st century (Part I): toward practice informed by epidemiology and the crisis of lifestyle conditions. Physiotherapy Theory and Practice 25(5–6): 330–353.

Dean E, Al-Obaidi S, De Andrade AD et al. (2011), The first physical therapy summit on global health: implications and recommendations for the 21st century. Physiotherapy Theory and Practice 27(8): 531–547.

Dimatteo MR, Haskard KB, Williams SL (2007), Health beliefs, disease severity, and patient adherence: a meta-analysis. Medical Care 45(6): 521–528.

Doyle C, Lennox L, Bell D (2013), A systematic review of evidence on the links between patient experience and clinical safety and effectiveness. BMJ Open 3(1): pii: e001570.

Dunn W (2009), Living Sensationally: Understanding Your Senses. Jessica Kingsley, London.

Easwaren E (1985), The Bhagavad Gita. Vintage Spiritual Classics, New York.

Easwaren E (2007), The Upanishads. Blue Mountain Center of Meditation, Tomales, CA.

Eisler RT (2007), The Real Wealth of Nations: Creating a Caring Economics. Berrett-Koehler, San Francisco, CA.

Eisler RT, Potter TM (2014), Transforming Interprofessional Partnerships: A New Framework for Nursing and Partnership-based Health Care. Sigma Theta Tau International, Indianapolis, IN.

Elenkov IJ, Iezzoni DG, Daly A (2005), Cytokine dysregulation, inflammation and well-being. Neuroimmunomodulation 12: 255–269.

Elliott AM, Smith BH, Hannaford PC et al. (2002), The course of chronic pain in the community: results of a 4-year follow-up study. Pain 99(1–2): 299–307.

REFERENCES

Erden ES, Genc S, Motor S et al. (2014), Investigation of serum bisphenol A, vitamin D, and parathyroid hormone levels in patients with obstructive sleep apnea syndrome. Endocrine 45(2): 311–318.

Fallone G (2002), Sleepiness in children and adolescents: clinical implications. Sleep Medicine Reviews 6(4): 287–306.

Folkins J (1992), Resource on Person-First Language. American Speech-Language-Hearing Association Skills for Calling and Caring Ministries – Learning the Language of Healing, developed by Kenneth J Mitchell and John S Savage of LEAD Consultants, Pittsford, New York (1979).

García-Lafuente A, Guillamón E, Villares A (2009), Flavonoids as anti-inflammatory agents: implications in cancer and cardiovascular disease. Inflammation Research 58(9): 537–552.

Garner G (2001), Professional Yoga Therapy, Level I Course Manual.

Garner G (2014), The role of relationship and creativity. In: M Taylor (ed.), Fostering Creativity in Rehabilitation. Nova Science Publishers, New York City, ch 6.

Glassel A, Coenen M, Kollerits B et al. (2014), Content validation of the International Classification of Functioning, Disability and Health core set for stroke from gender perspective using a qualitative approach. European Journal of Physical and Rehabilitation Medicine 50(3): 285–299.

Glocker C, Kirchberger I, Glassel A et al. (2013), Content validity of the comprehensive International Classification of Functioning, Disability and Health (ICF) core set for low back pain from the perspective of physicians: a Delphi survey. Chronic Illness 9(1): 57–72.

Goldberg DS, McGee SJ (2011), Pain as a global public health priority. BMC Public Health 11: 770.

Green JA, Gonzaga AM, Cohen ED et al. (2014), Addressing health literacy through clear health communication: a training program for internal medicine residents. Patient Education and Counseling 95(1): 76–82.

Groenewegen PP, Van den Berg AE, De Vries S et al. (2006), Vitamin G: effects of green space on health, well-being, and social safety. BMC Public Health 6: 149.

Hall AM, Ferreira PH, Maher CG et al. (2010), The influence of the therapist–patient relationship on treatment outcome in physical rehabilitation: a systematic review. Physical Therapy 90(8): 1099–1110.

Harris JE, Macdermid JC, Roth J (2005), The International Classification of Functioning as an explanatory model of health after distal radius fracture: a cohort study. Health and Quality of Life Outcomes 3: 73.

Hermsdorff HH, Zulet MA, Puchau B et al. (2010), Fruit and vegetable consumption and proinflammatory gene expression from peripheral blood mononuclear cells in young adults: a translational study. Nutrition and Metabolism 7: 42.

Hestbaek L, Leboeuf-Yde C, Kyvik KO (2006), Is comorbidity in adolescence a predictor for adult low back pain? A prospective study of a young population. BMC Musculoskeletal Disorders 7: 29.

Hoyez A (2007), The "world of yoga": the production and reproduction of therapeutic landscapes. Social Science and Medicine 65(1): 112–124.

Hughes P, Nienow D (2011), Courageous collaboration with Gracious Space: from small openings to profound transformation. June 2011, Center for Ethical Leadership, Seattle, WA, wwwethicalleadershiporg.

Institute of Medicine (US), Committee on Advancing Pain Research, Care, and Education (2011), Relieving Pain in America: A Blueprint for Transforming Prevention, Care, Education, and Research. National Academies Press, Washington DC.

International Association for the Study of Pain (IASP) and European Federation of IASP Chapters (2012), Unrelieved pain is a major global healthcare problem. http://wwwiasp-painorg/AM/Templatecfm?Section=Home&Template=/CM/ContentDisplaycfm&ContentID=2908 (last accessed August 8, 2012).

Iyengar BKS (1976), Light on Yoga: Yoga Dīpikā. Schocken Books, New York.

Jette AM (2006), Toward a common language for function, disability, and health. Physical Therapy 86(5): 726.

Jin R (2010), Inflammatory mechanisms in ischemic stroke: role of inflammatory cells. Journal of Leukocyte Biology 87(5): 779–789.

Jonsson G, Ekholm J, Schult ML (2008), The International Classification of Functioning, Disability and Health environmental factors as facilitators or barriers used in describing personal and social networks: a pilot study of adults with cerebral palsy. International Journal of Rehabilitation Research 31(2): 119–129.

Kaplan SA, Madden VP, Mijanovich T et al. (2013), The perception of stress and its impact on health in poor communities. Journal of Community Health 38(1): 142–149.

Kato K, Sullivan PF, Evengard B et al. (2006), Chronic widespread pain and its comorbidities: a population-based study. Archives of Internal Medicine 166(15): 1649–1654.

Kaufman A (2012), Linking university health resources to social determinants in the community: prioritizing health disparities in medical education to improve care. Lecture, New York Academy of Sciences, New York, October 2, 2012.

Keller A, Litzelman K, Wisk LE et al. (2012), Does the perception that stress affects health matter? The association with health and mortality. Health Psychology 31(5): 677–684.

Khalsa SB (2013), Your Brain on Yoga. Harvard Medical School Guide, RosettaBooks LLC, New York.

Khan F, Amatya B, Ng L et al. (2012), Relevance and completeness of the International Classification of Functioning, Disability and Health (ICF) comprehensive breast cancer core set: the patient perspective in an Australian community cohort. Journal of Rehabilitation Medicine 44(7): 570–580.

Kienreich K, Tomaschitz A, Verheyen N et al. (2013), Vitamin D and cardiovascular disease. Nutrients 5(8): 3005–3021.

Kitchenham A (2008), The evolution of John Mezirow's transformative learning theory. Journal of Transformative Education 6(2): 104–123.

Kochupillai V, Kumar P, Singh D et al. (2005), Effect of rhythmic breathing (Sudarshan Kriya and Pranayam) on immune functions and tobacco addiction. Annals of the New York Academy of Sciences 1056: 242–252.

Krein SL, Heisler M, Piette JD et al. (2005), The effect of chronic pain on diabetes patients' self-management. Diabetes Care 28(1): 65–70.

Kuntsevich V, Bushell WC, Theise ND (2010), Mechanisms of yogic practices in health, aging, and disease. Mount Sinai Journal of Medicine 77(5): 559–569.

Kutner MA, National Center for Education Statistics (2006), The health literacy of America's adults: results from the 2003 national assessment of adult literacy. US Department of Education, September 2006, NCES 2006-483, National Center for Education Statistics, Washington DC.

Lane IF (2010), Professional competencies in health sciences education: from multiple intelligences to the clinic floor. Advances in Health Sciences Education: Theory and Practice 15(1): 129–146.

Lasater JH (2000), Living Your Yoga. Rodmell Press, Berkeley, CA.

Lin YN, Chang KH, Lin CY et al. (2014), Developing comprehensive and Brief ICF core sets for morbid obesity for disability assessment in Taiwan: a preliminary study. European Journal of Physical and Rehabilitation Medicine 50(2): 133–134.

Lundahl B, Moleni T, Burke BL et al. (2013), Motivational interviewing in medical care settings: a systematic review and meta-analysis of randomized controlled trials. Patient Education and Counseling 93(2): 157–168.

Mafi JN, McCarthy EP, Davis RB et al. (2013), Worsening trends in the management and treatment of back pain. JAMA Internal Medicine 173(17): 1573–1581.

Mathur N, Pedersen BK (2009), Exercise as a means to control low-grade systemic inflammation. Mediators of Inflammation 2008: 109502, epub 2009, doi: 1020091155/2008/109502.

Mezirow J (2003), Transformative learning as discourse. Journal of Transformative Education 1(1): 58–63.

Miciak M, Gross DP, Joyce A (2012), A review of the psychotherapeutic "common factors" model and its application in physical therapy: the need to consider general effects in physical therapy practice. Scandinavian Journal of Caring Sciences 26(2): 394–403.

Mitchell KJ, Savage JS (1979), Skills for Calling and Caring Ministries – Learning the Language of Healing, developed by Kenneth J Mitchell and John S Savage of LEAD Consultants, Pittsford, New York.

Morris DM, Kitchin EM, Clark DE (2009), Strategies for optimizing nutrition and weight reduction in physical therapy practice: the evidence. Physiotherapy Theory and Practice 25(5–6): 408–423.

Nabi H, Kivimaki M, Batty GD et al. (2013), Increased risk of coronary heart disease among individuals reporting adverse impact of stress on their health: the Whitehall II prospective cohort study. European Heart Journal 34(34): 2697–2705.

Nathan C (2008), Epidemic inflammation: pondering obesity. Molecular Medicine 14(7–8): 485–492.

Noggle JJ, Steiner NJ, Minami T et al. (2012), Benefits of yoga for psychosocial well-being in a US high school curriculum: a preliminary randomized controlled trial. Journal of Developmental and Behavioral Pediatrics 33(3): 193–201.

Nosek M (2012), Nonviolent communication: a dialogical retrieval of the ethic of authenticity. Nursing Ethics 19(6): 829–837.

Nygaard E, Heir T (2012), World assumptions, posttraumatic stress and quality of life after a natural disaster: a longitudinal study. Health and Quality of Life Outcomes 10: 76.

Oberhauser C, Escorpizo R, Boonen A et al. (2013), Statistical validation of the brief International Classification of Functioning, Disability and Health core set for osteoarthritis based on a large international sample of patients with osteoarthritis. Arthritis Care and Research 65(2): 177–186.

Patel NK, Newstead AH, Ferrer RL (2012), The effects of yoga on physical functioning and health related quality of life in older adults: a systematic review and meta-analysis. Journal of Alternative and Complementary Medicine 18(10): 902–917.

Pergolizzi J, Ahlbeck K, Aldington D et al. (2013), The development of chronic pain: physiological change necessitates a multidisciplinary approach to treatment. Current Medical Research and Opinion 29(9): 1127–1135.

Pedersen BK (2006), The anti-inflammatory effect of exercise: its role in diabetes and cardiovascular disease control. Essays in Biochemistry 42: 105–117.

Pedersen BK (2011), Exercise-induced myokines and their role in chronic diseases. Brain, Behavior, and Immunity 25(5): 811–816.

Petersen AM, Pedersen BK (2006), The role of IL-6 in mediating the anti-inflammatory effects of exercise. Journal of Physiology and Pharmacology 57(Suppl. 10): 43–51.

Peterson PN, Shetterly SM, Clarke CL et al. (2011), Health literacy and outcomes among patients with heart failure. JAMA 305(16): 1695–1701.

Piette JD, Kerr EA (2006), The impact of comorbid chronic conditions on diabetes care. Diabetes Care 29(3): 725–731.

Pomeroy C (2012), Health disparities and social justice: a call to action for academic health centers: prioritizing health disparities in medical education to improve care. Lecture, New York Academy of Sciences, October 2, New York.

Pullen PR, Nagamia SH, Mehta PK et al. (2008), Effects of yoga on inflammation and exercise capacity in patients with chronic heart failure. Journal of Cardiac Failure 14(5): 407–413.

Quality Metric (2013), SF Health Surveys, http://wwwqualitymetriccom/WhatWeDo/GenericHealthSurveys/tabid/184/Defaultaspx(last accessed September 26, 2013).

Rollnick S, Miller WR, Butler C (2008), Motivational Interviewing in Health Care: Helping Patients Change Behavior. Guilford Press, New York.

Rosenbaum P, Stewart D (2004), The World Health Organization International Classification of Functioning, Disability, and Health: a model to guide clinical thinking, practice and research in the field of cerebral palsy. Seminars in Pediatric Neurology 11(1): 5–10.

Rosenberg MB (2003), Nonviolent Communication: A Language of Life. PuddleDancer Press, Encinitas, CA.

Ross A, Thomas S (2010), The health benefits of yoga and exercise: a review of comparison studies. Journal of Alternative and Complementary Medicine 16(1): 3–12.

Rudolf KD, Kus S, Chung KC et al. (2012), Development of the International Classification of Functioning, Disability and Health core sets for hand conditions – results of the World Health Organization international consensus process. Disability and Rehabilitation 34(8): 681–693.

Rutten GM, Harting J, Bartholomew LK et al. (2014), Development of a theory- and evidence-based intervention to enhance implementation of physical therapy guidelines for the management of low back pain. Archives of Public Health 72(1): 1.

Ryan JW, Anderson PH, Turner AG et al. (2013), Vitamin D activities and metabolic bone disease. Clinica Chimica Acta 425: 148–152.

Saha S (2006), Improving literacy as a means to reducing health disparities. Journal of General Internal Medicine 21(8): 893–895.

Saltychev M, Eskola M, Laimi K (2014), Lumbar fusion compared with conservative treatment in patients with chronic low back pain: a meta-analysis. International Journal of Rehabilitation Research 37(1): 2–8.

Scholl TO, Chen X, Stein TP (2013), Vitamin D, secondary hyperparathyroidism, and preeclampsia. American Journal of Clinical Nutrition 98(3): 787–793.

Scorza P, Stevenson A, Canino G (2013), Validation of the "World Health Organization Disability Assessment Schedule for children, WHODAS–Child" in Rwanda. PloS one 8(3): e57725.

Scott TL, Gazmararian JA, Williams MV et al. (2002), Health literacy and preventive health care use among Medicare enrollees in a managed care organization. Medical Care 40(5): 395–404.

Serafini M, Peluso I, Raguzzini A (2010), Flavonoids as anti-inflammatory agents. Proceedings of the Nutrition Society 69(3): 273–278.

Shochat T, Cohen-Zion M, Tzischinsky O (2014), Functional consequences of inadequate sleep in adolescents: a systematic review. Sleep Medicine Reviews 18(1): 75–87.

Streeter CC, Whitfield TH, Owen L et al. (2010), Effects of yoga versus walking on mood, anxiety, and brain GABA levels: a randomized controlled MRS study. Journal of Alternative and Complementary Medicine 16(11): 1145–1152.

Streeter CC, Gerbarg PL, Saper RB et al. (2012), Effects of yoga on the autonomic nervous system, gamma-aminobutyric-acid, and allostasis in epilepsy, depression, and post-traumatic stress disorder. Medical Hypotheses 78(5): 571–579.

Sudore RL, Yaffe K, Satterfield S et al. (2006), Limited literacy and mortality in the elderly: the health, aging, and body composition study. Journal of General Internal Medicine 21(8): 806–812.

Tawoda T (2012), Three pain specialists on shaping pain management healthcare policy. Becker Spine Review, April 26, 2012. http://beckersspinecom/pain-management/item/11705-3-pain-specialists-on-shaping-pain-management-healthcare-policy (last accessed July 29, 2013).

Tekur P, Nagarathna R, Chametcha S et al. (2012), A comprehensive yoga program improves pain, anxiety and depression in chronic low back pain patients more than exercise: an RCT. Complementary Therapies in Medicine 20(3): 107–118.

The Patient Patient (2013), The Biopsychosocial Model of Disease. wwwthepatientpatient2011blogspotcouk (last accessed July 28, 2015).

Turiano NA, Chapman BP, Agrigoroaei S et al. (2014), Perceived control reduces mortality risk at low, not high, education levels. Health Psychology 33(8): 883–890.

US Department of Health and Human Services, Office of Disease Prevention and Health Promotion (2010), National action plan to improve health literacy. http://wwwhealthgov/communication/hlactionplan/ (last accessed June 11, 2014).

Van Hecke O, Torrance N, Smith BH (2013), Chronic pain epidemiology and its clinical relevance. British Journal of Anaesthesia 111(1): 13–18.

Wahdan M (1996), The epidemiological transition. Eastern Mediterranean Health Journal 2(1): 8.

Watzl B (2008), Anti-inflammatory effects of plant-based foods and of their constituents. International Journal for Vitamin and Nutrition Research 78(6): 293–298.

White S, Chen J, Atchison R (2008), Relationship of preventive health practices and health literacy: a national study. American Journal of Health Behavior 32(3): 227–242.

Wilund KR (2007), Is the anti-inflammatory effect of regular exercise responsible for reduced cardiovascular disease? Clinical Science (London) 112: 543–555.

World Health Organization (1948), Preamble to the Constitution of the World Health Organization as adopted by the International Health Conference, New York, June 19–22, 1946; signed on July 22, 1946, by the representatives of 61 states (Official Records of the World Health Organization, no. 2, p. 100) and entered into force on April 7, 1948.

World Health Organization (2001), The International Classification of Functioning, Disability and Health. World Health Organization, Geneva.

World Health Organization (2002), Towards a Common Language for Functioning, Disability and Health: ICF. World Health Organization, Geneva.

World Health Organization (2005), Preventing Chronic Diseases – A Vital Investment: WHO Global Report. World Health Organization, Geneva.

World Health Organization (2010), Framework for Action on Interprofessional Education and Collaborative Practice. WHO Department of Human Resources for Health, WHO Press, Geneva.

Yang K (2007), A review of yoga programs for four leading risk factors of chronic diseases. Evidence-Based Complementary and Alternative Medicine: eCAM 4(4): 487–491.

Chapter 3

Adeeb N, Mortazavi MM, Tubbs RS et al. (2012), The cranial dura mater: a review of its history, embryology, and anatomy. Childs Nervous System 28(6): 827–837.

Ajimsha MS, Al-Mudahka NR, Al-Madzhar JA (2015), Effectiveness of myofascial release: systematic review of randomized controlled trials. Journal of Bodywork and Movement Therapies 19(1): 102–112.

Alfonse T, Masi AT, Nair K et al. (2010), Clinical, biomechanical, and physiological translational interpretations of human resting myofascial tone or tension. International Journal of Therapeutic Massage and Bodywork 3(4): 16–28.

Aligene K, Lin E (2013), Vestibular and balance treatment of the concussed athlete. NeuroRehabilitation 32(3): 543–553.

Allison GT, Morris SL (2008), Transversus abdominis and core stability: has the pendulum swung? British Journal of Sports Medicine 42(11): 930–931.

Alsalaheen BA, Mucha A, Morris LO et al. (2010), Vestibular rehabilitation for dizziness and balance disorders after concussion. Journal of Neurologic Physical Therapy 34(2): 87–93.

Anraku M, Shargall Y (2009), Surgical conditions of the diaphragm: anatomy and physiology. Thoracic Surgery Clinics 19(4): 419–429.

Arab AM, Behbahani RB, Lorestani L et al. (2010), Assessment of pelvic floor muscle function in women with and without low back pain using transabdominal ultrasound. Manual Therapy 15(3): 235–239.

Arendt E, Dick R (1995), Knee injury patterns among men and women in collegiate basketball and soccer NCAA data and review of literature. American Journal of Sports Medicine 23: 694–701.

Avison J (2015), Yoga: Fascia, Anatomy and Movement. Handspring Publishing, Pencaitland, UK.

Badel T, Savic-Pavicin I, Zadravec D et al. (2011), Temporomandibular joint development and functional disorders related to clinical otologic symptomatology. Acta Clinica Croatica 50(1): 51–60.

Bandy WD (1997), The effect of time and frequency of static stretching on flexibility of the hamstring muscles. Physical Therapy 77(10): 1090–1096.

Barber-Westin SD, Noyes FR, Smith ST et al. (2009), Reducing the risk of noncontact anterior cruciate ligament injuries in the female athlete. Physician and Sportsmedicine 37(3): 49–61.

Barker P, Briggs CA, Bogeski G (2004), Tensile transmission across the lumbar fasciae in unembalmed cadavers: effects of tension to various muscular attachments. Spine 29(2): 129–138.

Barker PJ, Freeman AD, Urquhart DM et al. (2010), The middle layer of lumbar fascia can transmit tensile forces capable of fracturing the lumbar transverse processes: an experimental study. Clinical Biomechanics (Bristol, Avon) 25(6): 505–509.

Ben M, Harvey LA (2010), Regular stretch does not increase muscle extensibility: a randomized controlled trial. Scandinavian Journal of Medicine and Science in Sports 20(1): 136–144.

Bi X, Zhao J, Zhao L et al. (2013), Pelvic floor muscle exercise for chronic low back pain. Journal of International Medical Research 41(1): 146–152.

Bialosky JE, Bishop MD, George SZ (2008), Regional interdependence: a musculoskeletal examination model whose time has come. Journal of Orthopaedic and Sports Physical Therapy 38(3): 159–160; author reply 160.

Bø K, Sherburn M (2005), Evaluation of female pelvic-floor muscle function and strength. Physical Therapy 85(3): 269–282.

Bolgla LA, Malone TR, Umberger BR et al. (2011), Comparison of hip and knee strength and neuromuscular activity in subjects with and without patellofemoral pain syndrome. International Journal of Sports Physical Therapy 6(4): 285–296.

Boling M, Padua D (2013), Relationship between hip strength and trunk, hip, and knee kinematics during a jump-landing task in individuals with patellofemoral pain. International Journal of Sports Physical Therapy 8(5): 661–669.

Bordoni B, Zanier E (2013), Anatomic connections of the diaphragm: influence of respiration on the body system. Journal of Multidisciplinary Healthcare 6: 281–291.

Bordoni B, Zanier E (2015), The continuity of the body: hypothesis of treatment of the five diaphragms. Journal of Alternative and Complementary Medicine 21(4): 237–242.

Brown RP, Gerbarg PL (2009), Yoga breathing, meditation, and longevity. Annals of the New York Academy of Sciences 1172: 54–62.

Bush HM, Pagorek S, Kuperstein J et al. (2013), The association of chronic back pain and stress urinary incontinence: a cross-sectional study. Journal of Women's Health Physical Therapy 37(1): 11–18.

Bushell WC (2009), Longevity: potential life span and health span enhancement through practice of the basic yoga meditation regimen. Annals of the New York Academy of Sciences 1172: 20–27.

Butler D (1991), Mobilisation of the Nervous System. Churchill Livingstone, Edinburgh, UK.

Cao TV, Hicks MR, Zein-Hammoud M et al. (2015), Duration and magnitude of myofascial release in 3-dimensional bioengineered tendons: effects on wound healing. Journal of the American Osteopathic Association 115(2): 72–82.

Casey E, Hameed F, Dhaher YY (2014), The muscle stretch reflex throughout the menstrual cycle. Medicine and Science in Sports and Exercise 46(3): 600–609.

Cashman GE (2012), The effect of weak hip abductors or external rotators on knee valgus kinematics in healthy subjects: a systematic review. Journal of Sport Rehabilitation 21(3): 273–284.

Chan SP, Hong Y, Robinson PD (2001), Flexibility and passive resistance of the hamstrings of young adults using two different static stretching protocols. Scandinavian Journal of Medicine and Science in Sports 11: 81–86.

Chapleau MW, Sabharwal R (2011), Methods of assessing vagus nerve activity and reflexes Heart Failure Reviews 16(2): 109–127.

Chiappa GR, Roseguini BT, Vieira PJ et al. (2008), Inspiratory muscle training improves blood flow to resting and exercising limbs in patients with chronic heart failure. Journal of the American College of Cardiology 51(17): 1663–1671.

Chung MJ, Wang M-JJ (2009), The effect of age and gender on joint range of motion of worker population in Taiwan. International Journal of Industrial Ergonomics 39(4): 596–600.

Cimen A, Celik M, Erdine S (2004), Myofascial pain syndrome in the differential diagnosis of chronic abdominal pain. Agri 16(3): 45–47.

Cipriani DJ, Terry ME, Haines MA et al. (2012), Effect of stretch frequency and sex on the rate of gain and rate of loss in muscle flexibility during a hamstring-stretching program: a randomized single-blind longitudinal study. Journal of Strength and Conditioning Research 26(8): 2119–2129.

Craig AD (2002), How do you feel? Interoception: the sense of the physiological condition of the body. Nature Reviews Neuroscience 3(8): 655–666.

Cresswell AG, Grundstrom H, Thorstensson A (1992), Observations on intra-abdominal pressure and patterns of abdominal intra-muscular activity in man. Acta Physiologica Scandinavica 144(4): 409–418.

Cretikos MA, Bellomo R, Hillman K et al. (2008), Respiratory rate: the neglected vital sign. Medical Journal of Australia 188(11): 657–659.

Da Silva RC, De Sá CC, Pascual-Vaca AO et al. (2013), Increase of lower esophageal sphincter pressure after osteopathic intervention on the diaphragm in patients with gastroesophageal reflux. Diseases of the Esophagus 26(5): 451–456.

Daban C, Martinez-Aran A, Cruz N et al. (2008), Safety and efficacy of vagus nerve stimulation in treatment-resistant depression. A systematic review. Journal of Affective Disorders 110: 1–15.

Dakwar E, Ahmadian A, Uribe JS (2012), The anatomical relationship of the diaphragm to the thoracolumbar junction during the minimally invasive lateral extracoelomic (retropleural/retroperitoneal) approach. Journal of Neurosurgery, Spine 16(4): 359–364.

Day JA, Copetti L, Rucli G (2012), From clinical experience to a model for the human fascial system. Journal of Bodywork and Movement Therapies 16(3): 372–380.

De Couck M, Nijs J, Gidron Y (2014), You may need a nerve to treat pain: the neurobiological rationale for vagal nerve activation in pain management. Clinical Journal of Pain 30(12): 1099–1105.

De Weijer VC, Gorniak GC, Shamus E (2003), The effect of static stretch and warm-up exercise on hamstring length over the course of 24 hours. Journal of Orthopaedic and Sports Physical Therapy 33: 727–733.

Delitto A, George SZ, Van Dillen LR et al., Orthopaedic Section of the American Physical Therapy Association (2012), Low back pain. Journal of Orthopaedic and Sports Physical Therapy 42(4): A1–A57.

Doebler M (2000), The effect of different static stretch hold times on hamstring muscle flexibility in active college students. Physical Therapy 80: 68.

Donatelli RA, Thurner MS (2014), The Young Athlete's Spinal Mechanics: Spinal Injuries and Conditions in Young Athletes. Springer, New York, pp. 17–25.

Downey R (2011), Anatomy of the normal diaphragm. Thoracic Surgery Clinics 21(2): 273–279.

Drake R, Vogl AW, Mitchell AWM (2009), Gray's Anatomy for Students, 2nd edition. Elsevier/Churchill Livingstone, New York.

Driscoll SW (2013), Concussion in children: what are the effects? Mayo Clinic, http://wwwmayocliniccom/health/concussion-in-children/AN02059, last accessed November 3, 2013.

Duong B, Low M, Moseley AM et al. (2001), Time course of stress relaxation and recovery in human ankles. Clinical Biomechanics (Bristol, Avon) 16: 601–607.

Dusek JA, Otu HH, Wohlhueter AL et al. (2008), Genomic counter-stress changes induced by the relaxation response. PloS one 3(7): e2576.

Dvorak J, Vajda EG, Grob D et al. (1995), Normal motion of the lumbar spine as related to age and gender. European Spine Journal 4(1): 18–23.

Dye D (2008), Vestibular rehabilitation: rehabilitation options for patients with dizziness and imbalance. American Speech-Language-Hearing Association Access Audiology 7(4).

Edmondston SJ, Henne SE, Loh W (2005), Influence of craniocervical posture on three dimensional motion of the cervical spine. Manual Therapy 10(1): 44–51.

Eherer A (2014), Management of gastroesophageal reflux disease: lifestyle modification and alternative approaches. Digestive Diseases (Basel, Switzerland) 32(1–2): 149–151.

Eherer AJ, Netolitzky F, Hogenauer C et al. (2012), Positive effect of abdominal breathing exercise on gastroesophageal reflux disease: a randomized, controlled study. American Journal of Gastroenterology 107(3): 372–378.

Eliasson K, Elfving B, Nordgren B et al. (2008), Urinary incontinence in women with low back pain. Manual Therapy 13(3): 206–212.

Epel E, Daubenmier J, Moskowitz JT et al. (2009), Can meditation slow rate of cellular aging? Cognitive stress, mindfulness, and telomeres. Annals of the New York Academy of Sciences 1172: 34–53.

Escamilla RF, Yamashiro K, Paulos L et al. (2009), Shoulder muscle activity and function in common shoulder rehabilitation exercises. Sports Medicine (Auckland, NZ) 39(8): 663–685.

Eyre H, Baune BT (2012), Neuroplastic changes in depression: a role for the immune system. Psychoneuroendocrinology 37(9): 1397–1416.

Fenton BW (2007), Limbic associated pelvic pain: a hypothesis to explain the diagnostic relationships and features of patients with chronic pelvic pain. Medical Hypotheses 69(2): 282–286.

Findley T, Chaudhry H, Stecco A et al. (2012), Fascia research – a narrative review. Journal of Bodywork and Movement Therapies 16(1): 67–75.

Folpp H, Deall S, Harvey LA et al. (2006), Can apparent increases in muscle extensibility with regular stretch be explained by changes in tolerance to stretch? Australian Journal of Physiotherapy 52(1): 45–50.

Franklin DW (2004), Impedance control balances stability with metabolically costly muscle activation. Journal of Neurophysiology 92(5): 3097–3105.

Fritz JM, Childs JD, Wainner RS et al. (2012), Primary care referral of patients with low back pain to physical therapy: impact on future health care utilization and costs. Spine 37(25): 2114–2121.

Fryer G, Morris T, Gibbons P (2004), Paraspinal muscles and intervertebral dysfunction: part 2. Journal of Manipulative and Physiological Therapeutics 27(5): 348–357.

Fuller RB (1975), Synergetics: Explorations in the Geometry of Thinking. Macmillan, London.

Gandevia SC, Mckenzie DK (2008), Respiratory rate: the neglected vital sign. Medical Journal of Australia 189(9): 532.

Gao F, Ren Y, Roth EJ et al. (2011), Effects of repeated ankle stretching on calf muscle-tendon and ankle biomechanical properties in stroke survivors. Clinical Biomechanics 26(5): 516–522.

Garner G (2001), Medical Therapeutic Yoga. Excerpt from Professional Yoga Therapy Studies Course Manuals, volumes I–IV. Living Well, Emerald Isle, NC.

Garner G (2013), Combining integrative medicine (yoga) with vestibular rehabilitation. Presentation, North Carolina Athletic Trainers' Association Annual Fall Symposium, November 9.

Garner G (2012), Medical Therapeutic Yoga. Vestibular case study. Module 4. Yoga as Medicine. Professional Yoga Therapy Studies, Professional Yoga Therapist Certification CE.

Garner Wood G (2004), Chronic pain and yoga: telling our story. International Journal of Yoga Therapy 14(1): 59–67.

Gellhorn AC, Chan L, Martin B et al. (2012), Management patterns in acute low back pain: the role of physical therapy. Spine, 37(9): 775–782.

Goldhill DR, McNarry AF, Mandersloot G et al. (2005), A physiologically-based early warning score for ward patients: the association between score and outcome. Anaesthesia 60: 547–553.

Goleman D (2013), The focused leader. Harvard Business Review, December 2013.

Goligher EC, Laghi F, Detsky ME et al. (2015), Measuring diaphragm thickness with ultrasound in mechanically ventilated patients: feasibility, reproducibility and validity. Intensive Care Medicine 41(4): 642–649.

Greenwood BN, Fleshner M (2011), Exercise, stress resistance, and central serotonergic systems. Exercise and Sport Sciences Reviews 39(3): 140–149.

Greenwood BN, Spence KG, Crevling DM et al. (2013), Exercise-induced stress resistance is independent of exercise controllability and the medial prefrontal cortex. European Journal of Neuroscience 37(3): 469–478.

Grewar H, Mclean L (2008), The integrated continence system: a manual therapy approach to the treatment of stress urinary incontinence. Manual Therapy 13(5): 375–386.

Griesbach GS, Tio DL, Nair S et al. (2013), Temperature and heart rate responses to exercise following mild traumatic brain injury. Journal of Neurotrauma 30(4): 281–291.

Groenewegen PP, Van Den Berg AE, De Vries S et al. (2006), Vitamin G: effects of green space on health, well-being, and social safety. BMC Public Health 6: 149.

Groves AK, Fekete DM (2012), Shaping sound in space: the regulation of inner ear patterning. Development (Cambridge, England) 139(2): 245–257.

Guimberteau J-C, Armstrong C (2015), Architecture of Human Living Fascia. Handspring Publishing, Pencaitland, UK.

Gurley JM, Hujsak BD, Kelly JL (2013), Vestibular rehabilitation following mild traumatic brain injury. NeuroRehabilitation 32(3): 519–528.

Harmon KG, Drezner JA, Gammons M et al. (2013), American Medical Society for Sports Medicine position statement: concussion in sport. British Journal of Sports Medicine 47(1): 15–26.

Hasebe K, Sairyo K, Hada Y et al. (2014), Spino-pelvic-rhythm with forward trunk bending in normal subjects without low back pain. European Journal of Orthopaedic Surgery and Traumatology 24(Suppl. 1): S193–S199.

Heller AS, Johnstone T, Shackman AJ et al. (2009), Reduced capacity to sustain positive emotion in major depression reflects diminished maintenance of fronto-striatal brain activation. Proceedings of the National Academy of Sciences of the United States of America 106(52): 22445–22450.

Hewett TE, Myer GD, Ford KR (2004), Decrease in neuromuscular control about the knee with maturation in female athletes. Journal of Bone and Joint Surgery American Volume 86-A(8): 1601–1608.

Hewett TE, Myer GD, Ford KR et al. (2007), Dynamic neuromuscular analysis training for preventing anterior cruciate ligament injury in female athletes. Instructional Course Lectures 56: 397–406.

Hides JA, Richardson CA, Jull GA (1996), Multifidus muscle recovery is not automatic after resolution of acute, first-episode low back pain. Spine 21(23): 2763–2769.

Hides JA, Jull GA, Richardson CA (2001), Long-term effects of specific stabilizing exercises for first-episode low back pain. Spine 26(11): E243–E248.

Hilton J (1863), On rest and pain: a course of lectures on the influence of mechanical and physiological rest in the treatment of accidents and surgical diseases, and the diagnostic value of pain, delivered at the Royal College of Surgeons of England in the years 1860, 1861, and 1862. Hilton, London.

Hodges PW, Cholewicki J (2007), Functional control of the spine. In: A Vleeming, V Mooney, R Stoeckart (eds), Movement, Stability and Lumbopelvic Pain. Elsevier, Edinburgh, ch. 33.

Hodges PW, Gandevia SC (2000), Activation of the human diaphragm during a repetitive postural task. Journal of Physiology 522(1): 165–175.

Hodges PW, Richardson CA (1996), Inefficient muscular stabilization of the lumbar spine associated with low back pain: a motor control evaluation of transversus abdominis. Spine 21(22): 2640–2650.

Hodges PW, Richardson CA (1999), Transversus abdominis and the superficial abdominal muscles are controlled independently in a postural task. Neuroscience Letters 265(2): 91–94.

Hodges P, Kaigle Holm A, Holm S et al. (2003), Intervertebral stiffness of the spine is increased by evoked contraction of transversus abdominis and the diaphragm: in vivo porcine studies. Spine 28(23): 2594–2601.

Hodgetts TJ, Kenward G, Vlachonikalis IG et al. (2002), The identification of risk factors for cardiac arrest and formulation of activation criteria to alert a medical emergency team. Resuscitation 54: 125–131.

Hoffman J, Gabel P (2013), Expanding Panjabi's stability model to express movement: a theoretical model. Medical Hypotheses 80(6): 692–697.

Hoge KM, Ryan ED, Costa PB et al. (2010), Gender differences in musculotendinous stiffness and range of motion after an acute bout of stretching. Journal of Strength and Conditioning Research 24(10): 2618–2626.

Holstege G, Bandler R, Clifford S (1996), The emotional motor system. Progress in Brain Research 107: 3–6.

Hujing PA (2009), Epimuscular myofascial force transmission: a historical review and implications for new research. International Society of Biomechanics Muybridge Award lecture, Taipei, 2007. Journal of Biomechanics 42(1): 9–21.

Intolo P, Milosavljevic S, Baxter DG et al. (2009), The effect of age on lumbar range of motion: a systematic review. Manual Therapy 14(6): 596–604.

Iosa M, Fusco A, Morone G et al. (2014), Development and decline of upright gait stability. Frontiers in Aging Neuroscience 6: 14.

Ismail MM, Gamaleldein MH, Hassa KA (2013), Closed kinetic chain exercises with or without additional hip strengthening exercises in management of patellofemoral pain syndrome: a randomized controlled trial. European Journal of Physical and Rehabilitation Medicine 49(5): 687–698.

Jacobs JV, Horak FB (2007), Cortical control of postural responses. Journal of Neural Transmission (Vienna, Austria) 114(10): 1339–1348.

Jacobs CA, Sciascia AD (2011), Factors that influence the efficacy of stretching programs for patients with hypomobility. Sports Health 3(6): 520–523.

Janssens L, Brumagne S, McConnell AK et al. (2013), Greater diaphragm fatigability in individuals with recurrent low back pain. Respiratory Physiology and Neurobiology 188(2): 119–123.

Jeanne M, Logier R, De Jonckheere J et al. (2009), Heart rate variability during total intravenous anesthesia: effects of nociception and analgesia. Autonomic Neuroscience 147: 91–96.

Jemmett RS, Macdonald DA, Agur AM (2004), Anatomical relationships between selected segmental muscles of the lumbar spine in the context of multi-planar segmental motion: a preliminary investigation. Manual Therapy 9(4): 203–210.

Jerath R, Edry JW, Barnes VA et al. (2006), Physiology of long pranayamic breathing: neural respiratory elements may provide a mechanism that explains how slow deep breathing shifts the autonomic nervous system. Medical Hypotheses 67(3): 566–571.

Jeter PE, Nkodo AF, Moonaz SH et al. (2014), A systematic review of yoga for balance in a healthy population. Journal of Alternative and Complementary Medicine 20(4): 221–232.

Jorgensen K, Nicholaisen T, Kato M (1993), Muscle fiber distribution, capillary density, and enzymatic activities in the lumbar paravertebral muscles of young men: significance for isometric endurance. Spine 18(11): 1439–1450.

Joseph CN, Porta C, Casucci G et al. (2005), Slow breathing improves arterial baroreflex sensitivity and decreases blood pressure in essential hypertension. Hypertension 46: 714–718.

Jull GA, Richardson CA (2000), Motor control problems in patients with spinal pain: a new direction for therapeutic exercise. Journal of Manipulative and Physiological Therapeutics 23(2): 115–117.

Jyotsna VP, Ambekar S, Singla R et al. (2013), Cardiac autonomic function in patients with diabetes improves with practice of comprehensive yogic breathing program. Indian Journal of Endocrinology and Metabolism 17(3): 480–485.

Kahkeshani K, Ward PJ (2012), Connection between the spinal dura mater and suboccipital musculature: evidence for the myodural bridge and a route for its dissection. A review. Clinical Anatomy 25(4): 415–422.

Kaltenborn FM, Evjenth O, Kaltenborn TB et al. (1999), Manual Mobilization of the Joints: The Kaltenborn Method of Joint Examination and Treatment: The Extremities, vol 1, Orthopedic Physical Therapy. Olaf Norlis Bokhandel, Oslo.

Kalyani BG, Venkatasubramanian G, Arasappa R et al. (2011), Neurohemodynamic correlates of "OM" chanting: a pilot functional magnetic resonance imaging study. International Journal of Yoga 4: 3–6.

Kapandji IA (2008), The Physiology of the Joints, 6th edition, vol 3. Churchill Livingstone, Edinburgh, UK.

Kemp WJ, 3rd, Tubbs RS, Cohen-Gadol AA (2012), The innervation of the cranial dura mater: neurosurgical case correlates and a review of the literature. World Neurosurgery 78(5): 505–510.

Kerr CE, Sacchet MD, Lazar SW et al. (2013), Mindfulness starts with the body: somatosensory attention and top-down modulation of cortical alpha rhythms in mindfulness meditation. Frontiers in Human Neuroscience 7: 12.

Johnson KO, Yoshioka T, Vega-Bermudez F (2000), Tactile functions of mechanoreceptive afferents innervating the hand. Journal of Clinical Neurophysiology 17: 539–558.

Khalsa SB (2013), Your Brain on Yoga. Harvard Medical School Guide. RosettaBooks LLC, New York.

Kibler WB, Ludewig PM, McClure PW et al. (2013), Clinical implications of scapular dyskinesis in shoulder injury: the 2013 consensus statement from the "scapular summit". British Journal of Sports Medicine 47(14): 877–885.

Kiecolt-Glaser JK, Christian L, Preston H et al. (2010), Stress, inflammation, and yoga practice. Psychosomatic Medicine 72(2): 113–121.

Kistemaker DA, Van Soest AJ, Wong JD et al. (2013), Control of position and movement is simplified by combined muscle spindle and Golgi tendon organ feedback. Journal of Neurophysiology 109(4): 1126–1139.

Kitada R (2010), Tactile sensation. In: The Corsini Encyclopedia of Psychology. Wiley, Hoboken, NJ.

Kjaer M, Hansen M (2008), The mystery of female connective tissue. Journal of Applied Physiology 105(4): 1026–1027.

Knudson DV, Magnusson P, McHugh MP (2000), Current issues in flexibility fitness. President's Council on Physical Fitness and Sports 3: 1–6.

Kolar P, Sulc J, Kyncl M et al. (2010), Stabilizing function of the diaphragm: dynamic MRI and synchronized spirometric assessment. Journal of Applied Physiology 109(4): 1064–1071.

Kolar P, Sulc J, Kyncl M et al. (2012), Postural function of the diaphragm in persons with and without chronic low back pain. Journal of Orthopaedic and Sports Physical Therapy 42(4): 352–362.

Kucyi A, Salomons TV, Davis KD (2013), Mind wandering away from pain dynamically engages antinociceptive and default mode brain networks. Proceedings of the National Academy of Sciences of the United States of America 110(46): 18692–18697.

Kumar K, Rizvi S (2014), Historical and present state of neuromodulation in chronic pain. Current Pain and Headache Reports 18(1): 387.

Kuntsevich V, Bushell WC, Theise ND (2010), Mechanisms of yogic practices in health, aging, and disease. Mount Sinai Journal of Medicine 77(5): 559–569.

Lakkireddy D, Atkins D, Pillarisetti J et al. (2013), Effect of yoga on arrhythmia burden, anxiety, depression, and quality of life in paroxysmal atrial fibrillation: the YOGA My Heart Study. Journal of the American College of Cardiology 61(11): 1177–1182.

Langevin HM, Bouffard NA, Fox JR et al. (2011), Fibroblast cytoskeletal remodeling contributes to connective tissue tension. Journal of Cellular Physiology 226: 1166–1175.

Laulan J, Fouquet B, Rodaix C et al. (2011), Thoracic outlet syndrome: definition, aetiological factors, diagnosis, management, and occupational impact. Journal of Occupational Rehabilitation 21(3): 366–373.

Le Bars D (2002), The whole body receptive field of dorsal horn multireceptive neurones. Brain Research Brain Research Reviews 40(1–3): 29–44.

Lederman E (2010), The myth of core stability. Journal of Bodywork and Movement Therapies 14(1): 84–98.

Lee D (2005), Pelvic stability and your core. Presented in whole or part at the American Back Society Meeting, San Francisco, 2005; BC Trial Lawyers Meeting, Vancouver, 2005; Japanese Society of Posture and Movement Meeting, Tokyo, 2006. Diane Lee and Associates.

Lee D (2006), An integrated model of "joint" function and its clinical application. Paper presented at the 4th Interdisciplinary

World Congress on Low Back Pain, March 29, 2006. http: // wwwphysioblastsorg/p/content/contentphp?content80 (last accessed September 9, 2015).

Lee D (2011), The Pelvic Girdle: An Integration of Clinical Expertise and Research, 4th edition. Churchill Livingstone/ Elsevier, Edinburgh, UK.

Lee SP, Powers C (2013), Description of a weight-bearing method to assess hip abductor and external rotator muscle performance. Journal of Orthopaedic and Sports Physical Therapy 43(6): 392–397.

Lee DG, Vleeming A (1998), Impaired load transference through the pelvic girdle – a new model of altered neutral zone function. Presented at the 3rd Interdisciplinary World Congress on Low Back Pain and Pelvic Pain, Vienna, Austria, November.

Lee DG, Lee LJ, McLaughlin L (2008), Stability, continence and breathing – the role of fascia in both function and dysfunction and the potential consequences following pregnancy and delivery. Journal of Bodywork and Movement Therapies 12: 333–348.

Lehrer PM, Vaschillo E, Vasschillo B et al. (2003), HRV in biofeedback increases baroreflex gain and peak expiratory flow. Psychosomatic Medicine 65: 796–805.

Levangie PK, Norkin CC (2011), Joint Structure and Function: A Comprehensive Analysis, 5th edition. FA Davis, Philadelphia, PA.

Levin SM (2012), Comments on Fascia Talkshow, episode 7, Biotensegrity (Avison). wwwbodyworkcpdcouk (190912 webinar).

Lewandowski W, Jacobson A (2013), Bridging the gap between mind and body: a biobehavioral model of the effects of guided imagery on pain, pain disability, and depression. Pain Management Nursing 14(4): 368–378.

Liakakosa T, Thomakosc N, Finec PM et al. (2001), Peritoneal adhesions: etiology, pathophysiology, and clinical significance, recent advances in prevention and management. Digestive Surgery 18: 260–273.

Liddell EGT, Sherrington CS (1924), Reflexes in response to stretch (myotatic reflexes). Proceedings of the Royal Society of London B 96: 212–242.

Littrell JL (2012), Taking the perspective that a depressive state reflects inflammation: implications for the use of antidepressants. Frontiers in Psychology 3: 297.

Lotrich FE, El-Gabalawy H, Guenther LC et al. (2011), The role of inflammation in the pathophysiology of depression: different treatments and their effects. Journal of Rheumatology 88(Suppl.): 48–54.

Loukas M, Shoja MM, Thurston T et al. (2008), Anatomy and biomechanics of the vertebral aponeurosis part of the posterior layer of the thoracolumbar fascia. Surgical and Radiolgic Anatomy 30(2): 125–129.

Luomajoki H, Moseley GL (2011), Tactile acuity and lumbopelvic motor control in patients with back pain and healthy controls. British Journal of Sports Medicine 45(5): 437–440.

MacDonald DA, Lorimer Moseley G, Hodges PW (2006), The lumbar multifidus: does the evidence support clinical beliefs? Manual Therapy 11(4): 254–263.

McGlone F, Reilly D (2010), The cutaneous sensory system. Neuroscience and Biobehavioral Reviews 34(2): 148–159.

McGonigal K (2013), The Upside of Stress. TEDGlobal 2013. http: //blogtedcom/2013/06/11/the-upside-of-stress-kelly-mcgonigal-at-tedglobal-2013/ (last accessed September 18, 2013).

McGrath N, Dinn WM, Collins MW et al. (2013), Post-exertion neurocognitive test failure among student-athletes following concussion. Brain Injury 27(1): 103–113.

McGregor AH, McCarthy ID, Hughes SP (1995), Motion characteristics of the lumbar spine in the normal population. Spine 20: 2421–2428.

McNair PJ, Dombroski EW, Hewson DJ et al. (2001), Stretching at the ankle joint: viscoelastic responses to holds and continuous passive motion. Medicine and Science in Sports and Exercise 33: 354–358.

Mafi JN, McCarthy EP, Davis RB et al. (2013), Worsening trends in the management and treatment of back pain. JAMA Internal Medicine 173(17): 1573–1581.

Magnusson SP, Simonsen EB, Aagaard P et al. (1995), Viscoelastic response to repeated static stretching in the human hamstring muscle. Scandinavian Journal of Medicine and Science in Sports 5: 342–347.

Magnusson SP, Simonsen EB, Aagaard P et al. (1996), A mechanism for altered flexibility in human skeletal muscle. Journal of Physiology 497: 291–298.

Magnusson SP, Aagard P, Simonsen E et al. (1998), A biomechanical evaluation of cyclic and static stretch in human skeletal muscle. International Journal of Sports Medicine 19: 310–316.

Magnusson SP, Mrici MV, Maganaris CN et al. (2008), Human tendon behavior and adaptation, in vivo. Journal of Physiology (London) 586: 71–81.

Maitland GD (1977), Peripheral Manipulation, 2nd edition. Butterworths, London.

Maitland GD (1986), Vertebral Manipulation, 5th edition. Butterworths, London.

Malone TR, Hardaker WT, Garrett WE et al. (1993), Relationship of gender to anterior cruciate ligament injuries in intercollegiate basketball players. Journal of the Southern Orthopaedic Association 2: 36–39.

Mancini F, Nash T, Iannetti GD et al. (2014), Pain relief by touch: a quantitative approach. Pain 155(3): 635–642.

Marcus EM, Jacobson S (2003), Integrated Neuroscience: A Clinical Problem Solving Approach, vol I. Springer, New York.

Mason H, Vandoni M, Debarbieri G et al. (2013), Cardiovascular and respiratory effect of yogic slow breathing in the yoga beginner: what is the best approach? Evidence-Based Complementary and Alternative Medicine eCAM 2013: 743504.

Meira EP, Brumitt J (2011), Influence of the hip on patients with patellofemoral pain syndrome: a systematic review. Sports Health 3(5): 455–465.

Melzack R (1990), Phantom limbs and the concept of neuromatrix. Trends in Neurosciences 13: 88–92.

Melzack R, Katz J (2013), Pain. Wiley Interdisciplinary Reviews: Cognitive Science 4(1): 1–15.

Melzack R, Loeser JD (1978), Phantom body pain in paraplegics: evidence for a central "pattern generating mechanism" for pain. Pain 4: 195–210.

Melzack R, Wall PD (1965), Pain mechanisms: a new theory. Science 150: 971–979.

Melzack R, Wall PD (1967), Pain mechanisms: a new theory. Survey of Anesthesiology 11(2): 89.

Mendell LM (2014), Constructing and deconstructing the gate theory of pain. Pain 155(2): 210–216.

Meng Q, Zhang W, Yang Y et al. (2008), Cardiovascular responses during percutaneous radiofrequency thermocoagulation therapy in primary trigeminal neuralgia. Journal of Neurosurgical Anesthesiology 20(2): 131–135.

Mense S (2010), Functional anatomy of muscle: muscle, nociceptors and afferent fibers. In: S Mense, RD Gerwin (eds), Muscle Pain: Understanding the Mechanisms. Springer-Verlag, Berlin, pp. 17–48.

Messlinger K, Fischer MJ, Lennerz JK (2011), Neuropeptide effects in the trigeminal system: pathophysiology and clinical relevance in migraine. Keio Journal of Medicine 60(3): 82–89.

Minett MS, Falk S, Santana-Varela S et al. (2014), Pain without nociceptors? Nav17-independent pain mechanisms. Cell Reports 6(2): 301–312.

Minshull C, Eston R, Bailey A et al. (2014), The differential effects of PNF versus passive stretch conditioning on neuromuscular performance. European Journal of Sport Science 14(3): 233–241.

Morinaka S (2009), Musculoskeletal diseases as a causal factor of cervical vertigo. Auris Nasus Larynx 36(6): 649–654.

Moriondo A, Bianchin F, Marcozzi C et al. (2008), Kinetics of fluid in the rat diaphragmatic submesothelial lymphatic lacunae. American Journal of Physiology Heart and Circulatory Physiology 295(3): H1182–H1190.

Morris SL, Lay B, Allison GT (2012), Corset hypothesis rebutted – transversus abdominis does not co-contract in unison prior to rapid arm movements. Clinical Biomechanics (Bristol, Avon) 27(3): 249–254.

Morris SL, Lay B, Allison GT (2013), Transversus abdominis is part of a global not local muscle synergy during arm movement. Human Movement Science 32(5): 1176–1185.

Moseley GL (2008), Tactile discrimination, but not tactile stimulation alone, reduces chronic limb pain. Pain 137(3): 600–608.

Moseley L (2014), It is not just the brain that changes itself – time to embrace bioplasticity? http: //wwwbodyinmindorg/time-to-embrace-bioplasticity/ (last accessed February 17, 2014).

Multon S, Schoenen J (2005), Pain control by vagus nerve stimulation: from animal to man … and back. Acta Neurologica Belgica 105(2): 62–67.

Myer GD, Ford KR, Hewett TE (2004), Rationale and clinical techniques for anterior cruciate ligament injury prevention among female athletes. Journal of Athletic Training 39(4): 352–364.

Myers T (2009), Anatomy Trains. Churchill Livingstone/Elsevier, Edinburgh, UK.

Myers T (2014), Anatomy Trains. Churchill Livingstone/Elsevier, Edinburgh, UK.

Nemeroff CB, Mayberg HS, Krahl SE et al. (2006), VNS therapy in treatment-resistant depression: clinical evidence and putative neurobiological mechanisms. Neuropsychopharmacology 31: 1345–1355.

Netter F (2014), Atlas of Human Anatomy, 6th edition. Elsevier/Saunders, Philadelphia.

Nilsson U (2008), The anxiety- and pain-reducing effects of music interventions: a systematic review. AORN Journal 87(4): 780–807.

O'Sullivan PB, Beales DJ (2007), Changes in pelvic floor and diaphragm kinematics and respiratory patterns in subjects with sacroiliac joint pain following a motor learning intervention: a case series. Manual Therapy 12: 209–218.

O'Sullivan K, Verschueren S, Van Hoof W et al. (2013), Lumbar repositioning error in sitting: healthy controls versus people with sitting-related non-specific chronic low back pain (flexion pattern). Manual Therapy 18(6): 526–532.

Olivo EL (2009), Protection throughout the life span: the psychoneuroimmunologic impact of Indo-Tibetan meditative and yogic practices. Annals of the New York Academy of Sciences 1172: 163–171.

Oyarce P (2013), Professional Yoga Therapy Studies course vestibular case study created in conjunction with Ginger Garner, submitted May 2013.

Pace TW, Negi LT, Adame DD et al. (2009), Effect of compassion meditation on neuroendocrine, innate immune and behavioral responses to psychosocial stress. Psychoneuroendocrinology 34(1): 87–98.

Panjabi MM (1992a), The stabilizing system of the spine. Part I. Function, dysfunction, adaptation, and enhancement. Journal of Spinal Disorders 5(4): 383–389; discussion 397.

Panjabi MM (1992b), The stabilizing system of the spine. Part II. Neutral zone and instability hypotheses. Journal of Spinal Disorders 5(4): 390–396.

Paoletti S (2006), The Fasciae: Anatomy, Dysfunction and Treatment. Eastland Press, Seattle, WA.

Parker MC, Wilson MS, Van Goor H et al. (2007), Adhesions and colorectal surgery – call for action. Colorectal Disease 9(Suppl. 2): 66–72.

Parshad O, Richards A, Asnani M (2011), Impact of yoga on haemodynamic function in healthy medical students. West Indian Medical Journal 60(2): 148–152.

Parsons J, Marcer N (2005), Osteopathy: Models for Diagnosis, Treatment, and Practice. Elsevier Health Sciences, Edinburgh, UK.

Peiper C, Junge K, Prescher A et al. (2004), Abdominal musculature and the transversalis fascia: an anatomical viewpoint. Hernia 8(4): 376–380.

Peters JS, Tyson NL (2013), Proximal exercises are effective in treating patellofemoral pain syndrome: a systematic review. International Journal of Sports Physical Therapy 8(5): 689–700.

Pickering M, Jones JF (2002), The diaphragm: two physiological muscles in one. Journal of Anatomy 201(4): 305–312.

Pinheiro CH, Medeiros RA, Pinheiro DG et al. (2007), Spontaneous respiratory modulation improves cardiovascular control in essential hypertension. Arquivos Brasileiros de Cardiologia 88: 651–659.

Pischinger A (1991), Matrix and Matrix Regulation: Basis for a Holistic Theory in Medicine. Haug International, Brussels.

Porges SW (1995), Orienting in a defensive world: mammalian modifications of our evolutionary heritage. A polyvagal theory. Psychophysiology 32(4): 301–318.

Porges SW (2007), The polyvagal perspective. Biological Psychology 74(2): 116–143.

Porges S (2011), Polyvagal Theory, Neurophysiological Foundations of Emotions, Attachment, Communication, and Self-Regulation. Norton Series on Interpersonal Neurobiology. WW Norton, New York.

Porges S (2012), The science of compassion: origins, measures, and interventions, ccarestanfordedu, lecture, July 19–22, 2012, Telluride, CO.

Porges S (2015a), The Polyvagal Theory, interview, http: // wwwyoutubecom/watch?v=8tz146HQotY (last accessed February 5, 2015).

Porges S (2015b), Personal interview, July 28, 2015.

Porges SW, Doussard-Roosevelt JA, Portales AL (1996), Infant regulation of the vagal "brake" predicts child behavior problems: a psychobiological model of social behavior. Developmental Psychobiology 29(8): 697–712.

Powers CM (2010), The influence of abnormal hip mechanics on knee injury: a biomechanical perspective. Journal of Orthopaedic and Sports Physical Therapy 40(2): 42–51.

Pruszynski JA, Scott SH (2012), Optimal feedback control and the long-latency stretch response. Experimental Brain Research 218(3): 341–359.

Puce A (2010), Somatosensory function. In: The Corsini Encyclopedia of Psychology, 4th edition. Wiley, Hoboken, NJ.

Purcell L (2009), What are the most appropriate return-to-play guidelines for concussed child athletes? British Journal of Sports Medicine 43(Suppl. 1): i51–i55.

Raison CL, Miller AH (2013), Do cytokines really sing the blues? Cerebrum 2013(July-August): 10.

Raison CL, Capuron L, Miller AH (2006), Cytokines sing the blues: inflammation and the pathogenesis of depression. Trends in Immunology 27(1): 24–31.

Rancour J, Holmes CF, Cipriani DJ (2009), The effects of intermittent stretching following a 4-week static stretching protocol: a randomized trial. Journal of Strength and Conditioning Research 23(8): 2217–2222.

Rao NP, Varambally S, Gangadhar BN (2013), Yoga school of thought and psychiatry: therapeutic potential. Indian Journal of Psychiatry 55(Suppl. 2): S145–S149.

Richardson C, Jull G, Hodges P et al. (1999), Therapeutic Exercise for Spinal Segmental Stabilization in Lower Back Pain. Churchill Livingstone, London.

Riechers RG, Ruff RL (2010), Rehabilitation in the patient with mild traumatic brain injury. Continuum (Minneapolis, Minn) 16(6 Traumatic Brain Injury): 128–149.

Ross A, Thomas S (2010), The health benefits of yoga and exercise: a review of comparison studies. Journal of Alternative and Complementary Medicine 16(1): 3–12.

Roudaut Y, Lonigro A, Coste B et al. (2012), Touch sense: functional organization and molecular determinants of mechanosensitive receptors. Channels (Austin, Texas) 6(4): 234–245.

Rumi (1995), The Essential Rumi, translated by Coleman Barks. Harper, San Francisco, CA.

Ryan ED, Beck TW, Herda TJ et al. (2008), The time course of musculotendinous stiffness responses following different durations of passive stretching. Journal of Orthopaedic and Sports Physical Therapy 38: 632–639.

Saatcioglu F (2013), Regulation of gene expression by yoga, meditation and related practices: a review of recent studies. Asian Journal of Psychiatry 6(1): 74–77.

Sakurai A, Atkins CM, Alonso OF et al. (2012), Mild hyperthermia worsens the neuropathological damage associated with mild traumatic brain injury in rats. Journal of Neurotrauma 29(2): 313–321.

Saladin K (2012), Anatomy and Physiology: The Unity of Form and Function. McGraw Hill, New York, pp. 607–608.

Sapsford RR, Hodges PW, Richardson CA et al. (2001), Co-activation of the abdominal and pelvic floor muscles during voluntary exercises. Neurourology and Urodynamics 20(1): 31–42.

Scarr G (2014), Biotensegrity: The Structural Basis of Life. Handspring Publishing, Pencaitland, UK.

Schleip R (2003), Fascial plasticity – a new neurobiological explanation. Journal of Bodywork and Movement Therapies 7(2): 104–116.

Schleip R (2009), Fascia as a Sensory Organ. World Massage Conference Webinar, 2009.

Schleip R (2015), Fascia in Sport and Movement. Handspring Publishing, Pencaitland, UK.

Schleip R, Muller DG (2013), Training principles for fascial connective tissues: scientific foundation and suggested practical applications. Journal of Bodywork and Movement Therapies 17(1): 103–115.

Schleip R, Klingler W, Lehmann-Horn F (2005), Active fascial contractility: fascia may be able to contract in a smooth muscle-like manner and thereby influence musculoskeletal dynamics. Department of Applied Physiology, Ulm University, Albert-Einstein-Allee 11, 89069 Ulm, Germany.

Schleip R, Mechsner F, Zorn A et al. (2014), The bodywide fascial network as a sensory organ for haptic perception. Journal of Motor Behavior 46(3): 191–193.

Schreinemacher MH, Ten Broek RP, Bakkum EA et al. (2010), Adhesion awareness: a national survey of surgeons. World Journal of Surgery 34(12): 2805–2812.

Schuenke MD (2012), A description of the lumbar interfascial triangle and its relation with the lateral raphe: anatomical constituents of load transfer through the lateral margin of the thoracolumbar fascia. Journal of Anatomy 221(6): 568–576.

Schuurmans J, De Vlugt E, Schouten AC et al. (2009), The monosynaptic Ia afferent pathway can largely explain the stretch duration effect of the long latency M2 response. Experimental Brain Research 193(4): 491–500.

Shemmell J, Krutky MA, Perreault EJ (2010), Stretch sensitive reflexes as an adaptive mechanism for maintaining limb stability. Clinical Neurophysiology 121(10): 1680–1689.

Singh S, Soni R, Singh KP et al. (2012), Effect of yoga practices on pulmonary function tests including transfer factor of lung for carbon monoxide (TLCO) in asthma patients. Indian Journal of Physiology and Pharmacology 56(1): 63–68.

Sizer PS (2007), Coupling behavior of the thoracic spine: a systematic review of the literature. Journal of Manipulative and Physiological Therapeutics 30(5): 390–399.

Skandalakis PN, Zoras O, Skandalakis JE et al. (2006), Transversalis, endoabdominal, endothoracic fascia: who's who? American Surgeon 72(1): 16–18.

Soljanik I, Janssen U, May F et al. (2012), Functional interactions between the fossa ischioanalis, levator ani and gluteus maximus muscles of the female pelvic floor: a prospective study in nulliparous women. Archives of Gynecology and Obstetrics 286(4): 931–938.

Standaert CJ, Herring SA (2007), Expert opinion and controversies in musculoskeletal and sports medicine: core stabilization as a treatment for low back pain. Archives of Physical Medicine and Rehabilitation 88(12): 1734–1736.

Staubesand J, Li Y (1996), Zum Feinbau der Fascia cruris mit besonderer Berücksichtigung epi- und intrafaszialer Nerven. Manuelle Medizin 34: 196–200.

Stecco C, Macchi V, Porzionato A et al. (2011), The fascia: the forgotten structure. Italian Journal of Anatomy and Embryology 116(3): 127–138.

Stokes IAF (2010), Intra-abdominal pressure and abdominal wall muscular function: spinal unloading mechanism. Clinical Biomechanics (Bristol) 25(9): 859–866.

Streeter CC Jensen JE, Perlmutter RM et al. (2007), Yoga asana sessions increase brain GABA levels: a pilot study. Journal of Alternative and Complementary Medicine 13: 419–426.

Streeter CC, Whitfield TH, Owen L et al. (2010), Effects of yoga versus walking on mood, anxiety, and brain GABA levels: a randomized controlled MRS study. Journal of Alternative and Complementary Medicine 16(11): 1145–1152.

Streeter CC, Gerbarg PL, Saper RB et al. (2012), Effects of yoga on the autonomic nervous system, gamma-aminobutyric-acid, and allostasis in epilepsy, depression, and post-traumatic stress disorder. Medical Hypotheses 78(5): 571–579.

Suarez-Roca H, Leal L, Silva JA et al. (2008), Reduced GABA neurotransmission underlies hyperalgesia induced by repeated forced swimming stress. Behavioural Brain Research 189: 159–169.

Sullivan MS, Dickinson CE, Troup JD (1994), The influence of age and gender on lumbar spine sagittal plane range of motion: a study of 1126 healthy subjects. Spine 19: 682–686.

Swenson R (2006), Review of clinical and functional neuroscience. Online version developed at Darmouth Medical School, https://wwwdartmouthedu/~rswenson/NeuroSci/indexhtml (last accessed September 9, 2015).

Tal M (1999), A role for inflammation in chronic pain. Current Review of Pain 3: 440–446.

Talasz H, Kremser C, Kofler M et al. (2011), Phase-locked parallel movement of diaphragm and pelvic floor during breathing and coughing – a dynamic MRI investigation in healthy females. International Urogynecology Journal 22(1): 61–68.

Tan G, Fink B, Dao TK et al. (2009), Associations among pain, PTSD, mTBI, and heart rate variability in veterans of Operation Enduring and Iraqi Freedom: a pilot study. Pain Medicine 10: 1237–1245.

Tan G, Jensen MP, Dao TK et al. (2011), Non-pharmacologic neuromodulatory approaches to pain management. In: MH Ebert, RD Kerns (eds) (2011), Behavioral and Psychopharmacologic Pain Management. Cambridge University Press, Boston, MA, ch. 13, pp. 201–213.

Taren AA, Gianaros PJ, Greco CM et al. (2015), Mindfulness meditation training alters stress-related amygdala resting state functional connectivity: a randomized controlled trial. Social Cognitive and Affective Neuroscience 10(12): 1758–1768.

Tateishi Y, Oda S, Nakamura M et al. (2007), Depressed heart rate variability is associated with high IL-6 blood level and decline in the blood pressure in septic patients. Shock 28: 549–553.

Taylor DC, Dalton JD, Seaber AV et al. (1990), Viscoelastic properties of muscle-tendon units: the biomechanical effects of stretching. American Journal of Sports Medicine 18: 300–309.

Ten Broek RP, Issa Y, Van Santbrink EJ et al. (2013), Burden of adhesions in abdominal and pelvic surgery: systematic review and meta-analysis. BMJ Clinical Research Edition 347: f5588.

Tharion E, Samuel P, Rajalakshmi R et al. (2012), Influence of deep breathing exercise on spontaneous respiratory rate and heart rate variability: a randomised controlled trial in healthy subjects. Indian Journal of Physiology and Pharmacology 56(1): 80–87.

Trew G, Cooke I, Lower A et al. (2009), Post-operative abdominal adhesions – awareness of UK gynaecologists – a survey of members of the Royal College of Obstetricians and Gynaecologists. Journal of Gynecologic Surgery 6: 25–37.

Trudelle-Jackson E, Ferro E, Morrow JR (2011), Clinical implications for muscle strength differences in women of different age and racial groups: the WIN Study. Journal of Women's Health Physical Therapy 35(1): 11–18.

Turankar AV, Jain S, Patel SB et al. (2013), Effects of slow breathing exercise on cardiovascular functions, pulmonary functions and galvanic skin resistance in healthy human volunteers – a pilot study. Indian Journal of Medical Research 137(5): 916–921.

Turvey MT, Fonseca ST (2014), The medium of haptic perception: a tensegrity hypothesis. Journal of Motor Behavior 46(3): 143–187.

Ullrich PM (2002), Journaling about stressful events: effects of cognitive processing and emotional expression. Annals of Behavioral Medicine 24(3): 244–250.

Vadiraja HS, Raghavendra RM, Nagarathna R et al. (2009), Effects of a yoga program on cortisol rhythm and mood states in early breast cancer patients undergoing adjuvant radiotherapy: a randomized controlled trial. Integrative Cancer Therapies 8: 37–46.

Van Herp G, Rowe P, Salter P et al. (2000), Three-dimensional lumbar spinal kinematics: a study of range of movement in 100 healthy subjects aged 20 to 60+ years. Rheumatology (Oxford) 39: 1337–1340.

Verrelst R, Willems TM, Clercq DD et al. (2014), The role of hip abductor and external rotator muscle strength in the development of exertional medial tibial pain: a prospective study. British Journal of Sports Medicine 48(21): 1564–1569.

Wainner RS, Whitman JM, Cleland JA et al. (2007), Regional interdependence: a musculoskeletal examination model whose time has come. Journal of Orthopaedic and Sports Physical Therapy 37(11): 658–660.

Wang XQ, Zheng JJ, Yu ZW et al. (2012), A meta-analysis of core stability exercise versus general exercise for chronic low back pain. PloS one 7(12): e52082.

Weber DJ (2011), Limb-state information encoded by peripheral and central somatosensory neurons: implications for an afferent interface. IEEE Transactions on Neural Systems and Rehabilitation Engineering 19(5): 501–513.

Weppler CH, Magnusson SP (2010), Increasing muscle extensibility: a matter of increasing length or modifying sensation? Physical Therapy 90(3): 438–449.

Willard FH (2015), The fascial system. Presentation at the University of New England, College of Osteopathic Medicine, http://wwwelsevierde/tools/showpdfphp?url=L13_Praesentation_Willardpdf (last accessed May 22, 2015).

Willard FH, Vleeming A, Schuenke MD et al. (2012), The thoracolumbar fascia: anatomy, function and clinical considerations. Journal of Anatomy 221(6): 507–536.

Willson JD, Dougherty CP, Ireland ML et al. (2005), Core stability and its relationship to lower extremity function and injury. Journal of the American Academy of Orthopedic Surgeons 13(5): 316–325.

World Health Organization (2001), The International Classification of Functioning, Disability and Health, WHO, Geneva.

Yahia L, Pigeon P, DesRosiers EA (1993), Viscoelastic properties of the human lumbodorsal fascia. Journal of Biomedical Engineering 15: 425–429.

Yavuz SU, Mrachacz-Kersting N, Sebik O et al. (2014), Human stretch reflex pathways reexamined. Journal of Neurophysiology 111(3): 602–612.

Zautra AJ, Fasman R, Davis MC et al. (2010), The effects of slow breathing on affective responses to pain stimuli: an experimental study. Pain 149(1): 12–18.

Zhang Z, Dellon AL (2008), Facial pain and headache associated with brachial plexus compression in the thoracic inlet. Microsurgery 28(5): 347–350.

Zhuo M (2007), A synaptic model for pain: long-term potentiation in the anterior cingulated cortex. Molecules and Cells 223: 259–271.

Chapter 4

Abu-Hijleh MF, Habbal OA, Moqattash ST (1995), The role of the diaphragm in lymphatic absorption from the peritoneal cavity. Journal of Anatomy 186(3): 453–467.

Adhana R, Gupta R, Dvivedii J et al. (2013), The influence of the 2:1 yogic breathing technique on essential hypertension. Indian Journal of Physiology and Pharmacology 57(1): 38–44.

Allison GT, Morris SL (2008), Transversus abdominis and core stability: has the pendulum swung? British Journal of Sports Medicine 42(11): 930–931.

Balasubramaniam M, Telles S, Doraiswamy M (2013), Yoga on our minds: a systematic review of yoga for neuropsychiatric disorders. Frontiers in Psychiatry 3: 117.

Barker PJ, Urquhart DM, Story IH et al. (2007), The middle layer of lumbar fascia and attachments to lumbar transverse processes: implications for segmental control and fracture. European Spine Journal 16(12): 2232–2237.

Barrall JP, Mercier P (2006), Visceral Manipulation, revised edition, vol I. Eastland Press, Seattle, WA.

Barrall JP, Mercier P (2007), Visceral Manipulation, revised edition, vol II. Eastland Press, Seattle, WA.

Beaule PE, O'Neill M, Rakhra K (2009), Acetabular labral tears. Journal of Bone and Joint Surgery American Volume 91(3): 701–710.

Bordoni B, Zanier E (2013), Anatomic connections of the diaphragm: influence of respiration on the body system. Journal of Multidisciplinary Healthcare 6: 281–291.

Brown RP, Gerbarg PL (2009), Yoga breathing, meditation, and longevity. Annals of the New York Academy of Sciences 1172: 54–62.

Byeon K, Choi JO, Yang JH et al. (2012), The response of the vena cava to abdominal breathing. Journal of Alternative and Complementary Medicine 18(2): 153–157.

Casartelli NC, Maffiuletti NA, Item-Glatthorn JF et al. (2011), Hip muscle weakness in patients with symptomatic femoroacetabular impingement. Osteoarthritis and Cartilage 19(7): 816–821.

Cherniack NS, Von Euler C, Glogowska M et al. (1981), Characteristics and rate of occurrence of spontaneous and provoked augmented breaths. Acta Physiologica Scandinavica 111(3): 349–360.

Chiappa GR, Roseguini BT, Vieira PJ et al. (2008), Inspiratory muscle training improves blood flow to resting and exercising limbs in patients with chronic heart failure. Journal of the American Collegte of Cardiology 51(17): 1663–1671.

Cibulka MT, Strube MJ, Meier D et al. (2010), Symmetrical and asymmetrical hip rotation and its relationship to hip rotator muscle strength. Clinical Biomechanics (Bristol, Avon) 25(1): 56–62.

Conti PB, Sakano E, Ribeiro MA et al. (2011), Assessment of the body posture of mouth-breathing children and adolescents. Jornal de Pediatria 87(4): 357–363.

Coulter D (2001), Anatomy of Hatha Yoga. Body and Breath, Honesdale, PA.

Crommert ME, Ekblom MM, Thorstensson A (2011), Activation of transversus abdominis varies with postural demand in standing. Gait and Posture 33(3): 473–477.

Defelice C, Toti P, Dimaggio G (2001), Absence of the inferior labial and lingual frenula in Ehlers–Danlos syndrome. Lancet 357(9267): 1500–1502.

Dusek JA, Otu HH, Wohlhueter AL et al. (2008), Genomic counter-stress changes induced by the relaxation response. PloS one 3(7): e2576.

Earl JE (2011), A proximal strengthening program improves pain, function, and biomechanics in women with patellofemoral pain syndrome. American Journal of Sports Medicine 39(1): 154–163.

Eherer AJ, Netolitzky F, Hogenauer C et al. (2012), Positive effect of abdominal breathing exercise on gastroesophageal reflux disease: a randomized, controlled study. American Journal of Gastroenterology 107(3): 372–378.

Ejnisman L, Philippon MJ, Lertwanich P et al. (2013), Relationship between femoral anteversion and findings in hips with femoroacetabular impingement. Orthopedics 36(3): e293–e300.

Friend L, Kelly BT (2009), Femoroacetabular impingement and labral tears in the adolescent hip: diagnosis and surgical advances. Current Opinion in Pediatrics 21(1): 71–76.

Gandevia SC, Mckenzie DK (2008), Respiratory rate: the neglected vital sign. Medical Journal of Australia 189(9): 532.

Garner G (2001), Professional Yoga Therapy Studies, vols I–IV. Continuing Education Course Manuals.

Ghiya S, Lee CM (2012), Influence of alternate nostril breathing on heart rate variability in non-practitioners of yogic breathing. International Journal of Yoga 5(1): 66–69.

Goleman D (2012), The sweet spot for achievement: what's the relationship between stress and performance? Psychology Today, March 29, 2012, https://wwwpsychologytodaycom/blog/the-brain-and-emotional-intelligence/201203/the-sweet-spot-achievement (last accessed July 30, 2015).

Grant AD, Sala DA, Schwarzkopf R (2012a), Femoro-acetabular impingement: the diagnosis – a review. Journal of Children's Orthopaedics 6(1): 1–12.

Grant AD, Sala DA, Davidovitch RI (2012b), The labrum: structure, function, and injury with femoro-acetabular impingement. Journal of Children's Orthopaedics 6(5): 357–372.

Harari D, Redlich M, Miri S et al. (2010), The effect of mouth breathing versus nasal breathing on dentofacial and craniofacial development in orthodontic patients. Laryngoscope 120(10): 2089–2093.

Hodges P (2008), Transversus abdominis: a different view of the elephant. British Journal of Sports Medicine 42(12): 941–944.

Hodges PW, Gandevia SC (2000), Activation of the human diaphragm during a repetitive postural task. Journal of Physiology 522(1): 165–175.

Hodges PW, Gandevia SC, Richardson CA (1997), Contractions of specific abdominal muscles in postural tasks are affected by respiratory maneuvers. Journal of Applied Physiology (Bethesda, Md: 1985) 83(3): 753–760.

Hodges P, Kaigle Holm A, Holm S et al. (2003), Intervertebral stiffness of the spine is increased by evoked contraction of transversus abdominis and the diaphragm: in vivo porcine studies. Spine 28(23): 2594–2601.

Hung HC, Hsiao SM, Chih SY et al. (2010), An alternative intervention for urinary incontinence: retraining diaphragmatic, deep abdominal and pelvic floor muscle coordinated function. Manual Therapy 15(3): 273–279.

Eng JJ, Chu KS (2002), Reliability and comparison of weight-bearing ability during standing tasks for individuals with chronic stroke. Archives of Physical Medicine and Rehabilitation 83(8): 1138–1144.

Janssens L, Brumagne S, McConnell AK et al. (2013), Greater diaphragm fatigability in individuals with recurrent low back pain. Respiratory Physiology and Neurobiology 188(2): 119–123.

Jerath R, Edry JW, Barnes VA et al. (2006), Physiology of long pranayamic breathing: neural respiratory elements may provide a mechanism that explains how slow deep breathing shifts the autonomic nervous system. Medical Hypotheses 67(3): 566–571.

Johnson S, Hoffman M (2010), Isometric hip-rotator torque production at varying degrees of hip flexion. Journal of Sport Rehabilitation 19(1): 12–20.

Jung J, Shim J, Kwon H (2014), Effects of abdominal stimulation during inspiratory muscle training on respiratory function of chronic stroke patients. Journal of Physical Therapy Science 26(1): 73–76.

Jyotsna VP, Ambekar S, Singla R et al. (2013), Cardiac autonomic function in patients with diabetes improves with practice of comprehensive yogic breathing program. Indian Journal of Endocrinology and Metabolism 17(3): 480–485.

Kolar P, Sulc J, Kyncl M et al. (2010), Stabilizing function of the diaphragm: dynamic MRI and synchronized spirometric assessment. Journal of Applied Physiology (Bethesda, Md: 1985) 109(4): 1064–1071.

Kolar P, Sulc J, Kyncl M et al. (2012), Postural function of the diaphragm in persons with and without chronic low back pain. Journal of Orthopaedic and Sports Physical Therapy 42(4): 352–362.

Kuntsevich V, Bushell WC, Theise ND (2010), Mechanisms of yogic practices in health, aging, and disease. Mount Sinai Journal of Medicine 77(5): 559–569.

Lin KH, Chuang CC, Wu HD et al. (1999), Abdominal weight and inspiratory resistance: their immediate effects on inspiratory muscle functions during maximal voluntary breathing in chronic tetraplegic patients. Archives of Physical Medicine and Rehabilitation 80(7): 741–745.

Lupien SJ, Fiocco A, Wan N et al. (2005), Stress hormones and human memory function across the lifespan. Psychoneuroendocrinology 30(3): 225–242.

Lupien SJ, Maheu F, Tu M et al. (2007), The effects of stress and stress hormones on human cognition: implications for the field of brain and cognition. Brain and Cognition 65(3): 209–237.

Marshall RS, Basilakos A, Williams T et al. (2014), Exploring the benefits of unilateral nostril breathing practice post-stroke: attention, language, spatial abilities, depression, and anxiety. Journal of Alternative and Complementary Medicine 20(3): 185–194.

Mason H, Vandoni M, Debarbieri G et al. (2013), Cardiovascular and respiratory effect of yogic slow breathing in the yoga beginner: what is the best approach? Evidence-Based Complementary and Alternative Medicine eCAM 2013: 743504.

Moriondo A, Bianchin F, Marcozzi C et al. (2008), Kinetics of fluid flux in the rat diaphragmatic submesothelial lymphatic lacunae.

American Journal of Physiology Heart and Circulatory Physiology 295(3): H1182–H1190.

Morris SL, Lay B, Allison GT (2012), Corset hypothesis rebutted – transversus abdominis does not co-contract in unison prior to rapid arm movements. Clinical Biomechanics (Bristol, Avon) 27(3): 249–254.

Morris SL, Lay B, Allison GT (2013), Transversus abdominis is part of a global not local muscle synergy during arm movement. Human Movement Science 32(5): 1176–1185.

Murphy KP (2009), Cerebral palsy lifetime care – four musculoskeletal conditions. Developmental Medicine and Child Neurology 51(Suppl. 4): 30–37.

Nakamura A, Yamada T, Goto A et al. (1998), Somatosensory homunculus as drawn by MEG. NeuroImage 7(4/1): 377–386.

Olivi G, Signore A, Olivi M et al. (2012), Lingual frenectomy: functional evaluation and new therapeutical approach. European Journal of Paediatric Dentistry 13(2): 101–106.

Porges S (2001), The polyvagal theory: phylogenetic substrates of a social nervous system. International Journal of Psychophysiology 42: 123–146.

Porges S (2011), Polyvagal Theory, Neurophysiological Foundations of Emotions, Attachment, Communication, and Self-Regulation. Norton Series on Interpersonal Neurobiology. WW Norton and Company, New York.

Porges S (2015), Personal interviews, July 14 and 28, 2015.

Pullen PR, Nagamia SH, Mehta PK et al. (2008), Effects of yoga on inflammation and exercise capacity in patients with chronic heart failure. Journal of Cardiac Failure 14(5): 407–413.

Qu S, Olafsrud SM, Meza-Zepeda LA et al. (2013), Rapid gene expression changes in peripheral blood lymphocytes upon practice of a comprehensive yoga program. PloS one 8(4): e61910.

Ramirez JM (2014), The integrative role of the sigh in psychology, physiology, pathology, and neurobiology. Progress in Brain Research 209: 91–129.

Reiman MP, Bolgla LA, Loudon JK (2012), A literature review of studies evaluating gluteus maximus and gluteus medius activation during rehabilitation exercises. Physiotherapy Theory and Practice 28(4): 257–268.

Restrepo CS, Eraso A, Ocazionez D et al. (2008), The diaphragmatic crura and retrocrural space: normal imaging appearance, variants, and pathologic conditions. Radiographics 28(5): 1289–1305.

Sakaguchi K, Mehta NR, Abdallah EF et al. (2007), Examination of the relationship between mandibular position and body posture. Cranio 25(4): 237–249.

Sapsford R (2004), Rehabilitation of pelvic floor muscles utilizing trunk stabilization. Manual Therapy 9(1): 3–12.

Sivakumar G, Prabhu K, Baliga R et al. (2011), Acute effects of deep breathing for a short duration (2–10 minutes) on pulmonary functions in healthy young volunteers. Indian Journal of Physiology and Pharmacology 55(2): 154–159.

Streeter CC, Gerbarg PL, Saper RB et al. (2012), Effects of yoga on the autonomic nervous system, gamma-aminobutyric-acid, and allostasis in epilepsy, depression, and post-traumatic stress disorder. Medical Hypotheses 78(5): 571–579.

Talasz H, Kofler M, Kalchschmid E et al. (2010), Breathing with the pelvic floor? Correlation of pelvic floor muscle function and expiratory flows in healthy young nulliparous women. International Urogynecology Journal 21(4): 475–481.

Telles S, Singh N, Yadav A et al. (2012a) Effect of yoga on different aspects of mental health. Indian Journal of Physiology and Pharmacology 56(3): 245–254.

Telles S, Joshi M, Somvanshi P (2012b), Yoga breathing through a particular nostril is associated with contralateral event-related potential changes. International Journal of Yoga 5(2): 102–107.

Telles S, Singh N, Puthige R (2013a), Changes in P300 following alternate nostril yoga breathing and breath awareness. BioPsychoSocial Medicine 7(1): 11.

Telles S, Yadav A, Kumar N et al. (2013b), Blood pressure and Purdue pegboard scores in individuals with hypertension after alternate nostril breathing, breath awareness, and no intervention. Medical Science Monitor 19: 61–66.

Tharion E, Samuel P, Rajalakshmi R et al. (2012), Influence of deep breathing exercise on spontaneous respiratory rate and heart rate variability: a randomised controlled trial in healthy subjects. Indian Journal of Physiology and Pharmacology 56(1): 80–87.

Tsai HJ, Kuo TB, Lee GS et al. (2015), Efficacy of paced breathing for insomnia: enhances vagal activity and improves sleep quality. Psychophysiology 52(3): 388–396.

Turankar AV, Jain S, Patel SB et al. (2013), Effects of slow breathing exercise on cardiovascular functions, pulmonary functions and galvanic skin resistance in healthy human volunteers – a pilot study. Indian Journal of Medical Research 137(5): 916–921.

Upadhyay Dhungel K, Malhotra V, Sarkar D et al. (2008), Effect of alternate nostril breathing exercise on cardiorespiratory functions. Nepal Medical College Journal 10(1): 25–27.

Urquhart DM, Hodges PW (2005), Differential activity of regions of transversus abdominis during trunk rotation. European Spine Journal 14(4): 393–400.

Urquhart DM, Barker PJ, Hodges PW et al. (2005), Regional morphology of the transversus abdominis and obliquus internus and externus abdominis muscles. Clinical Biomechanics (Bristol, Avon) 20(3): 233–241.

Vaschillo EG, Vaschillo B, Lehrer PM (2006), Characteristics of resonance in heart rate variability stimulated by biofeedback. Applied Psychophysiology and Biofeedback 31(2): 129–142.

Vaschillo EG, Vaschillo B, Buckman JF et al. (2015), The effects of sighing on the cardiovascular system. Biological Psychology 106: 86–95.

Vlemincx E, Taelman J, Van Diest I et al. (2010), Take a deep breath: the relief effect of spontaneous and instructed sighs. Physiology and Behavior 101(1): 67–73.

Vlemincx E, Abelson JL, Lehrer PM et al. (2013), Respiratory variability and sighing: a psychophysiological reset model. Biological Psychology 93(1): 24–32.

Yerkes RM, Dodson JD (1908), The relation of strength of stimulus to rapidity of habit-formation. Journal of Comparative Neurology and Psychology 18: 459–482.

Yoon TL, Park KM, Choi SA et al. (2014), A comparison of the reliability of the trochanteric prominence angle test and the alternative method in healthy subjects. Manual Therapy 19(2): 97–101.

Chapter 5

Banerjee P, McLean CR (2011), Femoroacetabular impingement: a review of diagnosis and management. Current Reviews in Musculoskeletal Medicine 4(1): 23–32.

Barker P, Briggs CA, Bogeski G (2004), Tensile transmission across the lumbar fasciae in unembalmed cadavers: effects of tension to various muscular attachments. Spine 29(2): 129–138.

Bordoni B, Zanier E (2013), Anatomic connections of the diaphragm: influence of respiration on the body system. Journal of Multidisciplinary Healthcare 6: 281–291.

Botser IB, Ozoude GC, Martin DE et al. (2012), Femoral anteversion in the hip: comparison of measurement by computed tomography, magnetic resonance imaging, and physical examination. Arthroscopy 28(5): 619–627.

Butler DS (1991), Mobilisation of the Nervous System. Churchill Livingstone, Edinburgh, UK.

Chakerian DL, Larson MA (1993), Effects of upper-extremity weight-bearing on hand-opening and prehension patterns in children with cerebral palsy. Developmental Medicine and Child Neurology 35(3): 216–229.

Chaudhry H (2011), Evaluation of the rotational stiffness and visco-elasticity of the low back and improving the low back visco-elasticity. International Journal of Experimental and Computational Biomechanics 1(4): 417.

Chaudhry H, Huang CY, Schleip R et al. (2007), Viscoelastic behavior of human fasciae under extension in manual therapy. Journal of Bodywork and Movement Therapies 11(2): 159–167.

Cook CE, Hegedus EJ (2013), Orthopedic Physical Examination Tests, An Evidence-Based Approach, 2nd edition. Pearson, Harlow, UK.

Cushing H (1927), The third circulation and its channels. Lancet 209(851).

Deutsch JE, Anderson EZ (2008), Complementary Therapies for Physical Therapy: A Clinical Decision-making Approach. Saunders, St Louis, MO.

Edelstein J (2009), Rehabilitating psoas tendonitis: a case report. HSS Journal 5(1): 78–82.

Edwards SL, Lee JA, Bell JE et al. (2010), Nonoperative treatment of superior labrum anterior posterior tears: improvements in pain, function, and quality of life. American Journal of Sports Medicine 38(7): 1456–1461.

Ejnisman L, Philippon MJ, Lertwanich P et al. (2013), Relationship between femoral anteversion and findings in hips with femoroacetabular impingement. Orthopedics 36(3): e293–e300.

Escamilla RF, Yamashiro K, Paulos L et al. (2009), Shoulder muscle activity and function in common shoulder rehabilitation exercises. Sports Medicine (Auckland, NZ) 39(8): 663–685.

Findley T, Chaudhry H, Stecco A et al. (2012), Fascia research – a narrative review. Journal of Bodywork and Movement Therapies 16(1): 67–75.

Findley T, Chaudhry H, Dhar S (2015), Transmission of muscle force to fascia during exercise. Journal of Bodywork and Movement Therapies 19(1): 119–123.

Gandevia SC, McKenzie DK (2008), Respiratory rate: the neglected vital sign. Medical Journal of Australia 189(9): 532.

Garner G (2001), Professional Yoga Therapy, Course Manuals.

Garner G (2011), Biomechanical precepts define 21st century yoga. Lower Extremity Review 3(3).

Gothe N, Pontifex MB, Hillman C et al. (2013), The acute effects of yoga on executive function. Journal of Physical Activity and Health 10: 488–495.

Hoffman J, Gabel P (2013), Expanding Panjabi's stability model to express movement: a theoretical model. Medical Hypotheses 80(6): 692–697.

Howle JM (2007), Neuro-Developmental Treatment Approach: Theoretical Foundations and Principles of Clinical Practice. NDTA, Laguna Beach, CA.

Huang TS, Ou HL, Huang, CY et al. (2015), Specific kinematics and associated muscle activation in individuals with scapular dyskinesis. Journal of Shoulder and Elbow Surgery 24(8): 1227–1234.

Hujing PA (2009), Epimuscular myofascial force transmission: a historical review and implications for new research. International Society of Biomechanics Muybridge Award lecture, Taipei, 2007. Journal of Biomechanics 42(1): 9–21.

Javadekar P, Manjunath NK (2012), Effect of Surya namaskar on sustained attention in school children. Journal of Yoga and Physical Therapy 2(110): 2.

Jover M, Schmitz C, Centelles L et al. (2010), Anticipatory postural adjustments in a bimanual load-lifting task in children with developmental coordination disorder. Developmental Medicine and Child Neurology 52(9): 850–855.

Kibler WB, Sciascia A, Wilkes T (2012), Scapular dyskinesis and its relation to shoulder injury. Journal of the American Academy of Orthopaedic Surgeons 20(6): 364–372.

Kibler WB, Ludewig PM, McClure PW et al. (2013), Clinical implications of scapular dyskinesis in shoulder injury: the 2013 consensus statement from the "scapular summit". British Journal of Sports Medicine 47(14): 877–885.

Langevin HM, Bouffard NA, Fox JR et al. (2011), Fibroblast cytoskeletal remodeling contributes to connective tissue tension. Journal of Cellular Physiology 226: 1166–1175.

Lee LJ (2012), The essential role of the thorax in whole body function and the "thoracic ring approach", assessment and treatment videos. Linda-Joy Lee Physiotherapist Corp (wwwljleeca).

Legaye J (2009), Influence of the sagittal balance of the spine on the anterior pelvic plane and on the acetabular orientation. International Orthopaedics 33(6): 1695–1700.

Lopes AD, Timmons MK, Grover M et al. (2015), Visual scapular dyskinesis: kinematics and muscle activity alterations in patients with subacromial impingement syndrome. Archives of Physical Medicine and Rehabilitation 96(2): 298–306.

McCreary EK, Provance PG, Rodgers MM et al. (2005), Muscles: Testing and Function, With Posture and Pain, 5th edition. Lippincott Williams and Wilkins, Baltimore, MD.

Masi AT, Nair K, Evans T et al. (2010), Clinical, biomechanical, and physiological translational interpretations of human resting myofascial tone or tension. International Journal of Therapeutic Massage and Bodywork 3(4): 16–28.

May-Benson T (2007), Use of a therapeutic brushing in best evidence statement (BESt): pressure proprioceptive protocols to improve sensory processing in children. Cincinnati Children's Medical Center, 2009.

Mihata T, McGarry MH, Tibone JE et al. (2008), Biomechanical assessment of type II superior labral anterior-posterior (SLAP) lesions associated with anterior shoulder capsular laxity as seen in throwers: a cadaveric study. American Journal of Sports Medicine 36(8): 1604–1610.

Myers T (2014), Anatomy Trains, 3rd edition. Churchill Livingstone, Edinburgh, UK.

Neumann DA, (2010), Kinesiology of the Musculoskeletal System: Foundations for Rehabilitation, 2nd edition. Mosby, St Louis, MO.

Onate JA, Dewey T, Kollock RO et al. (2012), Real-time intersession and interrater reliability of the functional movement screen. Journal of Strength and Conditioning Research 26(2): 408–415.

Page P (2011), Shoulder muscle imbalance and subacromial impingement syndrome in overhead athletes. International Journal of Sports Physical Therapy 6(1): 51–58.

Pluim BM (2013), Scapular dyskinesis: practical applications. British Journal of Sports Medicine 47(14): 875–876.

Porges SW (1995), Orienting in a defensive world: mammalian modifications of our evolutionary heritage. A polyvagal theory. Psychophysiology 32(4): 301–318.

Porges SW (2007), The polyvagal perspective. Biological Psychology 74(2): 116–143.

Porges S (2011), Polyvagal Theory, Neurophysioloical Foundations of Emotions, Attachment, Communication, and Self-Regulation. Norton Series on Interpersonal Neurobiology. WW Norton and Company, New York.

Radhakrishna S (2010), Application of integrated yoga therapy to increase imitation skills in children with autism spectrum disorder. International Journal of Yoga 3(1): 26.

Reese NB, Bandy WD (2002), Joint Range of Motion and Muscle Length Test. Saunders, Philadelphia, PA.

Rocha KK, Ribeiro AM, Rocha KC et al. (2012), Improvement in physiological and psychological parameters after 6 months of yoga practice. Consciousness and Cognition 21: 843–850.

Sahrmann S (2002), Diagnosis and Treatment of Movement Impairment Syndromes. Mosby, St Louis, MO.

Sakuma J, Kanehisa H, Yanai T et al. (2012), Fascicle-tendon behavior of the gastrocnemius and soleus muscles during ankle bending exercise at different movement frequencies. European Journal of Applied Physiology 112: 887–898.

Schleip R (2003), Fascial plasticity – a new neurobiological explanation. Journal of Bodywork and Movement Therapies 7(2): 104–116.

Schleip R, Klingler W, Lehmann-Horn F (2005), Active fascial contractility: fascia may be able to contract in a smooth muscle-like manner and thereby influence musculoskeletal dynamics. Department of Applied Physiology, Ulm University, Albert-Einstein-Allee 11, 89069 Ulm, Germany.

Seitz AL, McClure PW, Finucane S et al. (2012a), The scapular assistance test results in changes in scapular position and subacromial space but not rotator cuff strength in subacromial impingement. Journal of Orthopaedic and Sports Physical Therapy 42(5): 400–412.

Seitz AL, McClure PW, Lynch SS et al. (2012b), Effects of scapular dyskinesis and scapular assistance test on subacromial space during static arm elevation. Journal of Shoulder and Elbow Surgery 21(5): 631–640.

Smith CA, Chimera NJ, Wright NJ et al. (2013), Interrater and intrarater reliability of the functional movement screen. Journal of Strength and Conditioning Research 27(4): 982–987.

Stecco L (2004), Fascial Manipulation for Musculoskeletal Pain. PICCIN, Italy, p. 11.

Stecco A, Stern R, Fantoni I et al. (2016), Fascial disorders: implications for treatment. PM & R: The Journal of Injury, Function, and Rehabilitation 8(2): 161–168.

Stickler L, Finley M, Gulgin H (2015), Relationship between hip and core strength and frontal plane alignment during a single leg squat. Physical Therapy in Sport 16(1): 66–71.

Tate AR, McClure PW, Kareha S et al. (2008), Effect of the scapula reposition test on shoulder impingement symptoms and elevation strength in overhead athletes. Journal of Orthopaedic and Sports Physical Therapy 38(1): 4–11.

Teyhen DS, Shaffer SW, Lorenson CL et al. (2012), The functional movement screen: a reliability study. Journal of Orthopaedic and Sports Physical Therapy 42(6): 530–540.

Whedon JM, Glassey D (2009), Cerebrospinal fluid stasis and its clinical significance. Alternative Therapies in Health and Medicine 15(3): 54–60.

Wilson BN, Trombley CA (1984), Proximal and distal function in children with and without sensory integrative dysfunction: an EMG study. Canadian Journal of Occupational Therapy 51(1): 11–17.

Chapter 6

Alenezi F, Herrington L, Jones P et al. (2014), The reliability of biomechanical variables collected during single leg squat and landing tasks. Journal of Electromyography and Kinesiology 24(5): 718–721.

Bandy WD (1997), The effect of time and frequency of static stretching on flexibility of the hamstring muscles. Physical Therapy 77(10): 1090.

Beattie P (2010), The immediate reduction in low back pain intensity following lumbar joint mobilization and prone press-ups is associated with increased diffusion of water in the L5–S1 intervertebral disc. Journal of Orthopaedic and Sports Physical Therapy 40(5): 256.

Bolgla LA, Malone TR, Umberger BR et al. (2011), Comparison of hip and knee strength and neuromuscular activity in subjects with and without patellofemoral pain syndrome. International Journal of Sports Physical Therapy 6(4): 285–296.

Cashman GE (2012), The effect of weak hip abductors or external rotators on knee valgus kinematics in healthy subjects: a systematic review. Journal of Sport Rehabilitation 21(3): 273–284.

Chang A, Hurwitz D, Dunlop D et al. (2007), The relationship between toe-out angle during gait and progression of medial tibiofemoral osteoarthritis. Annals of the Rheumatic Diseases 66(10): 1271–1275.

Cook CE, Hegedus EJ (2013), Orthopedic Physical Examination Tests, An Evidence-Based Approach, 2nd edition. Pearson, Harlow, UK.

Cooper NA, Scavo KM, Strickland KJ et al. (2016), Prevalence of gluteus medius weakness in people with chronic low back pain compared to healthy controls. European Spine Journal 25(4): 1258–1265.

Crossley KM, Zhang WJ, Schache AG et al. (2011), Performance on the single-leg squat task indicates hip abductor muscle function. American Journal of Sports Medicine 39(4): 866–873.

Dolak KL, Silkman C, Medina Mckeon J et al. (2011), Hip strengthening prior to functional exercises reduces pain sooner than quadriceps strengthening in females with patellofemoral pain syndrome: a randomized clinical trial. Journal of Orthopaedic and Sports Physical Therapy 41(8): 560–570.

Flaxman TE, Speirs AD, Benoit DL (2012), Joint stabilisers or moment actuators: the role of knee joint muscles while weight-bearing. Journal of Biomechanics 45(15): 2570–2576.

Fujiya H, Kousa P, Fleming BC et al. (2011), Effect of muscle loads and torque applied to the tibia on the strain behavior of the anterior cruciate ligament: an in vitro investigation. Clinical Biomechanics (Bristol, Avon) 26(10): 1005–1011.

Fukuda TY, Rossetto FM, Magalhaes E et al. (2010), Short-term effects of hip abductors and lateral rotators strengthening in females with patellofemoral pain syndrome: a randomized controlled clinical trial. Journal of Orthopaedic and Sports Physical Therapy 40(11): 736–742.

Incavo SJ, Gold JE, Exaltacion JJF et al. (2011), Does acetabular retroversion affect range of motion after total hip arthroplasty? Clinical Orthopaedics and Related Research 469(1): 218–224.

Kerrigan DC, Lee LW, Collins JJ et al. (2001), Reduced hip extension during walking (healthy elderly and fallers versus young adults). Archives of Physical Medicine and Rehabilitation 82: 26–30.

Lee D (2011), The Pelvic Girdle: An Integration of Clinical Expertise and Research, 4th edition. Churchill Livingstone/Elsevier, Edinburgh, UK.

Lee SP, Powers C (2013), Description of a weight-bearing method to assess hip abductor and external rotator muscle performance. Journal of Orthopaedic and Sports Physical Therapy 43(6): 392–397.

Lynn SK, Costigan PA (2008), Effect of foot rotation on knee kinetics and hamstring activation in older adults with and without signs of knee osteoarthritis. Clinical Biomechanics (Bristol, Avon) 23(6): 779–786.

Neumann DA (2010), Kinesiology of the Musculoskeletal System: Foundations for Rehabilitation, 2nd edition. Mosby, St Louis, MO.

Patel AB, Wagle RR, Usrey MM et al. (2010), Guidelines for implant placement to minimize impingement during activities of daily living after total hip arthroplasty. Journal of Arthroplasty 25(8): 1275–1281e1.

Peters JS, Tyson NL (2013), Proximal exercises are effective in treating patellofemoral pain syndrome: a systematic review. International Journal of Sports Physical Therapy 8(5): 689–700.

Pollard CD, Sigward SM, Powers CM (2010), Limited hip and knee flexion during landing is associated with increased frontal plane knee motion and moments. Clinical Biomechanics (Bristol, Avon) 25(2): 142–146.

Reeves ND, Bowling FL (2011), Conservative biomechanical strategies for knee osteoarthritis. Nature Reviews Rheumatology 7(2): 113–122.

Reiman MP, Bolgla LA, Loudon JK (2012), A literature review of studies evaluating gluteus maximus and gluteus medius activation during rehabilitation exercises. Physiotherapy Theory and Practice 28(4): 257–268.

Ryan EE, Rossi MD, Lopez R (2010), The effects of the contract-relax-antagonist-contract form of proprioceptive neuromuscular facilitation stretching on postural stability. Journal of Strength and Conditioning Research 24(7): 1888–1894.

Stickler L, Finley M, Gulgin H (2015), Relationship between hip and core strength and frontal plane alignment during a single leg squat. Physical Therapy in Sport 16(1): 66–71.

Thorp LE, Wimmer MA, Foucher KC et al. (2010), The biomechanical effects of focused muscle training on medial knee loads in OA of the knee: a pilot, proof of concept study. Journal of Musculoskeletal and Neuronal Interactions 10(2): 166–173.

Trulsson A, Miller M, Hansson GA et al. (2015), Altered movement patterns and muscular activity during single and double leg squats in individuals with anterior cruciate ligament injury. BMC Musculoskeletal Disorders 16: 28.

Verrelst R, Willems TM, Clercq DD et al. (2014), The role of hip abductor and external rotator muscle strength in the development of exertional medial tibial pain: a prospective study. British Journal of Sports Medicine 48(21): 1564–1569.

Chapter 7

Delitto A, George SZ, Van Dillen LR et al., Orthopaedic Section of the American Physical Therapy Association (2012), Low back pain. Journal of Orthopaedic and Sports Physical Therapy 42(4): A1–A57.

Golanó P, Vega J, De Leeuw PA et al. (2010), Anatomy of the ankle ligaments: a pictorial essay. Knee Surgery, Sports Traumatology, Arthroscopy 18(5): 557–569.

Lee D (2014), Butt-grippers, back-grippers and chest grippers – are you one? http://wwwdianeleeca/article-butt-grippersphp (last accessed December 14, 2014).

Neumann DA (2010), Kinesiology of the musculoskeletal system: foundations for rehabilitation, 2nd edition. Mosby, St Louis, MO.

Sahrmann S (2011), Movement System Impairment Syndromes of the Extremities, Cervical, and Thoracic Spines. Elsevier/Mosby, St Louis, MO.

Sizer PS, Jr, Brismee JM, Cook C (2007), Coupling behavior of the thoracic spine: a systematic review of the literature. Journal of Manipulative and Physiological Therapeutics 30(5): 390–399.

Chapter 8

Anderzen-Carlsson A, Persson Lundholm U, Kohn M et al. (2014), Medical yoga: another way of being in the world. A phenomenological study from the perspective of persons suffering from stress-related symptoms. International Journal of Qualitative Studies on Health and Well-being 9: 23033.

Banerjee P, McLean CR (2011), Femoroacetabular impingement: a review of diagnosis and management. Current Reviews in Musculoskeletal Medicine 4(1): 23–32.

Chugh-Gupta N, Baldassarre FG, Vrkljan BH (2013), A systematic review of yoga for state anxiety: considerations for occupational therapy. Canadian Journal of Occupational Therapy 80(3): 150–170.

Cramer H, Rabsilber S, Lauche R (2015), Yoga and meditation for menopausal symptoms in breast cancer survivors – a randomized controlled trial. Cancer 121(13): 2175–2184.

Cushing H (1927), The third circulation and its channels. Lancet 209(851).

Gupta M (2015), Pelvic congestion syndrome. AOGD Bulletin 14–11(March): 10–12, http://wwwaogdorg/AOGD%20 Bulletin%20March%202015%20%281%29pdf (last accessed April 10, 2016).

May-Benson T (2007), Use of a therapeutic brushing in best evidence statement (BESt): pressure proprioceptive protocols to improve sensory processing in children. Cincinnati Children's Medical Center, 2009.

Whedon JM, Glassey D (2009), Cerebrospinal fluid stasis and its clinical significance. Alternative Therapies in Health and Medicine 15(3): 54–60.

Chapter 9

Ambegaonkar JP, Mettinger LM, Caswell SV et al. (2014), Relationships between core endurance, hip strength, and balance in collegiate female athletes. International Journal of Sports Physical Therapy 9(5): 604–616.

Demoulin C, Boyer M, Duchateau J et al. (2016), Is the Sorensen test valid to assess muscle fatigue of the trunk extensor muscles? Journal of Back and Musculoskeletal Rehabilitation 29(1): 31–40.

Escamilla RF, Yamashiro K, Paulos L et al. (2009), Shoulder muscle activity and function in common shoulder rehabilitation exercises. Sports Medicine (Auckland, NZ) 39(8): 663–685.

Key S (2013), Healing of painful intervertebral discs: implications for physiotherapy. Part 2 – pressure change therapy: a proposed clinical model to stimulate disc healing. Physical Therapy Reviews 18(1): 34–42.

San Juan JG, Suprak DN, Roach SM et al. (2015), The effects of exercise type and elbow angle on vertical ground reaction force and muscle activity during a push-up plus exercise. BMC Musculoskeletal Disorders 16: 23.

REFERENCES

Chapter 10

Brinjikji W, Luetmer PH, Comstock B et al. (2015), Systematic literature review of imaging features of spinal degeneration in asymptomatic populations. American Journal of Neuroradiology 36(4): 811–816.

Coulter D (2001), Anatomy of Hatha Yoga. Body and Breath, Honesdale, PA.

Drake JD, Aultman CD, McGill SM et al. (2005), The influence of static axial torque in combined loading on intervertebral joint failure mechanics using a porcine model. Clinical Biomechanics (Bristol, Avon) 20(10): 1038–1045.

Fejer R, Kyvik KO, Hartvigsen J (2006), The prevalence of neck pain in the world population: a systematic critical review of the literature. European Spine Journal 15(6): 834–848.

Foreman SM, Croft AC (2001), Whiplash Injuries: Cervical Acceleration/Deceleration Syndrome. Lippincott, Williams, and Wilkins, Baltimore.

Freburger PT, Holmes GM, Agans RP et al. (2009), The rising prevalence of chronic low back pain. Archives of Internal Medicine 169(3): 251–258.

Goel VK Clark CR, Gallaes K et al. (1988), Movement-rotation relationships of the ligamentous occipito-atlanto-axial complex. Journal of Biomechanics 21(8): 673–680.

Kolar P, Sulc J, Kyncl M et al. (2012), Postural function of the diaphragm in persons with and without chronic low back pain. Journal of Orthopaedic and Sports Physical Therapy 42(4): 352–362.

Mehnert MJ, Agesen T, Malanga GA (2005), "Heading" and neck injuries in soccer: a review of biomechanics and potential long-term effects. Pain Physician 8(4): 391–397.

Neumann DA (2010), Kinesiology of the musculoskeletal system: foundations for rehabilitation, 2nd edition. Mosby, St Louis, MO.

Nolan JP, Sherk HH (1988), Biomechanical evaluation of the extensor musculature of the cervical spine. Spine 13: 9–11.

Norkin CC, Levangie PK (1992), Joint Structure and Function, 2nd edition. FA Davis, Philadelphia, PA.

Panjabi M, Dvorak J, Duranceau J et al. (1988), Three-dimensional movements of the upper cervical spine. Spine 13(7): 726–730.

Panjabi MM, Cholewicki J, Nibu K et al. (1998), Critical load of the human cervical spine: an in vitro experimental study. Clinical Biomechanics (Bristol, Avon) 13(1): 11–17.

Patwardhan AG, Havey RM, Ghanayem AJ et al. (2000), Load-carrying capacity of the human cervical spine in compression is increased under a follower load. Spine 25(12): 1548–1554.

Swartz EE, Floyd RT, Cendoma M (2005), Cervical spine functional anatomy and the biomechanics of injury due to compressive loading. Journal of Athletic Training 40(3): 155–161.

White AA, Panjabi MM (1990), Clinical Biomechanics of the Spine, 2nd edition. Lippincott, Philadelphia, PA.

Yoganandan N, Kumaresan S, Pintar FA (2001), Biomechanics of the cervical spine. Part 2: cervical spine soft tissue responses and biomechanical modeling. Clinical Biomechanics (Bristol, Avon) 16(1): 1–27.

Chapter 11

Advanced Healthcare Network For Nurses (AHNN) (2011), Study ranks top 20 most commonly diagnosed conditions, February 10, 2011, http://NursingAdvancewebCom/News/National-News/Study-Ranks-Top-20-Most-Commonly-Diagnosed-ConditionsAspx (last accessed June 25, 2015).

American College of Sports Medicine (ACSM) (2014), ACSM Guidelines for Exercise and Prescription, 9th edition. Lippincott, Williams, and Wilkins, Philadelphia, PA, p. 456.

Balagué F, Mannion AF, Pellisé F et al. (2012), Non-specific low back pain. Lancet 379(9814): 482–491.

Brinjikji W, Luetmer PH, Comstock B et al. (2015), Systematic literature review of imaging features of spinal degeneration in asymptomatic populations. American Journal of Neuroradiology 36(4): 811–816.

Bunzli S, Gillham D, Esterman A (2011), Physiotherapy-provided operant conditioning in the management of low back pain disability: a systematic review. Physiotherapy Research International 16: 4–19.

Busseuil C, Freychat P, Guedj EB et al. (1998), Rearfoot-forefoot orientation and traumatic risk for runners. Foot and Ankle International 19: 32–37.

Carey T, Freburger JK, Holmes GM et al. (2009), A long way to go: practice patterns and evidence in chronic low back pain care. Spine 34(7): 718–724.

Cook CE, Hegedus EJ (2013), Orthopedic Physical Examination Tests: An Evidence–Based Approach, 2nd edition. Pearson, Harlow, UK.

Croft P (1993), Soft-tissue rheumatism. In: AJ Silman, MC Hochberg (eds), Epidemiology of the Rheumatic Diseases. Oxford University Press, Oxford, UK, pp. 375–421.

Delitto A, George SZ, Van Dillen LR et al., Orthopaedic Section of the American Physical Therapy Association (2012), Low back pain. Journal of Orthopaedic and Sports Physical Therapy 42(4): A1–A57.

Devan MR, Pescatello LS, Faghri P et al. (2004), A prospective study of overuse knee injuries among female athletes with muscle imbalances and structural abnormalities. Journal of Athletic Training 39(3): 263–267.

Fairclough J, Hayashi K, Toumi H et al. (2007), Is iliotibial band syndrome really a friction syndrome? Journal of Science and Medicine in Sport 10(2): 74–76; discussion 77–78.

Falvey EC, Clark RA, Franklyn-Miller A et al. (2010), Iliotibial band syndrome: an examination of the evidence behind a number of treatment options. Scandinavian Journal of Medicine and Science in Sports 20(4): 580–587.

Freburger PT, Holmes GM, Agans RP et al. (2009), The rising prevalence of chronic low back pain. Archives of Internal Medicine 169(3): 251–258.

Fredericson M, Wolf C (2005), Iliotibial band syndrome in runners: innovations in treatment. Sports Medicine 35: 451–459.

Fredericson M, Cookingham CL, Chaudhari AM et al. (2000), Hip abductor weakness in distance runners with iliotibial band syndrome. Clinical Journal of Sport Medicine 10: 169–175.

Fritz JM, Childs JD, Wainner RS et al. (2012), Primary care referral of patients with low back pain to physical therapy: impact on future health care utilization and costs. Spine 37(25): 2114–2121.

Gellhorn AC, Chan L, Martin B et al. (2012), Management patterns in acute low back pain: the role of physical therapy. Spine 37(9): 775–782.

Gellhorn AC, Katz JN, Suri P (2013), Osteoarthritis of the spine: the facet joints. Nature Reviews Rheumatology 9(4): 216–224.

Glockner SM (1995), Shoulder pain: a diagnostic dilemma. American Family Physician 51(7): 1677–1687.

Hamill J, Miller R, Noehren B et al. (2008), A prospective study of iliotibial band strain in runners. Clinical Biomechanics 23: 1018–1025.

Hestbaek L, Leboeuf-Yde C, Manniche C (2003), Low back pain: what is the long-term course? A review of studies of general patient populations. European Spine Journal 12(2): 149–165.

Hudson VJ (2010), Evaluation, diagnosis, and treatment of shoulder injuries in athletes. Clinics in Sports Medicine 29(1): 19–32.

Isabel De-la-Llave-Rincón A, Puentedura EJ, Fernández-de-las-Peñas C (2011), Clinical presentation and manual therapy for upper quadrant musculoskeletal conditions. Journal of Manual and Manipulative Therapy 19(4): 201–211.

Khaund R, Flynn, SH (2005), Iliotibial band syndrome: a common source of knee pain. American Family Physician 71(8): 1545–1550.

Kibler WB, McMullen J (2003), Scapular dyskinesis and its relation to shoulder pain. Journal of the American Academy of Orthopaedic Surgeons 11(2): 142–151.

Kibler WB, Ludewig PM, McClure PW et al. (2013), Clinical implications of scapular dyskinesis in shoulder injury: the 2013 consensus statement from the "scapular summit". British Journal of Sports Medicine 47(14): 877–885.

Kolber MJ, Beekhuizen KS, Cheng MS et al. (2010), Shoulder injuries attributed to resistance training: a brief review. Journal of Strength and Conditioning Research 24(6): 1696–1704.

Krogsgaard MR, Safran MR, Rheinlaedner P et al. (2009), Preventing shoulder injuries. In: R Bahr, L Engebretson (eds), Sports Injury Prevention. Blackwell Publishing, International Olympic Committee, Oxford, UK, ch. 9.

Lavine R (2010), Iliotibial band friction syndrome. Current Reviews in Musculoskeletal Medicine 3(1–4): 18–22.

Lininger MR, Miller MG (2009), Iliotibial band syndrome in the athletic population: strengthening and rehabilitation exercises. Strength and Conditioning Journal 31(3): 43–46.

Lucado A, Kolber M, Cheng MS et al. (2010), Subacromial impingement syndrome and lateral epicondylalgia in tennis players. Physical Therapy Reviews 15(2): 55–61.

Lucas K (2007), Effects of latent myofascial trigger points on muscle activation patterns during scapular plane elevation. Unpublished Phd dissertation, School Of Health Sciences, RMIT University, Melbourne, Australia.

MacMahon JM, Chaudhari AM, Andriacchi TP (2000), Biomechanical injury predictors for marathon runners: striding towards iliotibial band syndrome injury prevention. Conference of the International Society of Biomechanics in Sports, Hong Kong, June.

McQuade KJ, Smidt GL (1998), Dynamic scapulohumeral rhythm: the effects of external resistance during elevation of the arm in the scapular plane. Journal of Orthopaedic and Sports Physical Therapy 27(2): 125–133.

Mafi JN, McCarthy EP, Davis RB et al. (2013), Worsening trends in the management and treatment of back pain. JAMA Internal Medicine 173(17): 1573–1581.

Messier SP, Edwards DG, Martin DF et al. (1995), Etiology of iliotibial band friction syndrome in distance runners. Medicine and Science in Sports and Exercise 27: 951–960.

Miciak M, Gross DP, Joyce A (2012), A review of the psychotherapeutic "common factors" model and its application in physical therapy: the need to consider general effects in physical therapy practice. Scandinavian Journal of Caring Sciences 26(2): 394–403.

Miller R, Lowry J, Meardon S et al. (2007), Lower extremity mechanics of iliotibial band syndrome during an exhaustive run. Gait Posture 26: 407–413.

Noble C (1980), Iliotibial band friction syndrome in runners. American Journal of Sports Medicine 8: 232–234.

Noehren B, Davis I, Hamill J (2007), Prospective study of the biomechanical factors associated with iliotibial band syndrome. Clinical Biomechanics 22: 951–956.

Orchard J, Fricker P, Abud A et al. (1996), Biomechanics of iliotibial band friction syndrome in runners. American Journal of Sports Medicine 24: 375–379.

Paluska SA (2005), An overview of hip injuries in running. Sports Medicine 35(11): 991–1014.

Pedowitz RN (2006), Use of osteopathic manipulative treatment for iliotibial band friction syndrome. Journal of the American Osteopathic Association 12: 563–567.

Prins MR, Van Der Wurff P (2009), Females with patellofemoral pain syndrome have weak hip muscles: a systematic review. Australian Journal of Physiotherapy 55: 9–15.

Savage RA, Whitehouse GH, Roberts N (1997), The relationship between the magnetic resonance imaging appearance of the lumbar spine and low back pain, age and occupation in males. European Spine Journal 6: 106–114.

Sher I, Umans H, Downie SA et al. (2011), Proximal iliotibial band syndrome: what is it and where is it? Skeletal Radiology 40(12): 1553–1556.

Strauss EJ, Kim S, Calcei JG et al. (2011), Iliotibial band syndrome: evaluation and management. Journal of the American Academy of Orthopaedic Surgeons 19: 728–736.

Sueki DG, Chaconas EJ (2011), The effect of thoracic manipulation on shoulder pain: a regional interdependence model. Physical Therapy Reviews 16(5): 399–408.

Terry GC, Chopp TM (2000), Functional anatomy of the shoulder. Journal of Athletic Training 35(3): 248–255.

United States Department of Health and Human Services (USHHS) (2008), Physical Activity Guidelines for Americans. http://HealthGov/Paguidelines/Pdf/PaguidePdf (last accessed September 3, 2015).

World Health Organization (2003), Adherence to Long-Term Therapies: Evidence for Action. WHO Library Cataloguing-In-Publication Data.

Chapter 12

Aligene K, Lin E (2013), Vestibular and balance treatment of the concussed athlete. NeuroRehabilitation 32(3): 543–553.

Alsalaheen BA, Mucha A, Morris LO et al. (2010), Vestibular rehabilitation for dizziness and balance disorders after concussion. Journal of Neurologic Physical Therapy 34(2): 87–93.

Babu PV, Liu D, Gilbert ER (2013), Recent advances in understanding the anti-diabetic actions of dietary flavonoids. Journal of Nutritional Biochemistry 24(11): 1777–1789.

Barber MD, Walters MD, Bump RC (2005), Short forms of two condition-specific quality of life questionnaires for women with pelvic floor disorders. American Journal of Obstetrics and Gynecology 193: 103–113.

Binkley JM, Stratford PW, Lott SA et al. (1999), The lower extremity functional scale (LEFS): scale development, measurement properties, and clinical application. North American Orthopaedic Rehabilitation Research Network Physical Therapy 79(4): 371–383.

Bombardier C (2000), Outcome assessments in the evaluation of treatment of spinal disorders: summary and general recommendations. Spine 25(24): 3100–3103.

Brown C, Dunn W (2002), The Adolescent/Adult Sensory Profile Manual. Psychological Corporation, San Antonio TX.

Butler D (1991), Mobilisation of the Nervous System. Churchill Livingstone, Melbourne, Australia.

Chandra P, Sands RL, Gillespie BW et al. (2012), Predictors of heart rate variability and its prognostic significance in chronic kidney disease. Nephrology, Dialysis, Transplantation 27(2): 700–709.

Ciechanowski PS, Katon WJ, Russo JE (2000), Depression and diabetes: impact of depressive symptoms on adherence, function, and costs. Archives of Internal Medicine 27: 3278–3285.

De Michelis E (2005), A History of Modern Yoga. Continuum, London.

Debono DJ, Hoeksema LJ, Hobbs RD (2013), Caring for patients with chronic pain: pearls and pitfalls. Journal of the American Osteopathic Association 113(8): 620–627.

Delitto A, George SZ, Van Dillen LR et al., Orthopaedic Section of the American Physical Therapy Association (2012), Low back pain. Journal of Orthopaedic and Sports Physical Therapy 42(4): A1–57.

Dunn W (1997), The impact of sensory processing abilities on the daily lives of young children and families: a conceptual model. Infants and Young Children 9(4): 23–25.

Dunn W (2006), Sensory Profile School Companion. Psychological Corporation, San Antonio, TX.

Dunn W (2009), Living Sensationally: Understanding Your Senses. Jessica Kingsley Publishers, London, UK.

Fairbank JC, Pynsent PB (2000), The Oswestry Disability Index. Spine 25(22): 2940–2952; discussion 2952.

Garrity TF, Garrity AR (1985), The nature and efficacy of intervention studies in the national high blood pressure education research program. Journal of Hypertension (Suppl.)(3): S91–S95.

Grotle M, Garratt AM, Jenssen HK et al. (2012), Reliability and construct validity of self-report questionnaires for patients with pelvic girdle pain. Physical Therapy 92(1): 111–123.

Hermsdorff HH, Zulet MA, Puchau B et al. (2010), Fruit and vegetable consumption and proinflammatory gene expression from peripheral blood mononuclear cells in young adults: a translational study. Nutrition and Metabolism 7: 42.

Holman HR et al. (1997), Evidence that an education program for self-management of chronic disease can improve health status while reducing health care costs: a randomized trial. Abstract Book/Association for Health Services Research 14: 19–20.

Horne R, Weinman J (1998), Predicting treatment adherence: an overview of theoretical models. In: LB Myers, K Midence (eds), Adherence to Treatment in Medical Conditions. Harwood Academic, Reading, UK.

Horton C (2013), Yoga PhD. Kleio Books, Chicago, IL.

Iyengar BKS (1966, 1968, 1976), Light on Yoga: Yoga Dīpikā, Schocken, New York.

Kemp AH, Quintana DS (2013), The relationship between mental and physical health: insights from the study of heart rate variability. International Journal of Psychophysiology 89(3): 288–296.

Kim EJ, Choi JH, Kim KW et al. (2011), The impacts of open-mouth breathing on upper airway space in obstructive sleep apnea: 3-D MDCT analysis. European Archives of Oto-rhino-laryngology 268(4): 533–539.

Lai WH, Shih YF, Lin PL et al. (2012), Normal neurodynamic responses of the femoral slump test. Manual Therapy 17(2): 126–132.

Lee SH, Choi JH, Shin C et al. (2007), How does open-mouth breathing influence upper airway anatomy? Laryngoscope 117(6): 1102–1106.

Lehrer PM, Vaschillo E, Vaschillo B (2000), Resonant frequency biofeedback training to increase cardiac variability: rationale and manual for training. Applied Psychophysiology and Biofeedback 25(3): 177–191.

Lei-Rivera L, Sutera J, Galatioto JA et al. (2013), Special tools for the assessment of balance and dizziness in individuals with mild traumatic brain injury. NeuroRehabilitation 32(3): 463–472.

Leventhal H, Cameron L (1987), Behavioral theories and the problem of compliance. Patient Education and Counseling 10: 117–138.

Levy B (2014), Illness severity, trait anxiety, cognitive impairment and heart rate variability in bipolar disorder. Psychiatry Research 220(3): 890–895.

Liu HQ, Qiu Y, Mu Y et al. (2013), A high ratio of dietary n-3/n-6 polyunsaturated fatty acids improves obesity-linked inflammation and insulin resistance through suppressing activation of TLR4 in SD rats. Nutrition Research (New York, NY) 33(10): 849–858.

McCraty R, Shaffer F (2015), Heart rate variability: new perspectives on physiological mechanisms, assessment of self-regulatory capacity, and health risk. Global Advances in Health and Medicine 4(1): 46–61.

McEwen BS, Stellar E (1993), Stress and the individual: mechanisms leading to disease. Archives of Internal Medicine 153(18): 2093–2101.

McEwen BS, Eiland L, Hunter RG et al. (2012), Stress and anxiety: structural plasticity and epigenetic regulation as a consequence of stress. Neuropharmacology 62(1): 3–12.

McHorney CA, Ware JE, Jr, Lu JF et al. (1994), The MOS 36-item short-form health survey (SF-36): III. Tests of data quality, scaling assumptions, and reliability across diverse patient groups. Medical Care 32(1): 40–66.

McVicar A, Ravalier JM, Greenwood C (2014), Biology of stress revisited: intracellular mechanisms and the conceptualization of stress. Stress and Health 30(4): 272–279.

Mahalle NP, Garg MK, Kulkarni MV et al. (2013), Differences in traditional and non-traditional risk factors with special reference to nutritional factors in patients with coronary artery disease with or without diabetes mellitus. Indian Journal of Endocrinology and Metabolism 17(5): 844–850.

Maiese K (2010), Just in the nick of time: targeting acute versus chronic disease. Oxidative Medicine and Cellular Longevity 3(6): 359–360.

Massanari MJ (2000), Asthma management: curtailing cost and improving patient outcomes. Journal of Asthma 37: 641–651.

Mazzeo AT, La Monaca E, Di Leo R et al. (2011), Heart rate variability: a diagnostic and prognostic tool in anesthesia and intensive care. Acta Anaesthesiologica Scandinavica 55(7): 797–811.

Meeus M, Goubert D, De Backer F et al. (2013), Heart rate variability in patients with fibromyalgia and patients with chronic fatigue syndrome: a systematic review. Seminars in Arthritis and Rheumatism 43(2): 279–287.

Melillo P, Izzo R, De Luca N et al. (2012), Heart rate variability and renal organ damage in hypertensive patients. Proceedings of the Annual International Conference of the IEEE Engineering in Medicine and Biology Society, 2012, pp. 3825–3828.

Melzack R, Katz J (2013), Pain. Wiley Interdisciplinary Reviews: Cognitive Science 4(1): 1–15.

Minasny B (2009), Understanding the process of fascial unwinding. International Journal of Therapeutic Massage and Bodywork 2(3): 10–17.

Moore R, Wei Lum Y (2015), Venous thoracic outlet syndrome. Vascular Medicine (London, England) 20(2): 182–189.

Mustahsan SM, Ali SM, Khalid F et al. (2013), Sleep deprivation and its consequences on house officers and postgraduate trainees. Journal of the Pakistan Medical Association 63(4): 540–543.

National Institutes of Health (NIH), US National Library of Medicine (2013), Acute vs Chronic Condition. Linda J Vorvick, MD, Medical Director and Director of Didactic Curriculum, MEDEX Northwest Division of Physician Assistant Studies, Department of Family Medicine, UW Medicine, School of Medicine, University of Washington.

Nodine PM, Matthews EE (2013), Common sleep disorders: management strategies and pregnancy outcomes. Journal of Midwifery and Women's Health 58(4): 368–377.

Pearson TA, Mensah GA, Alexander RW et al. (2003), Markers of inflammation and cardiovascular disease: application to clinical and public health practice: a statement for healthcare professionals from the Centers for Disease Control and Prevention and the American Heart Association. Circulation (New York, NY) 107(3): 499–511.

Pinato DJ, North BV, Sharma R (2012), A novel, externally validated inflammation-based prognostic algorithm in hepatocellular carcinoma: the prognostic nutritional index (PNI). British Journal of Cancer 106(8): 1439–1445.

Put C, Van den Bergh O, Demedts M et al. (2000), A study of the relationship among self-reported noncompliance, symptomatology, and psychological variables in patients with asthma. Journal of Asthma 37: 503–510.

Quality Metric SF Health Surveys (2013), http://wwwqualitymetriccom/WhatWeDo/GenericHealthSurveys/tabid/184/Defaultasp (last accessed September 26, 2013).

Quartana PJ, Campbell CM, Edwards RR (2009), Pain catastrophizing: a critical review. Expert Review of Neurotherapeutics 9(5): 745–758.

Ramar K, Olson EJ (2013), Management of common sleep disorders. American Family Physician 88(4): 231–238.

Rohland BM, Rohrer JE, Richards CC (2000), The long-term effect of outpatient commitment on service use. Administration and Policy in Mental Health 27: 383–394.

Sammito S, Thielmann B, Zimmermann P et al. (2015), Influence of post-traumatic stress disorder on heart rate variability as marker of the autonomic nervous system – a systematic review. Fortschritte der Neurologie-Psychiatrie 83(1): 30–37.

Schleip R (2003), Fascial plasticity – a new neurobiological explanation. Journal of Bodywork and Movement Therapies 7(2): 104–116.

Shochat T, Cohen-Zion M, Tzischinsky O (2014), Functional consequences of inadequate sleep in adolescents: a systematic review. Sleep Medicine Reviews 18(1): 75–87.

Singleton M (2010), Yoga body: the origins of modern posture practice. Oxford University Press, New York.

Staud R (2008), Heart rate variability as a biomarker of fibromyalgia syndrome. Future Rheumatology 3(5): 475–483.

Stanton AM, Lorenz TA, Pulverman CS et al. (2015), Heart rate variability: a risk factor for female sexual dysfunction. Applied Psychophysiology and Biofeedback 40(3): 229–237.

Tuldra A, Fumaz CR, Ferrer MJ et al. (2000), Prospective randomized two-arm controlled study to determine the efficacy of a specific intervention to improve long-term adherence to highly active antiretroviral therapy. Journal of Acquired Immune Deficiency Syndromes 25: 221–228.

Turk DC, Okifuji A (2001), Pain terms and taxonomies. In: D Loeser, SH Butler, JJ Chapman et al., Bonica's Management of Pain, 3rd edition. Lippincott Williams and Wilkins, Philadelphia, pp. 18–25.

Valenti WM (2001), Treatment adherence improves outcomes and manages costs. AIDS Reader 11: 77–80.

Vaschillo EG, Vaschillo B, Lehrer PM (2006), Characteristics of resonance in heart rate variability stimulated by biofeedback. Applied Psychophysiology and Biofeedback 31(2): 129–142.

Walsh J, Hall T (2009), Reliability, validity and diagnostic accuracy of palpation of the sciatic, tibial and common peroneal nerves in the examination of low back related leg pain. Manual Therapy 14(6), 623–629.

Wang YM, Wu HT, Huang EY et al. (2013), Heart rate variability is associated with survival in patients with brain metastasis: a preliminary report. BioMed Research International 2013: 503421.

World Health Organization (2003), Adherence to Long-Term Therapies: Evidence for Action. WHO Library Cataloguing-in-Publication Data.

World Health Organization (2005), Preventing Chronic Diseases: A Vital Investment. WHO Global Report.

Xhyheri B, Manfrini O, Mazzolini M et al. (2012), Heart rate variability today. Progress in Cardiovascular Diseases 55(3): 321–331.

Yang M, Chung SJ, Floegel A et al. (2013), Dietary antioxidant capacity is associated with improved serum antioxidant status and decreased serum C-reactive protein and plasma homocysteine concentrations. European Journal of Nutrition 52(8): 1901–1911.

INDEX

Indexer: Laurence Errington

Note: Bold page references indicate glossary items.

INDEX

INDEX

R

radial nerve tension   324–5

raga   22, 25

raphe, lateral   54, 84, 116, 120

reach, roll and rise, child's pose and   144, 149, 150, 255–9

rectus abdominis diastasis   7

reflexes   30–2

regional interdependence theory/model   60, 305

religion and yoga   7–8
  see also spiritual inquiry

reproductive function   51
  therapeutic intentions and clinical prediction guidelines   73

resonation
  between three diaphragms   80
  teacher's voice   328

respiration   30, 48–54
  assessment   75–102
  physiology   49
  rate at rest   78
  see also cardiorespiratory function

rest (in acute phase)   314

retroversion, femoral/hip   74, 102, 104

reverse Phalen's test   118

"ringing the bell"   286, 287
  downward-facing dog with/without   141–2

Roland–Morris Disability Questionnaire   317

root lock
  anterior (*mula bandha*)   96, 100, **333**
  posterior (*ashwini mudra*)   96, 100, **333**

rotator cuff (RTC)
  hip, 61
    neuromuscular re-education   159
  shoulder (and problems incl. tear and impingement)   118, 121, 123, 124, 126, 133, 135, 305–9
    case study programs   308–9

Ruffini endings and receptors   53, 69, 322

RULE principle   19

S

sacroiliac joint (SIJ) dysfunction, 119, 135, 144, 169, 173, 183, 220, 234, 268, 269

safety, 315, 321, 326
  FMA algorithm use, 107
  inversion progression prerequisites for, 309–11
  see also danger

sage pose (*bharadvajasana*), 216–18

salabasana (locust), 267–8

salamba ardha urdhva dhanurasana, 238–41

salamba balasana (supported child's pose), 255–9

salamba sarvangasana (non-cervical-weight-bearing shoulderstands), 11, 293, 311

sandbag (breath), 90
  supine three-part breath with/without, 89

savasana (corpse and supine-to-sit transfer), 112, 226–7

scapula
  assistance test, 122
  repositioning test, 122

scapulothoracic stabilization, 60
  prayer hands plus *see* shoulder lock

sciatic nerve tension, 116, 136, 142, 249, 324

scoliosis, 119

screening/pre-screening, 102–4
  for inversions/semi-inversions, 277–8
  systemic dysfunction, 49

seated postures, 189–221
  arm spiral and float, 121–2
  level I, 189–210
  level II, 189, 190, 210–21
  transversus abdominis-assisted thoracodiaphragmatic breath, 130–6
  see also chair; sit-to-stand transfer

self-management, 5

semicircular canals, 36

semi-inversions, 277–90
  pre-screening, 277–8

sensorimotor integration *see* tissue extensibility and sensorimotor integration

sensory integration, 19, 23
  screening for patterns in (sensory profile measures), 318

sensory modulation, 30, 32, 39

sensory poetry, 34–5

sensory processing
  children, improving, 229, 231
  disorders, 114
  Dunn's model, 318
  in pain management, 45

sequencing   328–9

TATD compositions   136–49

setu bandha see bridge

sex *see* gender

sexual function   51

SF-36 (Short Form-36)   18, 318

shear forces in cervical spine with headstands   292

Short Form-36 (SF-36)   18, 318

shoulder (and shoulder complex)
  differential diagnosis of bony landmarks   113
  pain   305–9
  rotator cuff *see* rotator cuff

shoulder extension, three-tier approach   226

shoulder lock (*anjali mudra* plus active scapulothoracic stabilization)   96, 98–9, **333**
  supine   118

shoulder opener   130–3, **333**

shoulderstands, non-cervical-weight-bearing (*salamba sarvangasana*)   11, 293, 311

siddhasana (perfect pose)   189–93

side plank   265

single leg squat   159

sirsasanah see headstands

sit-to-stand transfer   158, 159, 160, 162, 163
  Five Times Sit-to-Stand test   159, 317
  see also seated

skin interruptions and adhesions   69–70, 300

sleep hygiene   314–15

"sleepy or kissing knees"   194, 214, 225, 226, 245

"slinky"   287
  downward-facing dog with/without   141–2

slump test   249, 325

snow angels   123, 206, 245

social support   313

somatosensory highway, mapping   40–8

somatosensory threshold, identifying   19

Sorenson trunk extensor test   267–8

sound (as therapy)   10–11
  see also orofacial phonation relaxation response

special tests   102–4
  rotator cuff case study programs   309

Sphinx *see* cobra and Sphinx

"spider legs" fingers   135, 136, 194, 195

U